DISEASES OF FISHES

DISEASES OF FISHES

C. van DUIJN, Jnr.,
Dip.Chem.E., M.Inst.P., M.I.Biol., M.I.P.T.
Fellow, Royal Microscopical Society

CHARLES C THOMAS · PUBLISHER
Springfield · Illinois · U.S.A.

CHARLES C THOMAS · PUBLISHER
BANNERSTONE HOUSE
301–327 East Lawrence Avenue, Springfield, Illinois, U.S.A.

ISBN 0-398-02718-8

First published in 1956
Second Edition 1967
Second Impression 1971
Third Edition 1973

© C. van Duijn, Jnr. 1973

*With THOMAS BOOKS careful attention is given to all
details of manufacturing and design. It is the Publisher's desire
to present books that are satisfactory as to their physical qualities and artistic
possibilities and appropriate for their particular use. THOMAS BOOKS
will be true to those laws of quality that assure a good name and good will*

Filmset and Printed in England by
Cox and Wyman Ltd.,
London, Fakenham and Reading

PREFACE

Scarcely four years had elapsed after publication of the second edition when the need for a new one became apparent. The increase of knowledge in the field of diseases of fishes, during that time, was considerable; accordingly, the text has again been extended and revised, where necessary. Some information with regard to marine aquaria has also been incorporated.

For prescriptions, the metric system (S.I. units) has now been given preference, but for the benefit of those users who are not yet accustomed to it, the Imperial and U.S. measures have been maintained as well.

A superscript R is used to denote some registered trade names throughout the text, but where a trade name appears several times in succession it is only indicated by an initial capital letter.

So many new bibliographical references are included in this new edition, that it has been decided to alter the referencing system from the previous method of footnoting the references on the page they occur. Now, the references are indicated in the text by a raised number and the complete list of numbered references are found at the end of each chapter.

As in the earlier editions, the main points in this treatise still concern diagnosis and therapy, rather than mere parasitology and pathology.

Zeist (Netherlands), 1972   C. van Duijn, Jnr.

CONTENTS

1

INTRODUCTION

All living beings can in certain circumstances become subject to disease and fishes make no exception. It is possible that at some time or other the aquarist or professional fish breeder has to deal with disease, and to do this properly it is necessary to know something about the illnesses likely to be contracted and how they can be cured.

You must not get the impression that it is difficult to keep fishes in a state of good health. Generally, fishes have a very great resistance to disease so long as they are not weakened by bad treatment, unsuitable food, lack of oxygen, too high or low temperature, or other adverse influences.

To avoid disease, the first thing to bear in mind is to keep your fishes in optimal conditions so that they have a good resistance when any infection occurs. Most infections, however, can be avoided. If a new tank has been set up with plants that have grown in water where there are no fish, and completely healthy fishes put into this tank, any parasite which causes disease later on will have been introduced from the outside, by means of new plants or living food (water fleas, mosquito larvae) or a new fish.

Generally, a fish parasite can only live in water where there are fishes. It is thus normally safe to add plants, snails, mosquito larvae and *Daphnia*, etc., from a ditch or pool in which no fish are present, after cleaning them under the tap. *Daphnia* and mosquito larvae will not be found abundantly in a pond with many fishes; as a rule these food supplies come from waters with no fishes and after some washing with fresh water they can be considered safe.

Plants and snails from suspected sources should be kept in quarantine for one to three weeks. If parasites were present, they will have died during this period, since they could not find a host to live on. With new fishes, it is generally sufficient to keep them in a separate tank for several weeks; if they show no sign of disease

1

after this time you can be certain that they are completely healthy. Such measures should not be necessary if you get plants or fishes from a reliable dealer or fellow-aquarist whose stock is known to be perfectly healthy.

Symptoms of disease in fish differ according to its nature, but there are several signs from which we may tell if a fish is healthy or suffering from any complaint.

A healthy fish will show good colours. Discoloration may be a sign of distress, although this is not always the case. It may also occur temporarily, e.g. if a strong light is put near the tank, when it has been in darkness for some time (Angel Fish behave in this way), while females of some species show discoloration after spawning. Some fishes may also temporarily lose their colours if they are frightened. But if discoloration occurs without apparent cause, and if it continues for some time, it should be taken as being a symptom of some disease.

Diseases of the skin will often show themselves not only by fading of the colours, but also by the formation of a slimy, grey excretion, covering small or greater areas. Such a symptom may be observed easily in dark-coloured fishes, while in others it does not show so clearly since there is less contrast between the grey slime and the parts of the body that are not yet affected. In other diseases of the skin, white, brownish or even black spots may show. Fungus growth can be recognised easily.

Often a disease of the skin may be recognised from the behaviour of the fish, when irritation causes it to rub its body against stones, plants or other surfaces. This also occurs when a fish has been attacked by one of the larger parasites, such as the fish louse, anchor worm or leech.

In many diseases, a fish will fold its fins while it lingers either near the bottom or the surface of the water. In tropicals this may be due to nothing more than too low temperature of the water. In diseases of the gills, breathing difficulties occur. The diseased fishes will open their gill coverings more widely than in normal respiration, while breathing frequency will become increased. The gill sheets are pale, while sometimes small red spots may show owing to inflammation. In some cases, the gill sheets are swollen and extend outside the gill coverings. Pale gills are always a sign of disease in living fish; the gills of healthy fishes will have a reddish colour unless they are pigmented, as is the case with Bettas and some other species, where the colour is dark.

Bacterial diseases are mostly characterised by red spots on the skin and in the muscles; these spots are called ecchymoses. Diseases of the eye may be recognised from a swelling of the organ, occurring in a disease called *Exophthalmus*, or from affection of the pupil (several kinds of cataract are known).

In judging the general health of a fish, a simple test may be made in which the eye plays an important rôle. If a completely healthy fish is taken in the hand (in the water) and turned to its side, the eye will not share this movement, but will remain in the normal position, so that from above the pupil remains invisible. If a fish is very sick, the ball of the eye will follow the turning of the body, when the pupil may be seen even when the fish is turned to its side. The simple experiment is a valuable aid in diagnosis in cases where more characteristic symptoms are lacking.

Diseases of the internal organs may cause either abnormal swelling of the belly (not to be confused with egg ripeness of females of spawning fishes or pregnancy of livebearers), or, on the contrary, the belly may go thin. The first-mentioned symptom may occur in dropsy and in some diseases of the reproductive organs, while the latter will generally be due to the activity of internal parasites. Worm parasites may cause either swelling of the belly or wasting. Formation of blood-flecked excrements is a sign of inflammation of the intestines.

Lack of appetite may be due to many causes; if it occurs together with some swelling of the belly but other symptoms are lacking the cause will probably be constipation. This complaint will be met

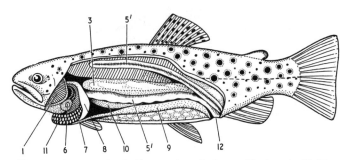

Fig. 1.1. Anatomy of male Trout (schematised). 1, gills. 3, swim bladder. 5, testicle. 6, heart. 7, liver. 8, stomach. 9, intestine. 10, spleen. 11. pylorus appendices of stomach. 12, anal vent

mostly in Veiltails and other varieties possessing a compressed body. Constipation usually results from incorrect feeding and is, therefore, avoidable.

Swim bladder disease may occur in tropicals, if they are kept for a period at excessively low temperatures. The victims have difficulty in keeping their equilibrium, sometimes they fall 'head over heels' or make tumbling movements. Finally, some will seek rest at the bottom, others will float near the surface. Other cases of swim bladder disease are due to pressure from some of the internal organs, such as may result from constipation or a disease in which the volume of the internal organs increases, or it may be due to fatty degeneration of the tissues of the bladder itself or to infections by *Bacteria*, *Sporozoa* or *Ichthyophonus*.

Several diseases may be recognised with sufficient accuracy from the general symptoms which can be determined by watching the behaviour and noting the appearance of the victims, but often closer investigation will be necessary. If there are symptoms of a disease of the skin, some slime may be taken with a lancet needle or a very small knife, going from the head to the tail, while holding the fish carefully in the hand in such way that its head remains in the water. In the same way, a sample of the slime of the gills may be taken, but one has to be very careful in doing this to avoid injury to the tender gill sheets. The slime is smeared upon a slide for microscopical examination, which may take place immediately, after a tiny drop of tap water has been added and the preparation has been covered with a cover-glass. If it is impossible to examine the smear at once under the microscope, no cover-glass is used.

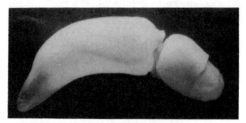

Fig. 1.2. Swim bladder of a Dace

One lets the smear dry in the air and then it can be investigated later on. If there is an opportunity for immediate examination, this is to be preferred, since many parasites will be much more easily recognisable when they are still alive. When the aquarist does not possess a microscope, however, the dried smear may be given to an expert for examination, but it is better to supply a living fish for expert examination whenever possible.

When a fish has died it is also advisable to make an investigation to find the cause of death. In most cases, this too calls for the aid of a microscope, but often a sufficiently accurate diagnosis may be acquired without such an instrument, although there may not be so great a certainty.

The investigation must begin as soon as possible after death. Some slime of the skin is taken and examined under the microscope, at first at a low magnification, then at a higher one (preferably with phase-contrast if this is available). We take the first sample from a spot of the skin that shows any abnormal appearance.

In dead fishes, the covering of the gills (operculum) is next removed and a small part of the gill is cut off and brought under the microscope or examined carefully with a good magnifying glass. After this, the dead fish is cut open with a sharp razor or dissection scissors, beginning with a cut along the belly from the anal opening to the head; then two cuts are made at each end of

this incision at about right-angles to it, so that the body wall can be
turned over and the entrails left free for the examination. Details
of pathological changes will be given in the later chapters. For
microscopical examinations a small part of each organ is brought on
a slide and rubbed out, making a thin smear. For more detailed

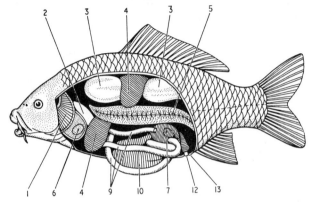

Fig. 1.3. Anatomy of a female Carp (schematised). Key to both
illustrations on this page: 1, gills. 2, gullet. 3. swim bladder.
4, kidney. 5 (1.3), ovary. 5 (1.4), testicle. 6, heart. 7, liver.
9, intestine. 10, spleen. 12, anal vent. 13, sexual vent. 14, urine
bladder. 15, brains. 16, peritoneum

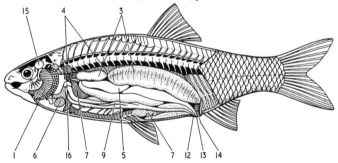

Fig. 1.4. Anatomy of a male Dace, L. leuciscus

investigations, organs should be excised, fixed in Bouin's fixative
and prepared for embedding in either paraffin wax or celloidin for
section cutting, followed by standard histological staining techniques. Small fishes may be fixed without dissection and total cutting
made with a microtome. Generally, longitudinal sections will give
most information, unless there are specific diseased regions recognisable.

The internal anatomy of a fish can be learned from Figs 1.1–1.5.
The length of the intestines differs according to the natural food

the fish is taking. Carnivorous fishes have short intestines while fishes that are taking less digestible foods can have a considerable length of intestine.

The swim bladder usually consists of two parts, united by a small course. The two parts can be of the same size, as in Carp (*Cyprinus carpio*), but often they are of different sizes, the part that is situated after the head being much smaller than the other.

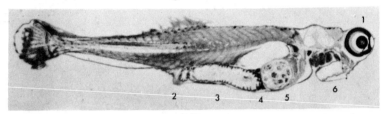

Fig. 1.5. Longitudinal section of a young Stickleback, showing: 1, eye. 2, anal vent. 3, intestine. 4, swim bladder. 5, stomach. 6, gills (macrograph by the author)

There are also fishes without a swim bladder, e.g. the Miller's Thumb (*Cottus gobio*). These animals cannot remain at the same depth of water without swimming and consequently they live near the bottom. Nevertheless, they can be good swimmers.

By means of its swim bladder a fish can regulate its density in accordance with that of the water so that it can remain at a certain depth without swimming. Most fishes do not swim with their fins, but by movements of their body in which the tail plays an important rôle (there are but few exceptions to this rule); the fins are used as steering organs, while the breast fins have largely the task of supplying the gills with fresh water and waving away the water from which the oxygen has already been taken.

2

SKIN PARASITES AND INFECTIONS

The skin of a fish consists of two layers of different composition (Fig. 2.1), namely, the epidermis (the upper part) and the cutis (the under-layer). The epidermis consists of epithelial cells with slime cells in between (Fig. 2.2). These slime cells excrete a slimy substance

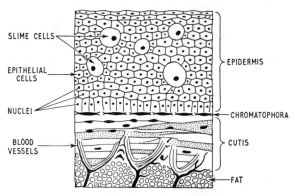

Fig. 2.1.
SECTION OF A FISH'S SKIN
Diagram (schematised) of a section through the skin of a fish to show its composition. In the epidermis are shown the epithelial and slime cells with the chromatophora arranged between the epidermis and the cutis layers

that covers the whole surface of the skin with a thin protective layer. Some fishes are more 'slimy' than others, e.g. the Tench (*Tinca tinca*) and the Eel (*Anguilla anguilla*) excrete much slime, while there is considerably less in white fish species.

7

The slime on the skin helps to protect the skin against bacterial infections and consequently fishes with a very slimy skin have a greater resistance to infections than others. The excretion of the slime cells becomes greater when they are irritated, as in the case when certain parasites are present. The abnormal slime excretion in such cases is an important symptom to be considered in diagnosing any trouble.

The cutis consists of fibres of connective tissue arranged in parallel layers. The cutis is rich in blood vessels. The upper part contains the scales, mounted in small pockets, analogous to the 'pockets' securing the hairs of mammals and the feathers of birds. Both sides

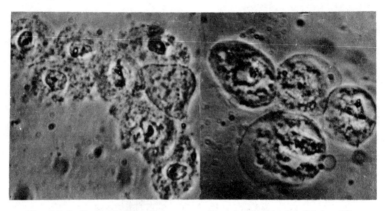

Fig. 2.2. Left: *Epithelial cells in a smear from the skin of a fish.* Right: *Slime cells in a similar smear. Phase-contrast photomicrographs. Magnification* × 500

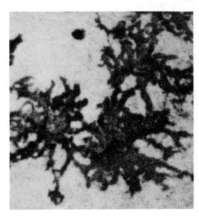

Fig. 2.3. Photomicrograph showing pigment cells extended to different degrees. Magnification approx. × 200

of this part of the scale are covered with connective tissue and the whole is covered once more by epithelial cells. If pathogenic bacteria penetrate into the scale pockets an inflammation is caused in which the pockets become filled with a watery exudate that presses tightly against the scales causing them to protrude.

Beneath the cutis fat cells are situated, while between cutis and epidermis chromatophora (pigment cells) are present. It is these which determine the colours of a fish. Different types may be distinguished, such as the small black chromatophora, called micromelanophora, and a larger variety, the macromelanophora; yellow and red pigment cells (xanthophora and erythrophora, respectively); and the iridocytes, which are the reflecting guanine-containing cells which give white fishes their iridescent appearance. The chromatophora may be more or less extended (Fig. 2.3), according to different conditions, and consequently the colours of a fish may vary within certain limits. A completely healthy fish will always be well coloured under normal conditions. The fading of its colours is in many cases a sign of disease. Fading can also be due to shock; if fishes are frightened they frequently go pale. The same phenomenon will occur when tropical fishes are kept at too low temperatures or when they are suddenly put under excessively strong artificial light.

The amount of pigment cells varies very much in different fishes, being very large in dark-coloured types, e.g. Fighting Fish (*Betta splendens*), and particularly in Black Mollies (*Mollienisia* species), while silvery-coloured fishes have but very little pigment. The photomicrograph in Fig. 2.3 shows pigment cells that are extended to different degrees. The degree of extension also depends on the colours of the surroundings. A fish will adapt itself as far as possible to these and consequently in a tank without plants its colours will tend to fade. Tench have a great power of adapting their colour to their surroundings; on a white ground they grow very pale so that the blood shows through the skin; while against a black mud bottom they grow nearly black. Naturally, such changes of colour have nothing to do with any illness. If, on the other hand, a fish fails to adapt itself to its surroundings, this may be a symptom of disease. In some fishes pigment is lacking; their colour, if any, is mainly dependent on the blood shining through the skin. An example among aquarium fishes is the blind Characin *Anoptichthys jordana* Hubbs & Innes, that is living in dark grottoes in Mexico.

While the uppermost part of the epidermis becomes horny in vertebrates that live in the air, this is not the case with fish. That of a fish always remains soft. Consequently, the skin is easily injured and, as such, has but little resistance to penetration of pathogenic organisms. As said before, however, the slime of the skin gives some protection against infections, since this has a more or less bactericidal power, while the scales protect the underlying skin against mechanical damage. The epidermis contains no blood vessels, consequently the skin may be injured badly without any bleeding showing.

Not all fishes have scales. Some have horny plates or shields instead, that give a still better protection against mechanical injury. Some examples are the Sticklebacks (*Gasterosteus* and *Pygosteus*), Sturgeons (*Acipenser*) and, of the exotic aquarium fishes, some of the Catfishes, namely *Corydoras* and related species.

FISH LOUSE

Turning now to the fish parasites, let us consider the fish louse (*Argulus*), one of the most well-known fish parasites. Two species usually found are *A. foliaceus* and *A. coregoni* (Fig. 2.4). The fish louse is a flattened creature, about as large as a water flea, belonging to the *Branchiura* or gill-tails, a Group of the *Crustacea*. The little animal has eight legs, with which it can swim through the water, and

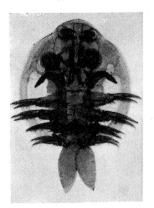 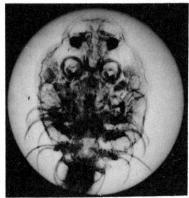

Fig. 2.4.
FISH LOUSE SPECIES
Two species of the fish louse (Argulus) *parasites which attack fishes. The photograph on the extreme left, by John Clegg, is of* A. coregoni. *The other, taken by the author, is* A. foliaceus. *Both occur in British waters*

a small fish-like tail, which acts like a rudder. The reproductive and breathing organs are situated in the tail. In the males there are two large testes, while the females possess two small receptaculae seminis, in which the sperm received from the male at the mating is preserved. There are two large suckers for attaching to the skin of its host. Above these suckers there are two facet eyes, while between them one simple eye is situated. Between the three eyes there is a large hollow 'sting' or proboscis. This 'sting' or tube-like extension is forced under the scale of the fish, penetrating to the cutis and by means of it the parasite feeds on the blood of its host.

The mouth is situated behind the proboscis on a small rostrum. The intestinal tube is very short, but the stomach is amply provided with branches. The intestine may be filled so full with the blood of a victim that the parasite may live without feeding for weeks. The heart lies hidden deep in the body. As previously said, the tail serves as a breathing organ, containing the gills; breathing, however, also takes place with the whole surface of the body. The colour of the fish louse ranges from light green to greenish yellow and brown. If the parasite is well fed its colour will be darker, due to filling with the blood of the host. Females will reach a length of about 6–7 mm while the males grow to about 4–5 mm.

Argulus foliaceus is widely distributed both in England and on the Continent and may be found on many species of fish, such as Carp (*Cyprinus carpio*), Tench (*Tinca tinca*), White Fish (*Leuciscus* sp.), Perch (*Perca fluviatilis*), Pike (*Esox lucius*), Bream (*Abramis brama*), Sticklebacks (*Gasterosteus*), Bitterling (*Rhodeus amarus*), Minnows (*Phoxinus phoxinus*), Trout (*Salmo fario*) and Sea Trout (*Salmo trutta*). Some other species of fish lice are known. *Argulus coregoni* Thorell [*A. phoxini* Leydig] is the largest, reaching a length of about 12 mm and a breadth of about 10 mm. On the Continent it is found on Pike-Perch (*Perca lucioperca*) and several Salmonids, viz. *Coregonus fera*, Grayling (*Thymallus thymallus*), Trout and Sea Trout, and there are reports of its having been found on fish in Britain. Further we know *Argulus pellucidus* Wagler [*A. viridis* Nettovich], with a length of up to 7 mm. Over the whole world about fifty other species occurring in fresh and salt waters are known.

The fish louse can only be introduced into tropical aquaria with supplies of *Daphnia* or other living food, obtained from waters in which fishes are present. There is but a very small chance of capturing a free-swimming fish louse, since this is only possible if this parasite is in search of a new host or if it has left its host for the purpose of reproduction. Consequently, in tropical tanks the fish louse will not often be met. However, the chance of getting them will be greatly increased during the time that the eggs of the fish louse are hatching and the small fry are in search of a suitable host.

Mating of the fish louse takes place from April to September. Before the spawning the females are strikingly swollen. The eggs have a citron-yellow colour and are deposited in long, flat lines on stones. In an aquarium they are often deposited on the glass. The females die after spawning and the eggs hatch about one month later. The fry have a shorter scale than the adults and the suckers are immature. Their length is about 0.75 mm. They have two eyes that are situated on movable stems (Fig. 2.5).

A first moult takes place about five days after hatching. In this second stage their length is about 1 mm. The antennae become shorter and the main attaching organ is formed, enabling the young parasites already in this stage to attack fish and occasionally larvae of frogs and newts. The legs at the thorax become straight and segmented. The tail begins to form. During the main part of this stage the larvae are attracted by light, but this tendency decreases when the time of the second moult is approached, which takes place 3–4 days later. During this period, several organs develop from the larval into mature state, e.g. the testes and the seminal receptacles increase in volume. Their length increases to about 1.4 mm. Segmentation of the thoracic leg proceeds further. The extensions of the antennae disappear and the larvae are no longer

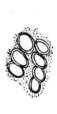 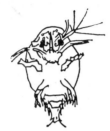

Fig. 2.5. Left: *Ova of* Argulus *(× 11)*. Right: *Newly hatched* Argulus *(× 25)   showing   its typical shape (after Claus)*

capable of floating in the water as in the preceding stages, but have now to swim actively. Further moults take place at intervals of about 3–7 days (according to water temperature) and during this period the young fish louse gradually increases in size, after the third moult up to about 1.9 mm and after the fifth one up to about 2.8 mm. Then the larva has become nearly identical with the adult. At an age of about one month, after the seventh moult, the fish louse is old enough for mating.

As is often the case in lower organisms females of the fish louse are more numerous than males. Although copulation sometimes takes place while the female is still holding to its host, it always leaves the fish for spawning. Reports in literature about the number of eggs do not agree. One states an amount of 100. Another investigator gives it as up to 400. Clifford Bower-Shore records the amount of eggs as averaging 185.

As typical skin parasites capable of free changing of host, fish lice may also act as transmitters of bacterial and virus infections from fish to fish. It has been experimentally established that in this way infectious dropsy is conveyed by infected fish lice.[1]

REMOVING FISH LICE FROM AFFECTED FISH

As the fish louse is quite a large creature, the parasites may be removed easily by means of a pair of forceps if you take the fish in your hand. If there are too many of them they can be removed by rubbing over the skin of the fish, always going from the head to the tail. Parasites that are sucking so strongly that it is impossible to remove them in this way, may be paralysed by dropping one or two drops of a strong solution of salt on them and then they may be rubbed off. Be careful, however, not to bring strong salt solution in direct contact with the skin of the fish. Using a small pencil or brush it will not be difficult to dislodge the parasite without doing injury to the fish.

Instead of using a strong salt solution for touching the parasites, a mixture of turpentine, iodine and kerosene has been recommended. Although this is also very effective, I do not advocate it since it is much more dangerous.

In most cases it will not be necessary to use such treatment, since the fish lice are generally easily removable by means of forceps or by rubbing only. The late Professor Bruno Hofer stated that Minnows in an aquarium had eaten fish lice, while other fishes tried to escape from the neighbourhood as soon as they saw the parasite.[2]

It has also been stated that the introduction of *Gambusia* into infested pools results in clearing up the fish lice from the infected fishes and from the pool itself.[3] Laboratory tests have shown that potential predators of *Argulus* are Flagfish (*Jordanella floridæ*), Golden Topminnow (*Fundulus chrysotus*), several *Centrarchidæ*, the fresh-water shrimp *Palæmonetes paludosus* and water scorpions (*Ranatra* sp.).[4]

TREATMENT OF PONDS

In ponds, it is impossible to remove all fish lice by individual treatment of the fishes and this would be ineffective, too, since the eggs and hatching young parasites are not removed so that new infections should occur very soon. In such cases a treatment with potassium permanganate may be tried. 4–5 mg/l is added (0.25–0.3 gr/Imp. gal, or 0.2–0.25 gr/U.S. gal). Never on any account add any crystals of permanganate directly to the water, but dissolve them first in a small amount of water and then pour the solution into the pond or tank that is to be treated. After 10 days the remedy should be repeated. Dosage of the chemical must be as accurate as possible, since too strong solutions are dangerous to the fish. Its activity depends on the liberation of oxygen in a very active state, which kills parasites. If the water is alkaline or only slightly acid, a precipitate of manganese may form which can damage the gills. Use artificial aeration during treatment.

Ponds that can be emptied and dried up, are most easily freed of even heavy infections with fish lice by letting the water off and keeping them unoccupied for a short time. Fish lice and their eggs and larvae will be killed within a period of 3 h of complete desiccation, or after 15–20 h if some adhering water remains in a moist surrounding.

NEGUVON TREATMENT

D. Bailösoff at the Research Institute for Veterinary Medicine in Sofia, Bulgaria, has applied the commercial drug 'Neguvon (Bayer)' for treatment of infected Carp, Prussian Carp and Trout.[5] Neguvon is the registered trade name of Messrs. Bayer AG, Leverkusen, Germany, for the chemical substance (2,2,2-trichloro-1-hydroxyethyl)–phosphonic acid-dimethyl ester. A 2–3.5% solution of this drug kills fish lice within 50–60 sec, whereas the recommended treatment is to dip the infected fish for 2–3 min in the solution. Ponds may be treated with a concentration of 1:1000 (1 g/l or 68 gr/Imp. gal, or 57 gr/U.S. gal) for a longer period. The water of the pond is changed as soon as inspection of the fish shows that no living fish lice are present.

Neguvon must not contact the human skin. If there is a risk of getting the solutions on the hands when handling a large number of fishes, rubber gloves should be worn. For further particulars see page 336.

TREATING CARP WITH LINDANE (GAMMEXANE)

Dr. Edward Hindle has successfully treated heavily infected tanks with lindane (1,2,3,4,5,6-hexachlorocyclohexane) in a dilution of 1:10 000 000 for 2–3 days. A 1% stock solution in absolute alcohol is prepared and 1 cm^3 of this solution is added to 100 l (approx. 20 Imp. gal or 25 U.S. gal) of water, with thorough stirring. When the solution is poured into the water, a slight milky precipitate may form which disappears almost at once when the water is stirred. After treatment the water has to be changed completely.

Dosage has to be very accurate, since lindane is very poisonous and if the solution is only slightly too concentrated, toxic effects may occur in the fish or they may even be killed. Lindane is also very toxic to human beings. It can cause them hyper-irritability, convulsions and death. Be careful not to get the stock solution in contact with your hands, since it is able to penetrate through the undamaged skin, causing irritation.

Further, Dr. Hindle emphasises that, with few exceptions, this treatment has only been applied to infected Carp and he considers it possible that other species of fish might be more susceptible to the toxic action. This treatment should only be used with the utmost caution. How dangerous the drug is can be demonstrated by the fact that it may kill Pike after 24 h in a 1:5 000 000 solution.

ANCHOR WORM

The females of this parasite, *Lernæa cyprinacea*, have a long body with anchor-like appendages at the head. Although the organism resembles a worm it is not one, however, but belongs to the *Copepoda* (a branch of the *Crustacea*) and is related to *Cyclops*, the well-known livefood. It reaches a length of about 20 mm ($\frac{3}{4}$ in), not including the appendages. By means of these appendages the adult female parasite sticks to the fish. Since the anchor penetrates deep under the skin into the muscles, the fish becomes badly injured. It is impossible to remove the parasites simply by means of forceps; in doing this serious wounds would be caused, open to bacterial and fungus infections. Such treatment would be worse than the effect of the attacks of the parasites. The male *Lernæa* does not attack fish and is rather different in shape.

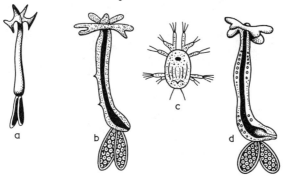

Fig. 2.6.
ANCHOR WORM PARASITES
(a) Lernæa cyprinacea *(after Seligo)*. (b) Lernæa cyprinacea *(after Roth)*. (c) *Nauplius larva (after Roth)*. (d) Lernæa esocina *(after Nordmann)*

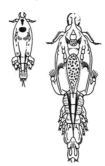

Fig. 2.7. Lernæa cyprinacea.
Larval and adult males (after H. van Laar)

The parasite has been known under the name of *Lernæocera cyprinacea* for over a century, but in recent years it has been shown by Wilson that some confusion of names has taken place, the true *Lernæocera* being a related Genus of larger (up to 4 cm) dark-red coloured parasites of the gills of marine fishes, particularly of Haddock, Plaice and Flounder (Figs 2.6, 2.7).

Reproduction of the parasite takes place in May. Two egg sacs are formed at the end of the female's body which reach a length of about 3 mm. From the eggs so-called nauplius larvae hatch, closely resembling those of *Cyclops* and other non-parasitic *Copepoda*. The larvae swim freely through the water for some time (growing in the meantime) till they meet a fish. The adults still preying on their host die at the end of May, leaving large holes with round

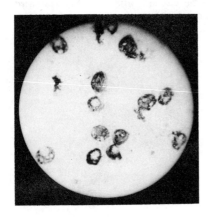

Fig. 2.8. Photomicrograph showing leucocytes in slime of the skin of a fish which has been attacked by worms, causing a secondary inflammation to be set up

openings in the muscles and skin of the fish. These wounds heal very slowly, if at all. They will often become infected with bacteria and fungus and the fish will die from these secondary infections (Fig. 2.8).

After reaching a fish, the young anchor worms penetrate through the skin of the victim into the underlying muscles. There they remain, feeding on the host and growing till they have reached a length of about 12 mm. The ends of their bodies become clearly visible outside the skin of the fish by the beginning of September. In the summer months the parasites cannot be noticed very easily, although they may be present and cause the victim much distress.

The female nauplii (plural of nauplius) reach sexual maturity in 2–3 weeks in summer, or in 3–6 weeks in spring and autumn. Development of the eggs depends very much on the temperature of the water. Under 14°C (57°F) no young will hatch, whereas at 25°C (77°F) development of the eggs is about thrice as fast, and at 33°C (91°F) even six times as fast as at 14°C. Consequently, the last generation of young females reaching the fish late in autumn will not reproduce during the same year, but hibernates in either of two ways. They may encyst in the epithelium of the fish, producing cysts of 2–3 mm, that fall off when size increases. A smaller number of parasites do not encyst, but bore themselves deep into the skin of the fish, where they hibernate in a free state. These specimens give rise to a new spread of the parasites in spring.

Lernæa cyprinacea is found on Goldfish (*Carassius auratus*), Crucian Carp (*Carassius carassius*), Golden Orfe (*Idus idus* var.) and, in tropical aquaria, in particular on Cichlids. Another species, *Lernæa esocina*, lives on Pike (*Esox lucius*), Perch (*Perca fluviatilis*), Stickle-backs (*Gasterosteus aculeatus* and *Pygosteus pungitius*), Miller's Thumb (*Cottus gobio*), Eelpout (*Lota vulgaris*), Tench (*Tinca tinca*) and Spined Loach (*Cobitis tænia*). In aquaria, however, this species seems to be very rare. A third European species is *Lernæa phoxinacea*

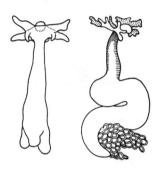

Fig. 2.9. Lernæa phoxinacea *and* Lernæocera branchialis *females (after Schäperclaus)*

(Fig. 2.9) with females reaching a length of about 6.5 mm, attacking Minnows (*Phoxinus phoxinus*). There are also some exotic species that have been imported with fishes.

If a few anchor worms are present on fishes in an aquarium, a good cure is to take each fish in the hand and touch the parasites with a small pencil or brush that has been dipped in a rather strong solution of potassium permanganate. Since only the parasites are touched with the permanganate, the solution may have a strength of 0.1% or more. With small fishes one must be careful not to touch the skin. The permanganate kills the anchor worms and makes them soft so that after this treatment they usually fall off. If they should still adhere to the fish they may be removed by means of forceps. The sore spots are then touched with Mercurochrome solution (strength 1 : 10) for disinfection.

Schäperclaus suggests the use of DDT for treatment of anchor worm infections. Fishes could be bathed for a short period of time in concentrations of 1 : 100 000 000 up to 1 : 50 000 000, which according to him they will stand for several days. Schäperclaus advocates making a more concentrated stock solution of DDT in alcohol and using small amounts of this to reach the final dilution required for treatment. Since in aquaria generally only a few parasites have to be coped with at one occasion, the present author would prefer local treatment again, by touching the parasite with a pencil dipped in a stock solution, or with a dry pencil dipped into the dry powder. The parasites are rapidly killed and can be removed easily. The fishes are then returned to well-aerated water.

If there is a possibility of new infections, as is the case when the parasites are in the breeding season (May), and are showing full egg sacs, it is advisable to transfer the fishes for some weeks into another tank so that the young parasites cannot find another host, and will therefore die. After a period of about 3–4 weeks, according to the water temperature (at higher temperatures the parasites will die sooner), the tank may be considered safe. It is also possible to disinfect a tank by means of the permanganate treatment, but if this is not absolutely necessary it is not advisable. In ponds, permanganate treatment has been the only way short of a complete clean-out and restocking and planting, until recent Japanese investigations suggested the use of salt in concentrations of 0.76–1.10%, provided the water temperature is not below 14°C (57°F); this salt concentration will kill the hatching nauplii. Treatment should continue for 2–3 weeks, during which period the water should be repeatedly changed and resalted after a few days, which still makes treatment a troublesome affair, except for reasonably small garden ponds.

INFECTION BY LARVAE OF FRESH-WATER MUSSELS

Bitterlings (*Rhodeus amarus*) deposit their eggs in fresh-water mussels, preferably *Unio pictorum*. The eggs are deposited by the female by means of an elongated ovipositor into the anal tube of the mussel and they are fertilised by the semen of the male that is discharged above the breathing crevice. The young hatch in the mantle cavity and between the gill sheets of the mussel, where they remain till they have reached a certain stage of further development, when the mussel gets rid of them. On the other hand the mussel uses the fish to take care of its brood.

The young specimens of the bitterling mussels (*Unio*), swan mussels (*Anodonta*), and fresh-water pearl mussel (*Margaritana margaritifera*) develop into a larval stage, called glochidium, between the gills of the mussel. From there they are released into the water after some weeks, mainly in the period from May to August. The glochidia open their valves and produce a long twisted thread with a sticky end. These threads exert undulatory movements until they contact each other, thus producing some kind of irregular net-work, acting as a matrix in which the animals are hanging with gaping valves. The edges of the small valves are barbed and enable the glochidia to attach to the skin or even the gill sheets of a fish that whirls the net-work up by its swimming movements (Fig. 2.10). The barbed valves grip into the epidermis and are then closed by the strong muscle. The epithelium tissue is irritated and reacts by proliferation of the cells in the vicinity of the glochidium, so that the latter is covered by a cyst, consisting of the epidermis (or gill epithelium if the glochidium is situated at a gill sheet) of the fish

(Fig. 2.11). The process of covering the glochidium takes only 2–4 h. The external appearance is that of a white or greyish bladder on the skin, or on a fin or a gill sheet of the attacked fish.

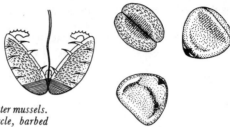

Fig. 2.10. Glochidia of fresh-water mussels. Left: *open, showing shell muscle, barbed hooks and byssus thread (after L. Reinhardt).* Right: *closed (after Hentschel)*

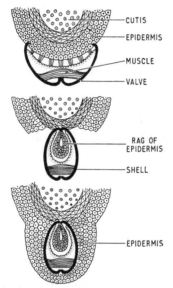

CUTIS
EPIDERMIS
MUSCLE
VALVE

RAG OF EPIDERMIS
SHELL

EPIDERMIS

Fig. 2.11. Upper: *First stage of glochidium attacking the skin of a fish.* Middle: *Glochidium attached to the skin after closure of its shell.* Lower: *Glochidium, encysted by proliferation of the epithelium of the skin of the fish (after H. van Laar)*

Inside this bladder the glochidium develops gradually into a small real mussel by changes and further development of the internal organs. This development takes several (up to 10) weeks. Then the young mussel bores through the epidermis bladder and leaves the fish.

Glochidia of the bitterling mussel and related species of the Genus *Unio* are most frequently found on Bitterlings (*Rhodeus amarus*) and Perch (*Perca fluviatilis*). Minnows (*Phoxinus phoxinus*) and Trout (*Salmo fario, Salmo salvelinus*, etc.) are more often attacked by the glochidia of the fresh-water pearl mussel (*Margaritana margaritifera*).

Big fish can stand the attack of even large numbers of glochidia. It has been reported that one-year-old Perch survived an invasion of about five hundred glochidia on the gills. However, at other occasions large numbers of glochidia infecting the gills may easily cause death from suffocation, whereas the general resistance of the fish to other infections is lowered, such as bacterial infections or to the parasites causing sliminess of the skin, *Costa necatrix* or *Cyclochæta domerguei* (see pages 67–76).

Occasionally the fish may be capable of coping with a heavy infection by immunological reactions leading to killing and resorption of the glochidia.

Obviously infection of fish by glochidia can only happen where fresh-water mussels are living at the bottom of the water. There is no way of removing the glochidia from the fish, since they are protected both by the layer of epidermis that grows over them and by their own shell. In the aquarium infection by glochidia can be avoided by keeping no more than one fresh-water mussel at a time, thus preventing intercourse between male and female mussels which must precede the production of brood. However, since a female mussel taken from free water may already contain brood during the period from spring to autumn, one should keep it in quarantine for several weeks, or one should collect the mussels at the end of autumn or in the winter season. As stated before, they are needed for breeding Bitterlings.

FISH LEECH

This is a worm-like creature with a membered body which has a large sucking disc at each end. One of these suckers is pierced by the mouth. The ordinary fish leech (*Piscicola geometra*) grows to about 20–50 mm (mean length about 1 in) and its body shows transverse stripes. Leeches lay their eggs in cocoons about 4 mm long on water plants, stones, and, in aquaria, on the glass. They are not obligatory parasites, but may leave their host for long periods. Thus they can be introduced into the aquarium with food and plants and by other means. Nevertheless, this does not seem to occur very often, and in several years' practice on fish pathology I did not meet with one single case in aquarium fishes. It is in ponds where they cause trouble.

Leeches belong to the Phylum *Annelida* (ringed worms), Class *Hirudinea*. This Class contains three Orders, but only in that of the *Rhynchobdellida* are fish parasites found. These lack botryoidal tissue

(tissue composed of branched canals, with walls of large cells containing black pigment, surrounding the gut in leeches of the Order *Gnathobdellida*) and have colourless blood. To the Family of fish leeches (*Piscicolidæ*) (Fig. 2.12) belong *Piscicola geometra, Cystobranchus respirans* and *Cystobranchus mammilatus*; further, a number of species that are parasites of marine fishes only, *Piscicola geometra* is not only

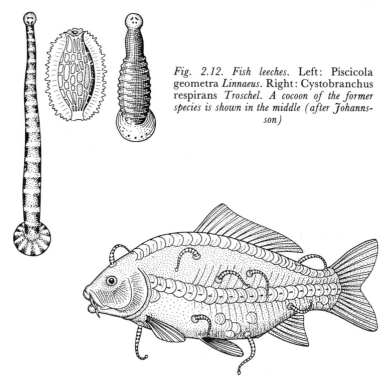

Fig. 2.12. Fish leeches. Left: Piscicola geometra *Linnaeus.* Right: Cystobranchus respirans *Troschel. A cocoon of the former species is shown in the middle (after Johannsson)*

Fig. 2.13. Carp attacked by Piscicola geometra

found in fresh water, but also in the Baltic (Fig. 2.13). In North America *Piscicola salmositica* Meyer (Fig. 2.14a) is found on Rainbow Trout (*Salmo gairdneri*) and on *Oncorhynchus kisutch*; it transfers the blood parasite *Cryptobia salmositica* Katz, which causes sleeping sickness (see p. 259). *Cystobranchus* is restricted to fresh water. *C. respirans* is found on Salmon (*Salmo salar*), Trout (*Salmo fario, S. salvelinus* a. o.), Grayling (*Thymallus thymallus*), Barbel (*Barbus barbus*), Perch (*Perca fluviatilis*) and some other fish. It reaches a length of 4 cm. *C. mammilatus* has been found on Eelpout (*Lota lota*) in Sweden and Germany; its length is up to 2 cm.

A second Family is that of the flat leeches (*Glossiphonidæ*) to which *Hemiclepsis marginata* (Fig. 2.14b) belongs. It parasitises freshwater fishes, amphibians, molluscs and worms. It reaches a length of 3 cm and it is characterised by a greenish or reddish-brown dorsal side on which a number of yellow spots are arranged in longitudinal and transverse series. The body is flat, whereas that of the members of the *Piscicolidæ* is cylindrical.

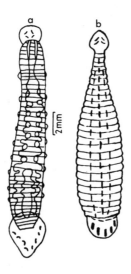

Fig. 2.14. Fish leeches. (a) Piscicola salmositica *Meyer (after Meyer)*. (b) Hemiclepsis marginata *(Müller) (after Johannsson)*

The leeches feed on the blood of their victims and can cause small fishes considerable harm. Places on the skin where leeches have been present are infiltrated with blood and show inflammation and can easily be affected by fungus. Fishes that are attacked by leeches swim restlessly and try by every means to get rid of their torturers, but usually in vain. Since the leeches adhere very securely they cannot be removed directly with forceps without causing serious damage to the skin of the fish. The best treatment is to place the fish in a $2\frac{1}{2}\%$ salt solution for 15 min. In this solution the fish will at first become restless, but this will do no harm. The parasites will be paralysed and the majority will fall off; if any remain on the fish they will be sufficiently affected to make it possible to remove them by means of forceps without injuring the skin of the fish. No special treatment for ponds is known at present.

It must be noted that although the salt solution paralyses the leeches it does not kill them. Thus do not throw them into any water.

Leeches can also be dangerous as bearers of blood parasites (*Cryptobia* and *Trypanosoma* species (see page 260)) that cause a sleeping sickness in fish. Leeches may sometimes be found on the gills and in the mouth of a fish and in such places they will do more harm than on the bodies.

YELLOW GRUB

The so-called yellow grubs are unsegmented flat worms of the Phylum *Platyhelminthes* and belong to the Class *Trematoda* and the Order *Digenea*. They occur frequently in the skin and the muscles of fresh-water fish; instances have been reported from all over the world. The worms are larval stages of the fluke *Clinostomum complanatum* (Rud. 1814) or *Clinostomum marginatum* (Rud. 1819).

Symptoms of the infection are the occurrence of small cream-coloured nodules or cysts, ranging from pinhead size up to 2.5 mm, depending on their age. These cysts are produced on the body, the head and the fins of the fishes. The number of cysts may vary from only one or two up to more than one hundred on one and the same fish. They have an oval or round shape.

The cysts, which contain the worms, are produced by the skin of the fish in reaction to the infection. This is to be regarded as a defensive measure, whereby the parasite is walled off and prevented from making further penetration into the body. If the cysts are opened, the worms will be found lying coiled up inside. They vary in length from $1\frac{1}{2}$ to 4 or even $6\frac{1}{2}$ mm. The larger ones may have a breadth of 2 mm. The worms are nearly white coloured, flat and able to change shape.

The infection does not seem to cause much discomfort to the victims, unless a large number of cysts with parasites is present, or unless the fish are very small. In some cases, the appearance of a cyst may be preceded by a greatly distended abdomen. It may take three weeks after the infection before the cysts become clearly visible, and seven weeks before they reach full size.

Clinostomum flukes have an intricate life cycle (Fig. 2.15). The adult parasites live in the throat and the mouth of fish-eating birds, such as herons and bitterns. The adult worms are hermaphrodites, but normally cross-fertilisation is practised. This takes place when they are in the bird. The ripe eggs are discharged by the parasite through its genital pore and reach the water either from the mouth or through the excreta of the bird.

The eggs hatch immediately after having reached the water, giving rise to the first larval stage, called miracidium. This is a free-swimming stage of very small dimensions, covered with a large number of fine hair-like cilia all over the body. Swimming is accomplished by the movement of the cilia.

The miracidia swim through the water till they find a snail of the Genus *Helisoma*. If they do not succeed in doing so within a few hours they are doomed to die. If, on the other hand, they do reach the right species of snail, they penetrate into the liver of this animal, where they change shape, losing their cilia and become so-called sporocysts. This change takes a period of three weeks. Then the sporocysts start an asexual reproduction process, consisting of a number of simple divisions, producing the third larval form, called

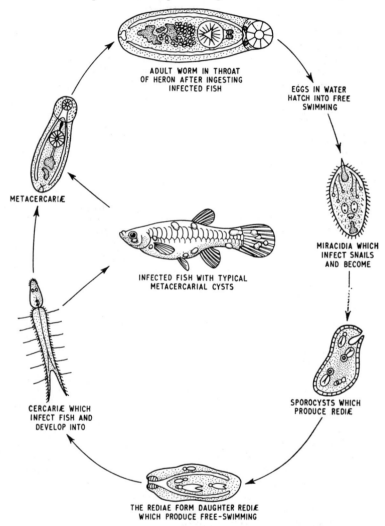

ADULT WORM IN THROAT
OF HERON AFTER INGESTING
INFECTED FISH

EGGS IN WATER
HATCH INTO FREE
SWIMMING

METACERCARIÆ

MIRACIDIA WHICH
INFECT SNAILS
AND BECOME

INFECTED FISH WITH TYPICAL
METACERCARIAL CYSTS

CERCARIÆ WHICH
INFECT FISH AND
DEVELOP INTO

SPOROCYSTS WHICH
PRODUCE REDIÆ

THE REDIAE FORM DAUGHTER REDIÆ
WHICH PRODUCE FREE-SWIMMING

Fig. 2.15. Life cycle of the yellow grub organism Clinostomum complanatum *(redrawn after Rosenthal). It passes through stages in snails and birds, as well as fish*

redia. The rediae themselves also multiply asexually, producing daughter rediae. These daughter rediae produce a fifth larval stage, called cercaria, consisting of a nearly cylindrical body with a forked tail and a covering of cilia.

The cercariae leave the snail and may swim through the water or they may float, hanging down from the surface of the water. When they contact a fish, they burrow into the skin of the head or the fins or beneath a scale of the body, dropping their tails before they have completed penetration. The skin of the fish is irritated by this infection and reacts by producing a cyst around the intruder. The encysted stage of the parasite in the fish is called metacercaria.

If an infected fish is eaten by a bird, the metacercariae are liberated from the cysts by the digestive juices dissolving the fish and the cyst wall. The worms are able to resist digestion and, once free, they migrate to the mouth and throat of the bird, where they attach themselves by means of a strong ventral sucker (acetabulum). In about four days they develop into the adult stage (Fig. 2.16). Then the complicated life cycle may start again.

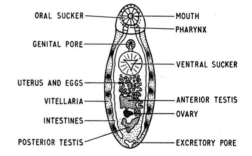

Fig. 2.16. Adult stage of C. complanatum (after Rosenthal)

ORAL SUCKER — MOUTH — PHARYNX
GENITAL PORE
VENTRAL SUCKER
UTERUS AND EGGS
VITELLARIA — ANTERIOR TESTIS
INTESTINES — OVARY
POSTERIOR TESTIS — EXCRETORY PORE

Since the infection cannot be transferred from fish to fish, it is not necessary to isolate diseased fish from the community tank. Snails, however, should be removed and quarantined for at least two months to avoid any risk of further infections originating from this source. It would be possible to introduce the parasites into the aquarium in the absence of snails; cercaria stages could be introduced with plants or livefood from natural waters. It is also possible that a new fish may already have been infected shortly before its introduction in the tank, since it could take three weeks before the cysts become visible.

Clinostomum has been found in a number of tropical fish including *Corynopoma riisei, Chriopeops goodei, Hypopomus artedi, Mollienisia velifera, Lebistes reticulatus* (Fig. 2.17), *Nannostomus trifasciatus, Piabucana* species and *Sternopygus macrurus*.

Infected fishes may be cured by careful opening of the cysts by means of a small scalpel (a small lancet-shaped knife, used for dissection), and removing the worms with a pair of fine-pointed tweezers. The incisions are disinfected by touching them with a small pencil or brush dipped into a solution of Mercurochrome to avoid bacterial or fungus infection. Then the fishes are placed in clean, fresh water where they soon recover completely.[6]

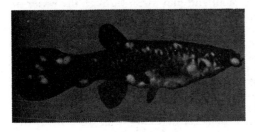

Fig. 2.17.
GUPPY
INFECTED WITH
YELLOW GRUB
Female Guppy (Lebistes reticulatus) *with numerous cysts containing metacercariae of* Clinostomum *(after Harold L. Rosenthal,* Aquarium Journal, *U.S.A.)*

Fishes that carry yellow grub infection must not be used for human consumption since its metacercariae may affect human health. A case of laryngopharingitis has been observed.[7]

SKIN FLUKES

In the first part of this chapter I have dealt with parasites that are easily visible to the naked eye and can be studied with the aid of a simple magnifying glass. We now consider some diseases which are caused by parasites of microscopical dimensions. Diagnosis of illness caused by them is not so easy, since absolute certainty as to the origin can only be obtained by means of a microscopical examination of the slime of the skin in which the parasites are present. However, by careful observation of the signs and symptoms, it is possible to recognise the trouble sufficiently accurately to allow suitable treatment being given.

There are closely related types of flukes that often attack aquarium fishes, namely, different species of the Families *Gyrodactylidæ* and *Dactylogyridæ*. The former, whilst they attack the gills, are frequently found on the skin of fish, while the latter are typical parasites of the gills. In many cases parasites of both kinds may be found on one and the same fish.

The most obvious symptoms of the condition of distress created by parasitic worms are, in the case of the Gyrodactylids, that at first the colours of the infected fish fade and the victim grows very pale; then the fins droop and fold and gradually become torn, while the skin becomes more slimy than normal and shows small blood spots. Small blood spots may also be seen at the base of the fins. Breathing generally is increased in frequency, even in cases where the gills are not affected. If all these signs and symptoms are present, it is advisable to treat the diseased fishes as having *Gyrodactyliasis*, even if you have no opportunity of confirming this diagnosis by a microscopical examination of the slime of the skin, as the probability is that it is one of the varieties of *Gyrodactylus* which is responsible.

The diseased fishes become dull and feeble, and rest frequently, mostly near the surface of the water, while every movement becomes more and more difficult until, in the end, the animals die from complete exhaustion. Since attacks are frequently fatal, treatment must begin as early as possible. If only the skin is affected, prognosis is not so bad, but if the gills are infected with one of the varieties of *Gyrodactylus* or, more likely, by *Dactylogyrus*, recovery is only possible with early and strong treatment, before the victims become too weak.

Fishes whose gills are infected by flukes gape for breath, their gill coverings being stretched open widely, while the gills are expanded and very pale. Parts of the gills often become protuberant and show as a small fleece outside the covering.

The flukes which attack the fish and cause the signs and symptoms described are unsegmented flat worms of the Phylum *Platyhelminthes* and belong to the Class *Trematoda*, the Order of *Monogenea* and the Super-family *Gyrodactyloidea*. They have an elliptical-shaped body that is flattened on the ventral side (on the 'belly'). At the front end there are two conical projections, which bear the openings of glands, secreting a thick, sticky liquid, enabling them to cling to the skin or the gills of a fish. At the hinder end a strong attachment organ is situated. This organ is disc-shaped and has two large hooks in the middle, surrounded by a ring of smaller hooks. In *Gyrodactylus* 16 small hooks are present, while in *Dactylogyrus* there are 14.

The parasite first attaches itself to the fish by means of the small hooks and then drives in the two large ones so that a firm hold is obtained. If the parasite wishes to move to another place it fastens its front end to the skin, then releases the hooks and swings its body to another part, where the hooks are refastened. Skin flukes feed on the epithelial cells, and in doing so they cause considerable damage to the skin of the fish. The mouth is situated on the ventral side, near the front end of the body.

Three species of *Gyrodactylus* generally known to aquarists are *Gyrodactylus elegans* (Fig. 2.18a, page 30), reaching a length of about 0.5–0.8 mm, the commonest form; *G. medius* (length about 0.3–0.35 mm); and *G. gracilis* (length about 0.18–0.32 mm). From these figures it may be seen that the parasites must be visible to the naked eye, but it is difficult to recognise them when they attack the fish's skin, as they soon become covered by the slime of the skin and by then are completely invisible. To study the parasite, it is therefore necessary to take some slime off the skin and smear this on a slide for microscopical examination. They are more easily seen when they attack the gills or, more accurately, the skin in the region of the gills. Other varieties recorded by Dr. Ben Dawes in his book 'The Trematoda',[8] in the Family *Gyrodactylidæ*, are *G. cobitis*, *G. grænlandicus*, *G. latus*, *G. parvicopula*, *G. rarus* and *G. atherinæ*.

The *Gyrodactylidæ* found in North America have been listed

by Putz and Hoffman.[9] These include *G. bullatarudis* (Fig. 2.18b, page 30), which is often found in aquaria on Guppies (*Lebistes reticulatus*), and members of the related Genera *Gyrodactyloides* and *Isancistrum* that are characterised by different constructions of their hook systems.

Gyrodactylus is a livebearing organism, and as such is remarkable, for not only can the young fluke be seen within the body of the adult, but in the body of this unborn young yet another embryo may be seen. Very often this 'grandchild' contains a 'great-grand-child', so that in one *Gyrodactylus* four generations may be preformed. At present, it is not yet known with absolute certainty how this remarkable phenomenon occurs. A most probable hypothesis is that the 'child' parasite (which has been procreated by a proper sexual process) produces an embryo by parthenogenesis before its own birth, while this embryo creates the 'great-grandchild' in the same manner. Such a parthenogenetical reproduction in the larval stage is called paedogenesis. The young parasites creep on the skin of the fish immediately after birth. They may remain on the same host or they may leave it and search for another. In the latter case, if they do not find a new host they die in a few days. Consequently, it is not necessary to disinfect a tank after the appearance of this disease, but it is sufficient to remove all fishes for a time. A week will be a completely safe period.

This holds also for cases of *Dactylogyrus* infection. However, this animal is not livebearing, but produces eggs, the young hatching as larvae.

Skin and gill flukes mostly attack members of the Carp Family (*Cyprinidæ*). This disease appears very often in Goldfish, Sticklebacks and Pike; members of the Trout Family (*Salmonidæ*) can also be subject to it. In tropical aquaria, Tooth-carps (*Cyprinodontidæ*) and *Characidæ* are the most common victims, but Labyrinth Fishes never appear to be affected, even if present in tanks with very badly infected other fishes. From my experience it seems also that the resistance of dark-coloured fishes is generally higher than of others.

ELIMINATING SKIN FLUKES

For curing diseased fishes, different chemicals can be used, but it is most important that the treatment is started as soon as possible, for if the fishes are already weak they possibly cannot be saved.

In early stages bathing the fishes for 10–15 min in a 2.5% salt (sodium chloride) solution can be effective.

An older treatment for skin flukes is to place the fishes for 5–15 min in a 1:2000 solution of ammonia. To prepare this, a dilution of 10 parts by volume of household ammonia (which has a strength of 10%) with 90 parts by volume of water is made; then 5 cm^3 of this solution are added to 1 l of water. For fishes with a strong skin, such as Goldfish, Tench and Carp, the solution may be made stronger, namely 1 : 1000; this is 10 cm³ of the aforementioned dilution per litre of water, or 45 cm³ per Imp. gal (or 37½ cm³ per U.S. gal).

Although this ammonia treatment has given good results when dealing with *Gyrodactyliasis*, it is not advisable for delicate fishes, since these can die in it from acute poisoning. In such cases methylene blue may be used which has also the advantage that it can be added directly to the tank. Good results have been obtained by this treatment.[10] A stock solution of methylene blue (medical quality) is made by dissolving 1 g (=15 gr) in 100 cm³ (about 0.09 qt) of water. Of this solution 0.2–0.4 cm³ (=3–6 drops) per litre of water are added (or 2–4 cm³/Imp. gal = 1.7–3.4 cm³/U.S. gal). The water becomes deep blue in colour, but this colour will fade gradually during the following days until it disappears completely. As long as the water shows the blue colouring the chemical is active. It is not necessary to repeat the treatment, since the activity remains long enough to kill any skin fluke either on the fish or in the water. Since it is not necessary to change the water after treatment, methylene blue may also be used for treatment of ponds in which the disease makes an appearance among the fish.

D. Bailösoff used Neguvon (Bayer) against *Gyrodactylus* infections in the same way as described on pages 14 and 336. In a 2–3.5% solution *Gyrodactylus elegans* was killed within 15 sec.

Quinine hydrochloride (1 g/50 l) has also been reported to be effective.

USE OF FORMALIN

The best treatment available at present may be the formaldehyde method recommended by Ian M. Rankin[11] (see Fig. 2.19). A stock solution is prepared of 1 cm³ of British Pharmacopæia grade formaldehyde solution to 99 cm³ of water. From 6–7 cm³ of this stock solution should be added to each litre of aquarium water, or 4 minims of undiluted formalin to each Imp. gal (3.5 minims/U.S. gal). The required dose of stock solution should be diluted with a large volume of water drawn from the tank which is to be treated and the solution can then be added slowly to the tank. Good mixing is essential and artificial aeration should be employed continuously during treatment. After three days, half the water must be removed and replaced by fresh water, and the same dose of formaldehyde solution as originally used added to the aquarium again. It is essential that the full dosage is given, because if a lower concentration is used resistant strains of parasites may be produced and then it would be very difficult to get rid of the infection.

The formaldehyde solution to be used in making the stock solution must be free from paraformaldehyde, which may be recognised as a 'white stuff' at the bottom and/or on the walls of the bottle. If this sediment or deposit should be present in any great quantity, the formaldehyde solution would be slightly weaker than it should be and dosage would be incorrect. Further, paraformaldehyde is toxic to fish. Therefore, a fresh supply of formaldehyde solution

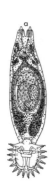 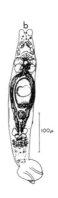 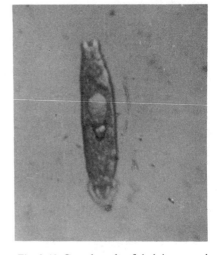

Fig. 2.18. Skin flukes. (a) Gyro-dactylus elegans *v. Nordmann (after Roth).* (b) Gyrodactylus bullata-rudis *Turnbull (after Turnbull)*

Fig. 2.19. Gyrodactylus *fluke being exposed to formalin. Embryo is clearly visible in the centre (photomicrograph by Ian M. Rankin)*

should be used always and this must be stored in a warm dark place, since the formation of paraformaldehyde is accelerated by light and low temperature. If a small amount of paraformaldehyde should be present, the solution should be filtered through a fine filter paper before use.

Formaldehyde must not be added to a tank or pond in which methylene blue or other dyes, which are adsorbed, have been em-ployed recently. Formaldehyde may act as an eluent (releasing agent) and the combination of formaldehyde with these other chemicals might result in toxic effects on the fish.

Although this formaldehyde treatment is excellent for tropicals, it may have a drawback in treatment of cold-water fish, since at temperatures below 18°C (approximately 65°F) there is some danger of fungus infection owing to the weakening of the mucous coat of the skin of the fish. If such secondary fungus infection should occur, the water has to be changed and a specific treatment for fungus started. As such, phenoxethol is recommended, as described on page 85.

OTHER CURES FOR FLUKES

Another highly effective cure for *Gyrodactyliasis*, suggested by Dr. C. van Dommelen, a Dutch physician, is with potassium antimonyl tartrate (Tartar Emetic) in a concentration of not more than 150 mg/100 l (0.1 gr/Imp. gal or 0.08 gr/U.S. gal). After two days the water must be slowly changed. Tartar Emetic has been found effective in treatment of yearling Goldfish, Veils and Fantails. During treatment no food must be given.

Chloramine treatment as described on page 322 may also be effective.

Prof. Schäperclaus has recommended the use of 'Zephirol' (benzalkonium chloride) 1 : 4000–1 : 2000. *Gyrodactylus* is killed within about 1–2 min. Therefore a 5-min treatment would be sufficient.

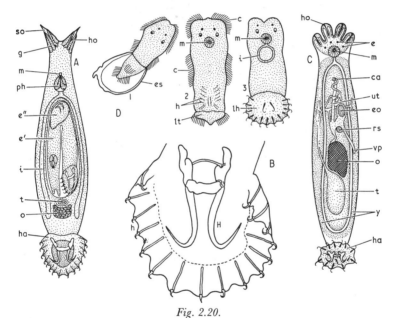

Fig. 2.20.
COMPARISON BETWEEN Gyrodactylus AND Dactylogyrus
A, Gyrodactylus, *adult containing two generations of embryos.* B, *posterior haptor of* A, *showing anchor-like hooks and sixteen hooklets.* C, Dactylogyrus, *adult with one egg in utero. Note haptor with fourteen hooklets (after Wilde).* D, *larvae of* C; 1, *hatching from egg.* 2, *free-living form with cilia.* 3, *juvenile taken from fish host (after Wilde).* c, *cilia;* ca, *copulatory apparatus;* e, *eyes;* e', *embryo of first generation;* eo, *egg in ootype;* es, *egg shell;* g, *glands of head organ;* h, *hooklets;* H, *hooks;* ha, *posterior haptor;* ho, *head-organ;* i, *intestine;* lh, *larval haptor;* lt, *larval tail;* m, *mouth;* o, *ovary;* ph, *pharynx;* rs, *receptaculum seminis;* so, *sense-organ;* t, *testis;* ut, *uterus;* vp, *vaginal pore;* y, *yolk follicles*

The chemical is much more toxic than formalin. Treatment exceeding 30 min could be lethal.

Other treatments include acriflavine (1 g/100 l, see p. 317) or acrinol (1 g/400–500 l, see p. 318) and hydrogen peroxide (not very effective, see p. 328).

In ponds potassium permanganate can be used (4–5 mg/l or 0.25–0.5 gr/Imp. gal or 0.2–0.4 gr/U.S. gal). Some aquarists have claimed the successful use of it in their tanks.

From time to time, other chemicals have been suggested for treatment of *Gyrodactylus* infection, such as immersing the fish for not more than 9 min in a solution of 'Dettol' containing about twelve drops in one Imp. gal of tap water (C. E. C. Cole). It is a drastic treatment, the fish dashing wildly after having been introduced to the bath. After some moments they slow down and turn on their sides with the gill coverings open to the fullest possible extent. These are Mr. Cole's observations. 'Dettol' originally contained 1.3% chloroxylenol, 0.4% dichloroxylenol and 9% terpineol in a soapy emulsion, but recently the composition was changed to 4.8% chloroxylenol and 9% terpineol in a soapy emulsion. Rankin found that chloroxylenol is ineffective against flukes, and in view of that, its high toxicity, and the change in the formula, I believe that the other treatments are safer and likely to be more efficacious.

Since fishes affected by flukes have a greater need of oxygen than normally it is advisable to aerate the water adequately by means of an air-pump.

For a description of gill flukes (*Dactylogyrus* and related organisms), see page 108 (also see Fig. 2.20).

BLACK SPOT

The symptom of black spot disease (*Diplostomiasis*) is the development of small brown or black spots on several parts of the body and fins. The specific sites are the cutis and the underlying muscles. Sometimes such spots can also be found in the eyes, the gills and the

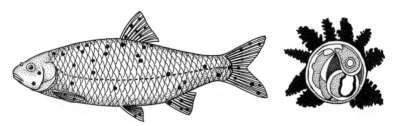

Fig. 2.21. Left: *Dace infected with black spot disease,* Diplostomiasis. Right: *Cyst of* Postho(Neo)diplostomum cuticola *with worm inside (after Nordmann)*

mouth. The size of the irregular spots is from 0.85–3.80 mm. Upon thorough examination of these dark spots, after dissection of the fish and with the aid of a microscope, it can be seen that they contain a light-coloured cyst of connective tissue in which a slowly moving worm lies rolled up. The cyst is surrounded by an accumulation of pigment cells, which causes the black spots to be seen from the outside. The worm in the cyst is a larval stage (metacercaria) of a sucking worm (*Trematoda*) and is known under the name of *Posthodiplostomum cuticola* Dubois (formerly *Neodiplostomum cuticola* Ciurea = *Neascus cuticola* v. Nordm), Fig. 2.21.

The adult of this parasite lives in the intestines of herons. The eggs of the worms reach the water with the excrement of the birds, where they hatch, and part of their life history takes place in aquatic snails. The parasites then infect fishes. If an infected fish is eaten by a water bird, the larvae penetrate into its intestines, where they change into the adult form.

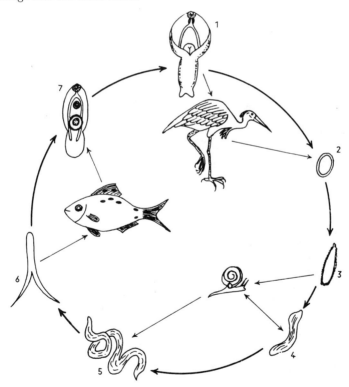

Fig. 2.22. Life cycle of Posthodiplostomum cuticola *Dubois (after Dönges)*: 1, *adult worm*. 2, *egg*. 3, *miracidium*. 4, *sporocyst*. 5, *daughter sporocyst*. 6, *cercaria*. 7, *metacercaria*

The parasite in the fish reaches a length of about 1–2 mm. It has a flat shape and oval outlines. The hind part has a sac-like prolongation. There are two suckers and an attachment organ on the body. The intestine is forked. If a few parasites are present on a big fish they will not do much harm, but if there are many, or if the fish is small, the disease is serious, and in such cases the scales may be damaged, too.

It must be noted that the colour of the spots may vary, according to the amount of pigment normally present in the skin of different species of fish. In fishes with little pigment, the spots will never be really black, but may remain a brownish colour. The cysts are normally present in the cutis of the fish, and the nearer to the surface of the skin, the darker the colour of the spots will appear.

As the life cycle of *Posthodiplostomum cuticola* (Fig. 2.22) relies on the presence of aquatic snails, the absence of these creatures from ponds and tanks removes the possibility of black spot disease appearing in the fishes. All species of *Planorbis* may be suspected in cases of infection. There is, of course, always the possibility of a fish being introduced to new quarters, after it has become infected, and in this instance the disease might manifest itself after a short time, even though snails were absent.

Since the disease is not infectious from fish to fish, it is sufficient to treat only the infected fishes without considering the others.

Fishes that show the signs of brown or black spots can be cured by bathing them in a solution of picric acid 2–7 : 100 000 for about 1 h. A stock solution is made by dissolving 1 g (15 gr) in 100 cm^3 of water, and of this solution 2–7 cm^3 should be added to 1 l of water (or about 9–30 cm^3 to 1 Imp. gal, 7.5–25 cm^3 per U.S. gal). For fishes with strong or very slimy skins, such as Goldfish, Carp and Tench, use the strongest concentration. After treatment, the fishes can be returned to the aquarium immediately.

BLACK GRUB

This infection is also characterised by the occurrence of black cysts in the skin, the gills and the muscles. The causative worm parasite is the metacercarian stage of *Crassiphiala bulboglossa* van Haitsma and its preferred victims are *Cyprinidæ* and *Percidæ* in North America. Intermediary hosts are snails of the Genus *Helisoma*. Final hosts are *Alcedinidæ*.

BLACK SCALE DISEASE

Black spots appear in the scales of affected *Cyprinidæ*. The causative organism is the metacercaria of *Metagonimus yokogawai* Katsurada (Fig. 2.23), belonging to the *Heterophyidæ*. The first intermediary hosts are *Melanoides, Fagotia* and related genera. The disease is also dangerous for human beings, who may contract it by consuming infected fish which have not been subjected to sufficient heat treatment.

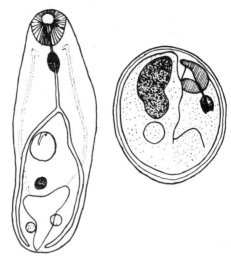

Fig. 2.23. Metacercaria of Metagonimus yokogawai *Katsurada.   Left: Free organism.* Right: *Cyst with worm (after Vojtkova)*

GREY PEARL DISEASE (*NEASCUSIASIS*)

This disease is related to black spot. Its symptoms are the occurrence of globular or ellipsoidal cysts, 1.8–2.3 mm in size, in the skin and the muscles. Sometimes cysts may also be found in the internal organs. The cysts in the skin look like a number of small grey pearls. They contain the metacercariae of the sucking worm *Neodiplostomum perlatum* Ciurea (*Neascus perlatus*)—see Fig. 2.24. The final hosts are water birds of prey.

Thus far, this infection has only been observed in Carp (*Cyprinus carpio*) and Prussian Carp in the Danube and surrounding regions.

Fig. 2.24. Metacercaria of Neodiplostomum perlatum *Ciurea (after Ciurea)*

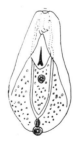

INK SPOT DISEASE

Another disease related to black spot, caused by encysted metacercariae of the sucking worm *Isoparorchis hypselobagri*, occurring under the skin, in the muscles and body cavity. The infection is common in Vietnam, where it is called 'Muc cá', in *Tylosurus annulatus* and *Ophicephalus striatus*.[12]

GREY SPOT DISEASE ('SUNBURN')

This condition is characterised by the appearance of large numbers of grey spots at the back of the fishes. It has no parasitary origin, but is apparently due to lack of nicotinic acid and may be healed by supplying adequate food containing this vitamin, such as liver, white meat, yeast or wholemeal flour (see p. 292).

WHITE SPOT (*ICHTHYOPHTHIRIASIS*)

One of the most prevalent diseases of fishes is the so-called white spot or 'Ich' (an abbreviation of the name of the parasite), which is characterised by the appearance of greater or smaller numbers of

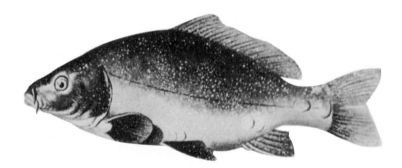

Fig. 2.25.
CARP WITH WHITE SPOT
Carp attacked by white spot protozoan (Ichthyophthirius) *(after colour plate by Hofer)*

'spots' of a white or greyish colour (Fig. 2.25), and having a diameter of about 0.5–1 mm, on the fins and the skin of the fish. Each 'spot' is in reality a small bladder (Fig. 2.26), containing one or more parasites that are rotating in lively fashion. The parasite is a protozoan (a unicellular organism) named *Ichthyophthirius multifiliis*, now classified in the Family *Ophryoglenidæ* of the Order *Holotricha* of the *Ciliata*.

The parasite penetrates the mucous coat and the upper layer of the epidermis. By its movements the epidermis is irritated and reacts by augmentation of the epithelial cells in the neighbourhood of the parasite, so that the latter is covered by a layer of the skin of

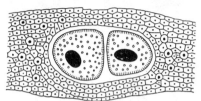

Fig. 2.26. Sketch (redrawn after Doflein) of section of fish skin with a complete white spot 'bladder' containing two protozoans

the fish. Thus the bladder is a pathological production of the fish skin in reaction to the activity of the parasite and not of the parasite itself. Often the young parasite reproduces itself by a simple division shortly after having penetrated into the skin, which is the reason that so many times two 'Ichs' are encountered inside one bladder. The 'Ich' is always situated between the epidermis and the cutis, where it feeds on red blood corpuscles, which it extracts from the superficial blood capillaries of the cutis, and on disintegrated epithelial cells. When after some days in the fish's skin the parasites are fully grown, they bore through the epidermis bladder and leave the fish for reproduction. Then they will have a diameter of 0.2–0.5 mm. In some cases still larger specimens, up to 1 mm, have been found.

The mature parasite, having left its host, sinks to the bottom of the water, where it secretes a soft, jelly-like covering about itself; a so-called 'cyst'. In this cyst the 'Ich' undergoes a rapid division into

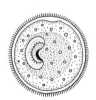

Fig. 2.27. These drawings by the author show (left) examples of organism Ichthyophthirius multifiliis. *Note the covering of cilia and the horseshoe-shaped nucleus in each. On the right are two white spot 'cysts' in which the protozoan undergoes rapid division into a number of young but complete parasites. From 500 to 1200 can be formed from one adult specimen*

numerous youngsters. The speed of this process depends on the temperature of the water; the higher the temperature, the higher the speed of reproduction. From 500 to 1200 young parasites (Fig. 2.27) may be produced from one adult. At a temperature of 18–20°C

(32–68°F) the division process takes about 12–18 h. The young parasites have a size of 0.03–0.04 mm. At first they do not move very much, but within 36 h of the mature parasite's leaving the fish they will be swimming freely through the water in search of a new host.

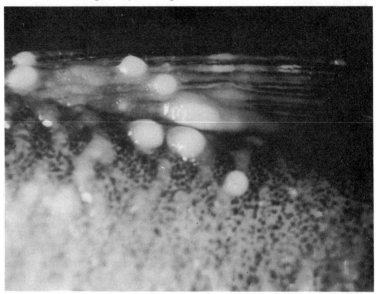

Fig. 2.28(a). Scardinius erythrophthalmus *(Rudd) infected with* Ichthyo-phthirius multifiliis *Fouquet.* × 2 *(photograph by Dr. E. Elkan)*

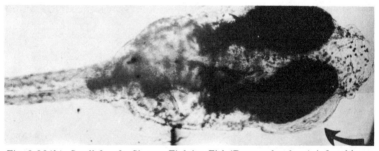

Fig. 2.28(b). Small fry of a Siamese Fighting Fish (Betta splendens) *infected by an* Ichthyophthirius *at the right eye. When living, the parasite was seen rotating lively in its specific way so that there could not be any doubt regarding its identity. Such infections of very young fishes are rare. Photomicrograph by the author.* × 80

Thus, in an aquarium the parasites leave the fishes periodically, but the animals become infected again and again by increasing numbers of parasites, till at last they are weakened so much that they die.

When the external conditions in the water are unfavourable for normal development of cysts, as is the case at low oxygen content or absence of suitable sites for settling, a deviation of the normal course of the reproductive process is observed (Fig. 2.29). In such conditions full-grown parasites having just left a fish do not encyst, but start dividing while still hovering in the water. The number of young parasites produced in this way by one mother parasite is less than in the normal process following cyst formation.

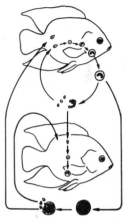

Fig. 2.29. Life cycle of Ichthyophthirius. Outer cycle: *Normal development with cyst formation.* Small inner cycle: *Deviating development with reproduction while hovering in the water without encysting (see text) (after Amlacher)*

The mature parasite is approximately sphere-shaped (see Fig. 2.27), but it can change its shape to a considerable extent, if necessary. The body bears a large number of cilia (little hairs) over the whole surface area, by the movement of which the parasite can swim through the water and penetrate into the skin of a fish. It has a tubular mouth, several vacuoles and a large nucleus. The 'Ich' is of a white colour and in a living state it is generally not very transparent. After killing the parasite with a suitable reagent on a microscopical slide (e.g. a drop of a solution of picric acid or a drop of formalin) the nucleus will show more clearly upon examination. Characteristic features of the parasite are the horseshoe-shaped nucleus, and its rotating movement when alive.

The development of *Ichthyophthirius* in the skin of a fish varies, depending on the temperature of the water. At temperatures between 21–26°C (70–80°F) three or four days after the white spot becomes visible to the naked eye, the parasite leaves the fish, while at a temperature of 10°C (50°F) this may take four weeks and more. Thus, raising the temperature will shorten the time that the parasites remain in the fish skin, but it also shortens the time before reinfection occurs and, since this new infection takes place by many more parasites, the results of this procedure will be disastrous, if it is not combined with suitable treatment for killing the young parasites that are leaving the cysts before they reach a fish.

The young parasites cannot live long in the water in a free state; if they cannot find a host, they die in a few days (Fig. 2.30). According to Schäperclaus, at a temperature of 20°C (68°F) no free-swimming young parasites will survive longer than 55 h. Thus, if all fishes are removed from an infected tank, after three days this tank will be safe again. Complete treatment of the diseased fishes will take a longer period, but after treatment in a separate tank they

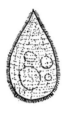 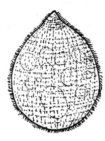

Fig. 2.30. Two diagrams (redrawn after Buschkiel) showing (left) the early stage in the life cycle of Ichthyophthirius before it has found a host and (right) soon after settling in the skin of a fish

can be put back into their own aquarium again quite safely. If possible, it is always better to treat fishes in a separate tank, since then complications through reactions of the chemical with organic substances present in the water that may decrease the activity of the medicine will not be of importance, while in a completely planted tank some chemicals soon lose their activity. Some chemicals will have a bad effect on the plants, too.

Ichthyophthirius is spread widely over the earth, both in Europe and North America as well as in tropical countries, and consequently it can stand high temperatures. The Dutch hydrobiologist, Dr. A. L. Buschkiel,[13] who has made thorough studies on Ichthyophthirius, both in Europe and in the former Dutch East Indies, mentions a white spot epidemic in fishponds on the island of Java, causing extensive losses.

It also occurs in brackish water and in the sea. It has been found on Coral Fishes, on Puffer Fish (Tetrodon fluviatilis), several species of Sea Bream in the Adriatic and the Mediterranean and on Mackerels.

In England Ichthyophthirius was not found in the wild until recently, and thus this parasite would not be introduced with livefood, plants, etc., from natural waters. All infections must be introduced with fishes or plants from other aquaria or artificial pools, the parasite being imported with fishes or plants from other countries. On the Continent of Europe and in the U.S.A. Ichthyophthirius is endemical in free waters. Aquarists in England were thus in a much more fortunate position than their fellow fishkeepers in other countries.

This happy state of affairs seems to have come to an end by now. In 1960, Mr. Raymond Jackson reported to me to have identified Ichthyophthirius parasites on Minnows (Phoxinus phoxinus) caught in the River Biss in Trowbridge U.D.C. Park, Wiltshire. He stated that the river at this point runs alongside a site frequently used by fair-grounds; in fact one was just moving away when the catch was made. He thinks it possible that the white spot disease could gain a hold in Britain by the indiscriminate dumping of diseased and dying Goldfish frequently given as prizes in these fairs; most of these fish are imported.

It is nearly always possible to avoid the infection. If plants, snails, etc., that have been obtained from a dealer or a fellow-aquarist are kept in quarantine for three days at a temperature of 20°C (68°F) or for about a week at lower temperatures, no young 'Ich' or cyst will survive. In England, cold-water fishes will not develop 'Ich' as often as tropicals, since introduction from free waters is less likely. In the U.S.A. and on the Continent of Europe, separating cold-water fishes before introducing them into the community tank does not give much security, except in summer, since at low temperatures development of the parasites in the skin of the fish goes on very slowly and consequently quarantine would have to continue for several weeks.

Experience shows that most cases of 'Ich' appear in autumn and winter, although the disease may occur in all four seasons. This may be due to the fact that in the seasons mentioned fishes will have less resistance to disease as a result of several circumstances, such as lack of light, causing less oxygen production by the plants, and lack of suitable live foods. If a completely healthy fish, living in very good conditions, is infected by one or two *Ichthyophthirius* parasites, it will not suffer much and, if the tank is not crowded, the chances of reinfection are not too great. In such cases the infection can remain latent for a long period, since the parasites in the skin of the fish will grow very slowly and consequently no symptoms of disease appear. But if the resistance of the fish is weakened by unsuitable conditions the parasites will get a better chance, and then an epidemic may occur. This explains why epidemics of *Ichthyophthirius* often appear when tropicals are kept at too low temperatures, while in cold-water fishes this can be the case when the water temperature is too high.

Cysts of *Ichthyophthirius* can often be found on water plants, which explains how these parasites can be smuggled into the aquarium by plants from an infected tank. *Ichthyophthirius* needs a good amount of oxygen, and if the oxygen content of the water is below a critical value, reproduction is greatly hindered. Instead of encysting itself, the parasite may divide directly in two parts (simple direct division) or it may even die.

RAISING THE TEMPERATURE

It is possible to cure diseased fishes that can stand considerable lack of oxygen in the water, namely Labyrinth Fishes, simply by putting them for a time in a tank without plants at a high temperature (up to 30°C = 86°F). The 'Ich' will die from lack of oxygen, while the fishes, due to their labyrinth system which enables them to breath atmospheric air, can stand this treatment. This is the reason why white spot can sometimes be cured by raising the temperature; warm water can hold less oxygen than cold, so that the oxygen content of the water becomes less at higher temperature. Except in the case of Labyrinth Fishes, treated in the way described above, temperature treatment will not give reliable results, for often the weakening effect on fishes will more than counterbalance the effect on the parasites. Heat treatment then, acts only indirectly; it is not the high temperature as such that harms the parasites, but only the lack of oxygen which can result from it. Thus, if the water is well aerated, or the plants are producing much oxygen under the influence of light, raising the temperature will have no effect whatsoever against the 'Ich', whilst it weakens the fishes.

There is, however, a limit to the heat resistance of the parasite, depending on the actual stage of development. According to Dr. A. Stolk, mature parasites in the skin of the fish are killed at a temperature of 32–33°C (90°F), but the cysts can withstand this heat, although development is retarded. Later, as soon as the temperature drops, development of the parasites inside the cysts recommences. New infections of fish can occur, unless the temperature is suddenly raised again to kill the young parasites that have just left the cysts. From these considerations, Stolk derived an improved heat treatment consisting of the intermittent raising and lowering of the temperature of the water, up to 33°C (90°F) and down to 21°C (75°F). The maximum temperature has to be reached within a few hours early in the morning and then it has to be maintained during the day. Towards the evening the tank is allowed to cool down to 21°C. The process is repeated from three to five times (or more, if necessary). Good results have been obtained with Livebearing Tooth-carps and with Flame Fish (*Hyphessobrycon flammeus*).

Although this treatment can safely be applied to tropical fish, it cannot be recommended for cold-water fish. Temperatures exceeding 30°C (86°F) are fatal for most cold-water species, whilst some may die from lack of oxygen before this temperature is reached.

With tropical tanks, it may be difficult to raise the temperature to the required level within the course of a few hours. In wintertime, a powerful heater would be needed for a large tank. The problem can be solved by transferring the fish to a smaller aquarium for treatment.

To make sure that newly obtained fishes have no latent *Ichthyophthirius*, a long quarantine period is necessary; four to eight weeks for cold-water fishes, two to four weeks for tropicals. It is also possible to give the fishes a prophylactic treatment either with quinine or with methylene blue.

There is no chemical available that enables us to kill the *Ichthyophthirius* in the skin of the fish, without killing the fish too. This is due to the fact that the parasite is protected by the layer of epidermis that grows over it so that the chemicals cannot penetrate directly to it. Thus we have to wait for the moment when the 'Ich' must leave the fish. The unprotected parasite, the cysts and the young parasites in search of a host can be successfully attacked. Treatment must always be extended over a period long enough to ensure that all parasites have left the fish, and consequently we have to use permanent baths in which the fish are kept until they are cured.

QUININE SALTS EFFECTIVE

Different medicaments have been tried with negative, or unreliable, results, but some have been found that show a very good activity. The most important ones are quinine salts and methylene blue. The quinine treatment was introduced in 1931 by the Swiss pharmacist W. Jung.[14] He used concentrations of 1 : 100 000. The investigations of Buschkiel proved that this is too low for killing all free-swimming young parasites, while the cysts are not attacked. A strength of 3 : 100 000, however, is sufficient to kill all young parasites and cysts, without having bad effects on adult fishes. Schäperclaus has reported, however, that Prussian Carp of 3–6 cm length were killed within 9–18 h in a 1 : 50 000 solution and within 24–48 h in a 1 : 100 000 solution.[15] There are reports that young fishes that had been treated with quinine salts were less fertile, but their health was not affected.

In strengths of 3–4 : 100 000 quinine salts have a bad effect on several water plants and this is the disadvantage of the cure. To avoid this it is advisable to remove all fishes from the planted tank and to put them in a separate unplanted tank, in which they are treated with the quinine salt. This has also the advantage that the quinine does not disappear by chemical reactions with substances present in the water as fast as is the case in a fully planted tank with old water. The activity of quinine salts also depends to some extent on the pH of the water; the activity is at its best if the water is slightly acid (about pH 6.5). It is helpful, therefore, to use a pH testing outfit. Alkaline water (pH above 7) can be made slightly acid by adding drops of phosphoric acid till, after a thorough stirring, a new test shows that the desired reaction is reached. Such additions are made after adding the quinine salt to the water and before putting the fishes in the tank.

The best quinine salt that can be used is quinine chloride (quinine hydrochloride). Let your chemist make you a solution of 3 g quinine hydrochloride in 300 cm^3 of water, or buy 3 g of the chemical and dissolve it in the same amount of water yourself. This solution is sufficient for a tank containing 100 l (approx. 20 Imp. gal or 24 U.S.

gal) of water. For smaller tanks, it is 15 cm^3/Imp. gal (or 13 cm^3/ U.S. gal). This amount is not added at once, but in three equal parts with a mean time of half a day. The fishes must remain in this bath till every white spot has disappeared. The time this will take depends on the temperature; the higher the temperature the quicker the parasite will grow to mature size and leave the fish.

I do not find it advisable to raise the temperature very much, as this has a weakening effect on most fishes. Since at temperatures between 21°C and 26°C (70–80°F) the parasites leave the host 3–4 days after the white spot first becomes visible to the naked eye, it is certainly not necessary to raise the normal temperature for tropicals. For cold-water fishes, however, it is advisable to raise it to 15–20°C (60–68°F) if it should be lower, since at still lower temperatures development of the parasite in the skin of the fish goes much too slowly (it may take four weeks and more at a temperature of 10°C (50°F)).

The shortest period after which the fishes may be replaced in the original tank, or, if they were treated in it, the period after which the water must be changed, is one week. In most cases, however, it is advisable to leave them for two weeks in the quinine bath, since it is possible that at the moment no white spot is to be seen, but that there are still some small parasites in the skin which have

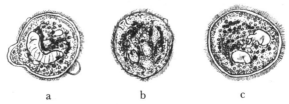

a   b   c

Fig. 2.31. Diagrams showing an Ichthyophthirius *parasite dying in a solution of quinine hydrochloride. In stages* (a) *and* (b) *the parasite was lively. Beginning of degeneration of nucleus is seen in* (b) *;* (c) *is dead parasite*

not yet developed into such a size that they may be recognised from the exterior. At temperatures between 15°C and 20°C (60–68°F) the period must be three weeks. Changing of the water after treatment is necessary, since too long a contact with quinine has a bad effect on the fishes, especially on their fertility. The quinine bath, as described, kills free-swimming *Ichthyophthirius* parasites, that have just left a fish, within about 3 h (Fig. 2.31); the long period of treatment is thus only due to the fact that not all parasites will leave the fish at the same time.

MEDICAL QUALITY OF METHYLENE BLUE

Methylene blue was used first of all in the U.S.A. Methylene blue
is a dye used for staining textile fibres and for staining tissues in
microscopical technique, while it is also used for medicinal purposes.
To ensure success it is important to use a good quality, which in
England means medical quality.

Dye substances are often produced in dilutions with other substances, such as glucose or amylum or salts, and using such a product the dosage will be too low. I have tried methylene blue for
treatment of 'Ich' in many experiments with very good results, and
I introduced this treatment first in Holland in 1936, and, later on,
in England as preferable to quinine.[16] I have used methylene blue,
quality 'A', from Brocapharm, a Dutch manufacturer of pharma-
ceutical products, but experiments with another quality from an
unknown manufacturer gave the same good results.

Reading the reports on methylene blue that have been published
in the U.S. magazine *The Aquarium*, it seems that the qualities they
have used there had a less strong effect than that which we had in
Holland, since I obtained good results with lower concentration.
I used methylene blue as a permanent bath of 1 : 500 000 and at
temperatures between 21°C and 26°C (70–80°F); in most cases the
disease disappeared in five days. This strength is about half that
advocated by the two well-known American aquarists, W. T. Innes
and F. H. Stoye. Except for some of the lower plants, namely *Chara*
and *Nitella*, I could not see any bad effect on the plants. This is
contradictory to several statements in U.S. literature saying that
methylene blue has a very bad effect on plants, but this can be
explained by the fact that I used it for my experiments in a lower
concentration.

The methylene blue treatment according to these prescriptions
has been used in England over a lengthy period with good success.
Dr. P. W. Godfrey, a medical specialist who tried out several methods
of treatment, stated: 'I have come to the conclusion that your
contributor Mr. van Duijn's methylene blue method is by far the
simplest and best.'[17] Donald W. Johnson, M.D., a U.S. physician,
also preferred methylene blue as a harmless treatment for fish.[18]

Methylene blue may be added directly to the aquarium and the
fishes may remain in it for an indefinite period without any harm.
The water becomes deep blue coloured but this colour fades
gradually as the dye is reduced by bacterial processes and reactions
with substances present in the water. The best method for use is to
make a 1% stock solution. At first, 0.2 cm^3/l (1 cm^3/gal) of water
is added, and after one or two days this is repeated. If necessary,
the strength may be increased to 4 cm^3/Imp. gal (3.5 cm^3/U.S. gal)
but if medical quality methylene blue is used, this will not be necessary. A methylene blue treatment can also be used for ponds, and this
is much cheaper than quinine.

It is possible to state on which phenomena its activity depends. Experiments of the Dutchman, Dr. A. A. van der Kroon[19] have shown that a methylene blue solution hinders the reproduction, forcing the parasite to simple division, when after a short period the 'Ich' dies. This shows that methylene blue has a direct poisoning effect on *Ichthyophthirius*. I have also given attention to the effect of methylene blue on the oxygen content of the water. Plants will only produce oxygen under the influence of long-wave (red) light rays and the water is coloured dark blue so that no red can penetrate to them. Due to this, the oxygen production of the plants will decrease to a very large extent and consequently the oxygen content of the water will decrease. This, too, has a bad effect on the parasites, as explained before, and this will indirectly have some effect on the parasites that are still living in the skin of the fish. It can also be shown that methylene blue is absorbed in the skin and other tissues of the fish, so that these get a little blue colour. From this it seems possible that local higher concentrations can occur, which might affect the parasites while they are still in the skin of the fish (Fig. 2.32). However, this has not yet been proved.

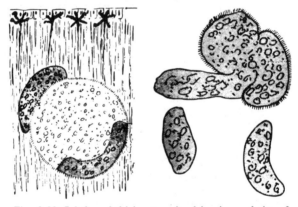

Fig. 2.32. Ichthyophthirius *parasite dying in a solution of methylene blue.* Left: *Parasite with a small part of the skin of the fish from which it was removed. The 'Ich' was lively rotating and tried to get rid of the parts that had been penetrated by the dye by rapid division.* Right: *Dead parasite (after Dr. A. A. van der Kroon)*

It is certain that methylene blue has a direct poisoning effect on free-swimming parasites while it also acts, indirectly, by hindering the oxygen production of the plants so that the oxygen content of the water decreases, which in turn affects the parasites, as already explained. This has no weakening effect on the fishes, since methylene blue is adsorbed in the cells of the fishes and there it acts in a way similar to the haemoglobin of the red blood corpuscles, viz., as a transmitter of oxygen in the respiratory cycle, therewith enabling the fishes to live in water with a very low oxygen content. It has also been shown that injections with methylene blue produce a significant increase of the haemoglobin content of the blood, thus improving severe cases of anaemia.

Bacteria can also profit by this effect of methylene blue; acetic acid bacteria cannot grow in a culture medium that is not in contact with air, but if methylene blue is added they can grow without oxygen, using the dye as a respiratory substratum instead. Protozoans seem to have no respiration system in which methylene blue could be of use. In all cases where fishes suffer from lack of oxygen (e.g. due to a disease of the gills) a methylene blue treatment will have a palliative effect, even if it does not affect the cause of the disease.

Since methylene blue is adsorbed by many organic substances, it is important that the aquarium in which it is used is kept clean. Before adding the dye, remove the dirt from the bottom of the tank. Filters should not be used, while aeration generally is inadvisable too; only large bubble aeration near the surface is allowable. This is to avoid undue increase in the oxygen content at greater depth of water.

MALACHITE GREEN

This dye has been recommended for treatment of Carp and Trout in breeding ponds in which the water can easily be changed by means of a pump.[20, 21] It should not be used for fishes destined for human consumption, and it is too toxic for treatment of small aquarium fishes; *Hyphessobrycon* species and others cannot even stand 0.1 mg/l. Its activity is thought to depend on specific destruction of one of the respiratory enzymes, namely, cytochrome C, as well as on a stimulating effect inducing the parasites to leave the fish sooner. For further particulars see pages 331–333.

MEPACRINE (QUINACRINE) HYDROCHLORIDE FOR PERSISTENT CASES

Whilst, generally, white spot infections can be eradicated by either the methylene blue or the quinine hydrochloride treatment, there have been a few occasions where persistent infections occurred. One of these was described by Mr. D. C. Slater,[22] who succeeded in eradicating the infection and its relapses by treatment with mepacrine (quinacrine) hydrochloride.

This drug had already been suggested as a cure for 'Ich' by the Dutch physician Dr. C. van Dommelen, but Mr. Slater used it independently. On the Continent, mepacrine hydrochloride is known by the name of atebrine hydrochloride. There have also been reports from America and Germany of successful treatments of stubborn cases of 'Ich' with this chemical.

Mr. Slater used a concentration of mepacrine hydrochloride up to 0.28 gr per Imp. gal, which was built up by adding one-third of the total amount at a time, at intervals of 48 h. One week after the last portion was added, the water was changed. After this period, however, signs of intoxication were observed in Guppies, but not in other fish. The Guppies became thin and wasted away.

These observations are in agreement with those by Prof. Schäperclaus (1954), who found that Guppies of 2 cm length died within 6 h in a solution of 1 g in 10 l, and within 2 days in a solution of 1 g in 100 l of water, whereas they survived at a concentration of 1 g in 1000 l of water.

As a result of further experience it is now recommended that mepacrine hydrochloride should be used in a concentration not exceeding 300 mg/100 l (0.2 gr/Imp. gal or 0.17 gr/U.S. gal). The drug is commercially available in tablets containing $1\frac{1}{2}$ gr (100 mg). A stock solution can be prepared by dissolving three of these tablets in 350 cm^3 of water. This solution is sufficient for a tank containing 20 Imp. gal (or 24 U.S. gal) of water. For smaller tanks, it is 15 cm^3/Imp. gal (or 13 cm^3/U.S. gal). As with quinine, the total amount is not added at once, but in three equal portions at intervals. With mepacrine, however, intervals of 48 h are advisable. Use of artificial aeration is strongly recommended.

The temperature of the water has to be between 21°C and 26°C (70–80°F). The tank must not receive strong sunlight during treatment. Treatment should not be extended over long periods. Generally, 8–10 days should be sufficient.

Since mepacrine is more toxic than quinine, not to speak of methylene blue, one should not use it unless it is necessary. Application of mepacrine should be restricted to stubborn cases of 'Ich' only after methylene blue and quinine hydrochloride have both failed to do the job.

MERCUROCHROME[R] (MERBROMIN)

Other treatments that have been advocated include Mercurochrome which was used on a large scale in the U.S.A. before the introduction of methylene blue. It has also been used in England. On the Continent of Europe it has never become an established treatment owing to the quinine treatment having been in general practice much earlier. Although Mercurochrome is effective against white spot, its use is not recommended now that we have the quinine hydrochloride and methylene blue treatments available. Mercurochrome is a mercury compound with rather high toxicity to fish, causing renal and liver damage. Its effectiveness does not surpass that of methylene blue or quinine hydrochloride.

The biologist Lewis M. Dorsey isolated several specimens of

Ichthyophthirius from a fish and brought them on to a slide under the microscope, adding a rather heavy dose of Mercurochrome. After several hours, no effect could be observed. The parasite is only susceptible to the action of the dye in certain stages of its development. Comparing the result of this experiment with similar ones in which quinine salts and methylene blue were used, one would come to the conclusion that Mercurochrome is inferior to the other two medicaments.

As to the toxic effects, these may even cause casualties. Lloyd C. Wademan, M.D., described a case of 50% mortality due to delayed effects of Mercurochrome in his own tanks.[23] Tetras, Danios, Barbs, *Corydoras* and Cichlids were among the victims, while Dwarf Gouramies, Pearl Gouramies and Fighting Fish were not affected. Dr. Wademan describes the symptoms of poisoning as follows: 'A fish that appeared healthy would suddenly begin to swim in a slow, aimless, lazy manner as though going nowhere and having all day to do it. Sense of balance seemed disturbed. The apparent muscle weakness progressed so that the aimless swimming resulted in the fish being on and off the bottom. At this stage there might be occasional brief but violent efforts to swim, but soon the fish would be on the bottom again, moving and breathing feebly. After the first signs of illness, death occurred within twelve to twenty-four hours.'

In England the commercial 2% Mercurochrome solution is a scheduled poison. The dosage which has been used is from 3–6 drops of this solution per Imp. gal. It is much better, however, to use a further dilution of one part by volume of commercial 2% solution with nine parts by volume of water, thus making a stock solution of 0.2%. This dilution can be prepared by your chemist and you can obtain it without any restriction. Using this stock solution, dosage can be much more accurate than with the 2% commercial solution; 2·cm^3 of the 0.2% diluted Mercurochrome solution is added per Imp. gal (or 1.65 cm^3/U.S. gal).

A complete cure should be obtained within five to nine days, provided that the water temperature is not below 21°C (70°F), and not exceeding 24°C (75°F). After that time a complete change of water has to be made. It should be pointed out that Mercurochrome is not dependably stable at temperatures higher than 21°C (70°F). Raising the temperature appreciably when treating fish with Mercurochrome would, therefore, be a serious mistake. During treatment, the tank must be protected from strong sunlight. The maximum dosage is double the amount as mentioned above, but this should never be added at one time. Mercurochrome has a bad effect on plants, and this is especially true with *Aponogeton*.

As stated previously, I do not recommend this treatment, however, because the after-effects of mercury poisoning may impair the health of the fish for a long time after recovery from the white spot infection. With delicate fishes, casualties may occur.

ACRIFLAVINE AND ANTIBIOTICS NOT RECOMMENDED

In France, a treatment with acriflavine has been advocated. Although this chemical is valuable in the treatment of certain other infectious diseases, it cannot be recommended for treatment of white spot. Mr. P. W. Godfrey found it less effective than methylene blue, whilst it has toxic effects, although according to Schäperclaus its toxicity is less than that of quinine salts. Acriflavine treatment should be confined to specific cases where no better cure is available. Details of acriflavine treatment are described on page 317.

Some antibiotics seem to be effective against *Ichthyophthirius*, even when it is in the skin of the fish. Penicillin in a concentration of 40 000 I.U./100 l (1800 I.U./Imp. gal or 1500 I.U./U.S. gal) is said to clear the condition in 6 h. Aureomycin[R] has also been reported to be effective, but Chloromycetin[R] had no effect.

Although it would seem that some antibiotics are very effective, I do not think it advisable to use them for treatment of an infection which can be cured with cheaper substances. The indiscriminate use of antibiotics for all kinds of infections, including those that can be successfully cured by other methods, is not without its drawbacks. Owing to their expensiveness, there is a great risk that people would try them in relatively low concentrations, which might be sufficient to kill protozoans, but not bacteria. Thus, resistant strains of bacteria may be produced which cannot be afterwards killed by the same antibiotic.

CHLORAMINE TREATMENT

Under the names of Chloramine-B and Chloramine-T some organic chlorine compounds are known, that are in general use for disinfection purposes and were also found to be effective against white spot and some other infections in fish. In Holland both compounds are sold under the trade name Halamid, whereas in other countries many other commercial names are used. A stock solution of 1 g (15 gr) in 100 cm^3 of tap water is prepared, and of this 1 cm^3/l of water in the tank is added (or $4\frac{1}{2}$ cm^3/Imp. gal, or $3\frac{1}{2}$ cm^3/U.S. gal). Fishes are treated in this solution for 24 h.

Since the effective amount of this drug depends on the quantity of organic substances present in the water and on the bottom, dirt should be removed prior to treatment; therefore it will even be better to apply this treatment in a separate clean glass tank. On no account may a Chloramine treatment be given in a tank or container where there is contact with any bare metal, since this may cause severe metal poisoning. During treatment no coal filters may be used, but afterwards such filters may be applied to remove the remaining drug instead of making a complete change of water.

NEGUVON TREATMENT

Bailösoff found the commercial drug Neguvon (Bayer) effective for killing *Ichthyophthirius*, but the optimum conditions have still to be found. Owing to the fact that this parasite is entirely surrounded by the proliferating skin tissue of the fish, Neguvon cannot kill it rapidly when still on the fish. Some kind of permanent treatment as with other medicaments would have to be developed. For further particulars see page 336.

PSETTUS AS DESTROYER OF WHITE SPOT

On several occasions it has been observed that *Monodactylus* (*Psettus*) *argenteus* has the habit of attacking white spot appearing in other fishes and eating it away.[24] It might be good policy always to keep some specimens of *Psettus* in tropical tanks together with other fishes if one fears risk of introducing white spot, just to help keeping an occasional infection in check.

WHITE SPOT DISEASE IN MARINE FISHES

Ichthyophthirius may also occur in sea-water aquaria. In such cases, methylene blue in the higher concentration of $1 : 125\,000$ (4 cm^3 of 1% stock solution per Imp. gal, added in two parts) has proved efficacious, whereas quinine and mepacrine are useless at the relatively high pH values of sea-water.

A longer period of treatment is required than for fresh-water fishes, namely at least 10 days after the second dose has been added. At water temperatures below 15°C (60°F) even longer duration of treatment may be necessary.

However, apart from this 'salt-water Ich', apparently similar symptoms of white spot are caused in marine fishes by another infusorian of the *Ciliata*, called *Cryptocaryon irritans* Brown (Fig. 2.33).

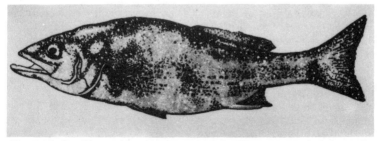

Fig. 2.33. Sea Trout with white spot caused by Cryptocaryon irritans *(after Sikama, from Sindermann)*

This parasite causes excessive production of slime by the skin of the fish (as in sliminess of the skin in fresh-water fishes), petechial lesions on the body and the gills, together with erosion of the tissues of the gill sheets, and blindness as well as the whitish pustules after which the disease is named.

Effective cures have been obtained by acriflavine[25] and by either formalin, copper treatment in the form of cupric acetate, or tris(hydroxymethyl)aminomethane dissolved in sea-water.[26]

VELVET, RUST OR GOLD-DUST DISEASE

Fishes suffering from velvet or rust disease have a 'dusty' appearance on the skin. It looks like a surface which has been dusted with powdered sulphur or with talcum powder of a dark shade. The 'dust' is of a pale yellowish colour, and may move over the skin surface. Owing to this colour, the disease is sometimes called 'gold dust'. Symptoms may resemble those of white spot ('Ich') so it is sometimes confused with *Ichthyophthirius*.

If some of the 'dust' is scraped off and examined under the microscope with a high-power objective, a number of small unicellular parasites can be found, which belong to the Dinoflagellates. These are protozoans, generally characterised by the possession of a scale, consisting of two valves and having a cross-fold or groove.

The causative organism of velvet disease was detected in 1946 by Jacobs; it is named *Oodinium limneticum*. This creature may appear in a free-living, motile stage, conforming to the general appearance of Dinoflagellates. The average length is about 13 μm (1 μm = 0.001 mm) and the shape is more or less ellipsoidal. There are two flagella, a longer one directed backwards and used for locomotion and another which is shorter and concealed in the transverse groove.

When a motile *Oodinium* comes in contact with the skin of a fish, it adheres with its long flagellum, but this is only a temporary stage. Several outgrowths are produced (pseudopodia), resembling those of certain species of *Rhizopoda* (a group of protozoans to which also the well-known *Amœba* belongs). The pseudopodia grow into the skin or the gills of the fish and in this way the parasite gets a firm hold. The flagella and the transverse groove disappear and the shape of the body becomes pear-like.

Both the free-swimming and the parasitic forms of the organism contain some chlorophyll, enabling it to obtain food by the process of photosynthesis, as in green plants. This chlorophyll gives the organisms a yellowish colour. However, the parasitic form derives most of its food from the epidermal cells of its host. At the expense of the fish the parasite may grow from five to seven times its original diameter. When reaching maturity, the organism loses its pseudopodia and encysts itself for multiplication. Inside the cyst a series of equal divisions take place, which may give rise to more than 200 (generally 256) young parasites in the course of a few days.

These young parasites develop into the free-swimming, flagella-bearing stage and leave the cyst and the fish. They swarm out into the water and, after some time, may settle again on the skin or the gills of a fish. In this way the infection spreads. It is not yet known for how long the motile parasites may survive before finding a suitable host (Fig. 2.34).

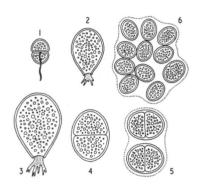

Fig. 2.34. Various stages on the development of the organism causing velvet disease, Oodinium limneticum. *× 270. 1, free-swimming stage. 2 and 3, parasitic forms. 4, first division in cyst. 5 and 6, cysts with parasites (drawings modified after Kozloff)*

Oodinium limneticum has been found in its parasitic form on White Cloud Mountain Minnows, Barbs, Danios, Labyrinth Fish and livebearers. The infection is most dangerous for young fish; adult specimens, having a higher resistance, may carry the parasites for long periods without showing distress. Consequently, most casualties will occur in batches of young fish, unless the victims are treated immediately signs of the disease have become apparent.

Fortunately velvet disease is not difficult to cure.[27] There are treatments available, which have proved very effective, such as methylene blue and acriflavine or Trypaflavine neutral (the latter two are different trade names for the same chemical substance 3,6-diamino-10-methylacridinium chloride).

TREATING VELVET DISEASE

For the methylene blue treatment make a 1% stock solution of methylene blue (medical quality) in water. At first, 1 cm³/Imp. gal of water is added, and after one or two days this is repeated. Except for some of the lower plants (*Chara* and *Nitella*) this concentration will not affect the plants.

If necessary, the strength of the methylene blue solution may be increased to 4 cm³ of stock solution per Imp. gal (or 3.5 cm³/U.S. gal).

However, this higher concentration may be more harmful to the plants.

Before adding the methylene blue to a tank, it is necessary to siphon the dirt from the bottom since that would adsorb the dye, rendering it ineffective. A filter with active coal must not be used during the cure, for the same reason. Ordinary aeration, or the use of a jet pump without a coal filter, are allowable.

Treatment has to be prolonged for two or three days more than is required for cleaning the skin of the diseased fishes from the yellowish 'dust'. Six to ten days will generally be sufficient. The temperature in the tank should not be too low during treatment, but excessive heat is to be avoided, too. A temperature of 24–27°C (75–80°F) is recommended for tropicals.

Methylene blue treatment is completely harmless even to young fish. It is also effective against white spot, *Gyrodactylus*, as a general palliative medicament in cases of diseases of the gills and in some cases of fungus.

Acriflavine (Trypaflavine neutral), a yellow dye, is sold by chemists in tablets containing 3 mg (0.46 gr) to be used for disinfection of the mouth and throat in human beings. These tablets are also a very useful form for treatment of diseased fish. The normal dosage is one tablet per 33 Imp. gal (or 40 U.S. gal) of water whilst, for obstinate cases, the strength may be doubled.

The tablets must not be added directly to the water, but should be dissolved first. Therefore, it is recommended that a stock solution of one tablet in 330 cm^3 of water (use hot water for dissolving the substance) be made; then 10 cm^3 of this stock solution per Imp. gal are added. Stir the water whilst adding the chemical. The use of artificial aeration during the cure is strongly recommended but a coal filter must not be used, since this would remove the dye from the water. The temperature of the water has to be raised to 27°C (about 80°F).

The tank should be kept in subdued light to avoid adverse effects on the fish due to photosensitisation by the dye, by which is meant a process where a substance absorbing light energy transfers this to a substratum to which it is adsorbed, thereby inducing chemical reactions which would not have been exerted by the same light energy if the dye had not been present. Many toxic effects of dyestuffs have been found to be due to photosensitisation instead of to toxicity of the dyes itself.

Treatment is extended over a period of three days, then the water is changed and, at the sixth day, the treatment is repeated for another two or three days. The repetition is necessary to avoid reinfections, because the encysted parasites are not affected by the medicament. Excessively long contact by the fish with the dye must be avoided since it is not completely harmless like methylene blue. It has been said that acriflavine produces a temporary sterility in both egglaying and livebearing fish. In egglayers, although spawning may take place normally, most of the eggs fail to hatch, while such fry as may still emerge from some eggs, are weak and generally die within a week of attaining the free-swimming stage, according to a publication under the name of Earle E. Patterson.[28] In the same paper it was mentioned that female livebearers, after treatment with acriflavine, produced only 1–3 youngsters at two subsequent deliveries and these lived only a brief time. However, normal fertility is restored after a period of several months.

In a personal communication of 1956, soon after the publication of the first edition of this book, Mr. Patterson denied the observations published under his name. He then stated that acriflavine does not make fish sterile, and wrote: 'We have spawned many fish in solutions of acriflavine at a strength of 1 gr to 15 U.S. gal. The quantity and quality of the fry was above average.'

In the meantime, however, independent information on effects of acriflavine and other acridine derivatives has become available from the fields of cytogenetics and biochemistry. It has been shown that these substances combine with nucleic acids, including those in the cell nucleus of which the units of hereditary information are composed, thus increasing the incidence of mutations. Further, certain enzymes of cellular metabolism are inhibited. The effects are enhanced in presence of light and oxygen. From these observations alone one would predict at least the possibility of harmful effects on reproduction and quality of offspring.

It is quite likely that young fish would be affected more seriously in this respect than adults. It would consequently seem advisable to restrict the acriflavine treatment to adult fish and then only in such cases where methylene blue does not have the required effect. Against velvet disease, methylene blue will generally be efficacious. Acriflavine affects some aquatic plants. *Cabomba* and *Anacharis* die, whilst *Vallisneria*, *Sagittaria* and *Nitella* can stand it. Blue-green algae will die, too.

In a personal communication (July 1956) Mr. Earle E. Patterson described results obtained with a combined treatment with potassium permanganate and rock salt. He says that 'one teaspoon' of rock salt per U.S. gal will effect a complete and lasting cure in about ten days, whereas the combination with $\frac{1}{8}$ gr of potassium permanganate per U.S. gal generally was effective in 24 h. However, in one case of heavily infected *Rasbora heteromorpha* it took three such dosages of potassium permanganate, added every other day, to completely clear the fish.

Permanganate alone would remove the parasites from the fish, but would not prevent new infections, so its combination with salt is required for a rapid cure, according to Mr. Patterson. A difficulty is the inexact measure given for the salt; teaspoons in different countries have no identical dimensions, and one can charge even the same spoon with different loads. To provide a fairly gradual addition of the salt, Patterson puts the measured quantity of salt in the outside filter, with which all his tanks are equipped. According to my experience, quantities to be used should be higher. I would recommend the addition of 7 g of salt per litre (or 1 oz/Imp. gal = 0.8 oz/U.S. gal) and 40–45 mg of potassium permanganate per litre (or 0.3 gr/Imp. gal = 0.25 gr/U.S. gal). After the addition of the permanganate (dissolved separately and put directly in the tank) any coal filter should be put out of operation till the next day. A change of water is made after 3–5 days to remove the excess salt.

In the U.S.A., the antibiotic Chloromycetin[R] (chloramphenicol) has been used also as a cure for velvet. A dosage of 25 mg/U.S. gal (30 mg/Imp. gal) has been effective.

Reichenbach-Klinke has also mentioned a treatment with quinine hydrochloride 1.5 g/100 l during 2–3 days; and bathing in 3.5% sodium chloride (salt) for 1–3 min only.[29]

COPPER CURE

It has been claimed that the infection can be cured by placing copper gauze in the tank at a rate of 1 cm^2 area per litre (about $\frac{3}{4}$ in^2 for every Imp. gal). It is said that usually the disease is cured within three days, whilst most fish can stand at least three days of this treatment and usually even five days before showing signs of distress.[30] However, some fish, such as *Barbus tetrazona* and *B. nigrofasciatus*, are more susceptible to copper poisoning. If the fish should 'hang' near the surface or swim along the surface for some time, the copper should be removed and at least one-third of the water changed. The effect depends on some of the copper dissolving into the water and killing the parasites by its oligodynamic activity.

This seems to be a very simple method of getting rid of an infection indeed, but there are some complications. Copper is very poisonous to fish, an amount as small as 0.5 mg/l killing large Trout within a few hours. This is approximately equivalent to a dilution of 1 : 500 000 of copper sulphate. The rate at which copper dissolves in water depends on actual conditions, such as the oxygen content, pH value, concentration of carbonates and free carbon dioxide, ammonium compounds and others. It may vary from about 1 mg/dm^2 per day up to 10–67 mg/dm^2 per day in natural waters saturated with air and carbon dioxide.[31] If we take a value of 10 mg/dm^2 per day as a safe average, then we can expect a copper concentration in the water amounting to 0.1 mg/l, after having been in contact for one day with a solid piece of copper with a surface area of $\frac{3}{4}$ in^2/gal. In copper gauze, the actual surface area in contact with the water is greatly increased by its consisting of rather thin wires, having a large area/volume ratio. After three days, the amount of dissolved copper could be of the order of 0.3 mg/l which is sufficient to cause severe copper poisoning and death.

If conditions are more favourable, so that a corrosion rate of the copper of only 1 mg/dm² per day occurs, the copper concentration would be of the order of 0.03 mg/l after three days, and of the order of approximately 0.05 mg/l after five days. The latter concentration is approximately equivalent to an addition of copper sulphate of 1 : 5 000 000. Even this low concentration is known to have been lethal to some species of tropical fish, 1 : 10 000 000 being the maximum concentration to be regarded as safe.

In the writer's opinion, it would be preferable to know exactly what amount of copper is introduced into the water rather than depending on unpredictable corrosion rates. This would require the addition of a copper salt instead of placing metallic copper in the water.

A stock solution should then be prepared by dissolving 400 mg of copper sulphate in 1 l of water. This solution is used at a ratio of 1 cm³/Imp. gal (4.56 l). Dosage has to be very accurate; for measuring the volume to be added a calibrated pipette is to be preferred to a measuring glass.

For U.S. measures, the stock solution should be made by dissolving 320 mg in 1 l of water to allow 1 cm³ of this per U.S. gal to be added.

When using tap water for preparing the stock solution, this may turn cloudy owing to the formation of copper carbonate which is only slightly soluble. If this occurs, the solution should be shaken before using it. In any case, the water in the aquarium must be stirred vigorously when adding the chemical. It is advisable to take a rather large volume out of the tank in an enamelled, glass or porcelain, but not metal, vessel adding the required amount of stock solution to this and then returning the contents of the vessel to the aquarium. In this way the risk of uneven distribution through the water is eliminated.

After treatment, a complete change of water has to be made. During treatment, no *Daphnia* or other Crustaceans should be fed, since these will be killed within a day. Copper treatment will also kill blue-green algae.

PILLULARIS DISEASE

In 1951 Schäperclaus[32] observed an infectious disease in *Colisa lalia*, caused by *Oodinium pillularis* (Fig. 2.35), as he afterwards named the parasitic organism. The parasite resembles *Oodinium limneticum* but there are sufficient differences for a separate treatment.

Symptoms of the infection differ from that of velvet or gold-dust disease in the 'dust' on the skin not being of a pale yellowish colour, but greyish; furthermore, parts of the skin may come off in tatters. With a powerful magnifying glass small greyish-white to yellowish-brown dots may be observed. Schäperclaus first observed the disease in *Colisa lalia* of one month old, 1.3–1.8 cm of length. The course

of the disease was very slow; one week after the appearance of
symptoms of the disease only 20 specimens out of a stock of 1170
had died and after two weeks only 60. However, after three months,
66% of the original number had died. On the survivors all symptoms
of the infection disappeared when they had reached a length of
2.5 cm and when the labyrinth organ had become fully developed.

Youngsters of Neon Fish (*Paracheirodon innesi*), of Angel Fish
(*Pterophyllum scalare*) and of Wagtail Platys were not affected.

The infection has since also been observed in *Colisa labiosa*,
Trichopsis (*Ctenops*) *vittatus*, Paradise Fish (*Macropodus opercularis* and
M. cupanus dayi), Siamese Fighting Fish (*Betta splendens*), *Tanichthys*

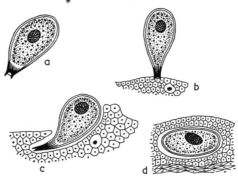

Fig. 2.35. Oodinium pillularis: (a) *free-swimming
parasite.* (b) *parasite adhering to the skin surface.*
(c) *parasite penetrating into the epidermis; epithelial
cells begin to proliferate.* (d) *parasite surrounded by
epithelial cells. In stages* (b) *and* (c) *one slime cell is
shown between the epithelial cells (after Reichenbach-
Klinke)*

albonubes, *Barbus phutunio*, *B. pentazona*, *B. tetrazona*, *Brachydanio rerio*,
Rasbora heteromorpha, *Aphyosemion arnoldi*, *A. sjoestedti*, *A. spurelli*, *A.
multicolor*, *Hyphessobrycon flammeus*, *Pristella tholdlei*, Guppies (*Lebistes
reticulatus*), Sword Tails (*Xiphophorus helleri* and *X. montezumæ*) and
Xiphophorus (*Platypoecilus*) *variatus*; further in Carp (*Cyprinus carpio*),
Prussian Carp (*Carassius carassius*) and Sea Trout (*Salmo trutta*).

Hirschmann and Partsch studied the life history of the parasite in
detail.[33] A few minutes after a mature parasite has left the fish it
becomes globular in shape, sinks to the bottom and changes to a
so-called 'palmella' stage. Within a few hours a stricture is formed,
followed by nuclear division and division of the chromatophores.
Then the two parts separate into two new individuals, that again
get a globular shape, then produce a new membrane and proceed
with further divisions till finally 32 or 64 young cells have come into
being (compare the development of *Oodinium limneticum*, as represented in the drawings on page 53). Each young parasite now

develops further into the free-living, motile stage, characterised by a cross-fold or groove, a red eye-spot and two flagella, a short one which is concealed in the transverse groove, and a longer one directed backwards. This stage is called dinospore. The dinospores swim freely through the water with great speed till they contact a fish. They seem to prefer such parts that have already been damaged by the older parasites. On the other hand, on fish that had not yet been infected, such parts are preferred where the epidermis is at a higher level, such as at the junctures of the fins. According to observations by Reichenbach-Klinke,[34] the parasite not only bores itself mechanically into the epidermis of the fish, but it is also able to macerate the epithelium cells by means of certain secretions. As a result of this destruction of cells the parasite penetrates into deeper layers of the skin. Just as in *Ichthyophthirius* infections the skin reacts by augmentation, resulting in a covering of the parasite by a layer of the skin of the fish. Since *Oodinium pillularis* is much smaller than *Ichthyophthirius*, these spots (cysts) are also much smaller and can only be recognised by the aid of a good magnifier. *Oodinium pillularis* may also be found on the gills.

The life cycle of the parasite depends very much on the temperature of the water and the illumination level. At 23–25°C (73–77°F) under (for the parasite) optimal illumination development from the 'palmella' stage to the final dinospore takes 50–70 h. In darkness, or at a temperature of 15–17°C (59–63°F) this takes more than 11 days.

At 23–25°C the dinospores may keep alive in the free-swimming stage of 12–24 h. On the fish a dinospore changes within 3–4 days into a mature palmella stage (at the same temperature) and the cycle may start anew.

The mature parasites may have a length of 30–140 μm (generally 50–70 μm) and they have a globular or oval-shaped nucleus of about 12 μm, according to Schäperclaus.

TREATMENT OF PILLULARIS DISEASE

Oodinium pillularis appears to be much more resistant to medication than *O. limneticum*. Schäperclaus tried very strong formalin baths (1 cm³/l) for 15–20 min, but even after eight days surviving parasites were found on the treated fishes, although the number of casualties among the latter appeared to be less than in a group of untreated specimens. Acriflavine, potassium permanganate and salt also failed to do the job.

Hirschmann and Partsch found a treatment with a 3–5% salt bath, for 1–3 min only, successful.

Considering the whole information on the life history of the parasite, the following procedure is suggested. All fish should be removed from the infected tank and treated with a 3% salt bath for 5–15 min. Then they should be put in a separate clean tank without plants and bottom covering; the tank should be kept in darkness, but the water should be well aerated and preferably filtered as well. In this way the chance of reproduction of any surviving parasite and reinfection will be very small. In the meantime the infected tank is put under full illumination and the temperature of the water is raised up to about 30°C (86°F) for 24 h; then it may cool down and after 48 h the fish may be put back. If there is any doubt as to the complete clearance of the infection, the salt bath should be repeated just prior to reinsertion.

The heat and light treatment of the tank without fish will speed up the development of the free parasites and reduce the period of time during which they are able to keep alive without finding a fish.

From the high degree of dependence of the life cycle on light and temperature it could be expected that the alternating heat treatment advocated by Stolk for coping with white spot infection (see page 42) may be effective, too. During the heat period the tank should be kept fully illuminated, if possible by direct sunlight, whereas during the low temperature parts of the cycle, light should be excluded.

CORAL FISH DISEASE

In sea-water aquaria another species of *Oodinium* has been observed. It is called *Oodinium ocellatum* (Figs 2.36, 2.37). This parasite was first detected and named by E. M. Brown in 1934 and further studied by Nigrelli in 1936.[35]

In Germany, Schäperclaus has found this parasite on Coral Fish and he named it *Branchiophilus maris*, in 1935. Later it could be demonstrated that the organism was identical with *Oodinium ocellatum*, described one year earlier. This parasite has been observed on the skin and the gills of *Prochilus* (*Amphiprion* or *Premnas*) *percula, Dascyllus*

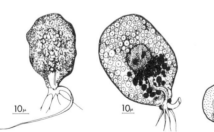

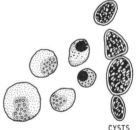

CYSTS

Fig. 2.36. Parasitic stages (tropho-
zoites) of Oodinium ocellatum
Brown (after Brown and Hovasse,
from Sindermann)

Fig. 2.37. Oodinium ocellatum *as seen in stained slides.
Cysts (0.3 mm long) are shown
to the right*

aruanus, Monodactylus (Psettus) argenteus, Chætodon capistratus and *Balistes vetula*, where it caused a large number of casualties. Other species that have suffered from the infection in sea-water aquaria are *Balistapus rectangularis, Chætodontoplus mesoleucus, Heniochus acuminatus, Platax orbicularis, Pl. vespertilio, Pterois radiata, Pt. russeli* and *Scatophagus argus*. Brackish water fishes such as Scats and Malayan Angels, when kept in sea-water, are apparently more resistant.

On the fish the parasite appears to have a globular shape and is not transparent when living. Its dimensions are generally from 20 to 70 µm, but they may reach 115 µm. By staining, a nucleus can be found with a diameter of 5–15 µm surrounded by small granules of starch.

In the gills of the diseased fishes oval-shaped cysts of about 0.3 mm long could be identified. These cysts have a higher resistance to chemical treatments than the parasites themselves.

Whereas *Oodinium limneticum* and *O. pillularis* are primarily parasites of the skin and only spread from there on to the gills, *Oodinium ocellatum* is in the first place a gill parasite, although it may also be found on the skin. The life cycle of the parasites is identical with that of the other *Oodinium* species, described before.

After the mature parasite has left the fish, division in two parts starts at once. At temperatures exceeding 25°C (77°F) in three days 256 dinospores are produced, which have a size of 9–15 µm. At temperatures below 10°C (50°F) no divisions take place, whereas between 10°C and 20°C (68°F) the process is very slow. The dinospores are highly motile. Optimal conditions for the development of the dinospores were shown to exist at pH 8.0, a density for the sea-water of 1.012–1.021 and the presence of a relatively large amount of dissolved nitrates (these are always produced as one of the final products of the aerobic breakdown of proteins).

The parasites cause haemorrhages, inflammation and necrosis in the gills, which open the way to secondary bacterial infections. The first signs of the disease are gasping and rising to the surface of the water, followed by weakness and apathy.

Coral fish disease has been observed mostly in November, which could be due to decreased resistance of a related kind to that observed with autumn sickness in fresh-water tanks.

TREATMENTS

Treatment must start as soon as possible, because once serious damage is done to the gills, recovery is unlikely. Heavy spread of the parasites on the body may generally be taken as a sign that the infection has already advanced too far for cure, but even then treatment should be applied for at least eradicating the infection from the tank.

If applied in time, before the infection has proceeded too far, most cases can be cured with the methylene blue treatment as prescribed for treating velvet disease (p. 53), keeping the tank in darkness (but with good aeration) and at as low a temperature as the fish will stand. This will increase the resistance of the fish by maintaining a higher oxygen concentration than at higher temperatures, whereby the life cycle of the parasite is slowed down. No more food should be given than is immediately eaten. Wasted food and dirt should be siphoned off every day. Treatment must be continued for at least 10 days after the addition of the second dose.

According to R. A. Riseley,[36] in East Africa good results have been obtained by alternating the heat treatment, darkening the tank and raising the temperature slowly to 32°C (90°F), followed by a slow drop to normal temperature after a short time. Strong aeration is required to compensate for the drop in oxygen tension; this treatment has to be carried out on two successive days. Probably the efficacy of this method can be further improved by allowing strong illumination during the high temperature period.

Copper treatment has been advocated by Lee Chin Eng (mentioned by Riseley). 1 cm^3 of a 0.1% stock solution of copper sulphate is administered per litre of aquarium water, divided into three equal doses over 24 h. For treatment a clean, empty tank is to be used and the fish have to be watched carefully for signs of distress. Full aeration should be given. The fishes must not be fed. In case of distress, decrease the concentration at once. *Chelmon rostratus* has been reported to be particularly sensitive. Corals and sea anemones are killed rapidly.

Normally, treatment takes four days, the fishes are then put into clean water and kept in quarantine for a further 10 days in fresh sea-water. The main tank must stay unoccupied for 14 days. As in other copper treatments, results are often varying. Generally, methylene blue or heat treatments are to be preferred.

ICHTHYOCHYTRIUM AND MUCOPHILUS INFECTIONS

These are parasites of vegetable origin, that are now considered to belong to the unicellar algae.

Ichthyochytrium vulgare Plehn, often attacks the cells of the skin and the gills of fresh-water fishes. The general shape resembles that of the parasite stage of *Oodinium*, while it has also a yellowish colour, due to the presence of chlorophyll. The dimensions vary from 5 to 20 μm. Inside the body of the parasite a number of highly refractive granules can be observed. The parasites may be found either singly or in groups of 20–30 individual cells on the skin and the gills of fish. In stained slides the nucleus of the organisms is clearly shown.

Mucophilus cyprini Plehn has occasionally been found on the skin of Carps and other *Cyprinidæ*, although it is mainly a gill parasite. *Mucophilus* is larger than *Ichthyochytrium*, varying from 60–70 μm (Fig. 2.38).

Neither parasite seems to do much harm, provided there are not large numbers. If numbers are excessive they may give rise to distress and complications due to secondary infections caused by fungus or bacteria. Treatments with acriflavine, Aureomycin^R,

Fig. 2.38. Mucophilus cyprini
specimens

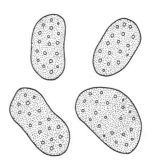

copper sulphate, formalin, methylene blue, potassium dichromate, salt, sulphamethazine sodium, and Terramycin^R have been tried and were all ineffective, according to a personal report by the U.S. biologist Don Estes (1960).

CHLOROCHYTRIUM INFECTION

Occasionally infections with unicellular green algae have been observed which are characterised by inflammations, secondary fungus infection and cyst formation, or poor growth and emaciation. The causative organisms belong to the Class *Chlorophyceæ*, Order *Volvocales*, Family *Protococcaceæ*. Best known is *Chlorochytrium piscicolens* Link.

The parasites penetrate deep into the skin and the epithelium of the gills, reaching the connective tissue, where they are encysted. *Chlorochytrium* cells have a round or oval shape, 9–120 μm in size. The larger specimens can be observed in the living fish as tiny dark pin-points, when the fish is held against the light. The parasites have a green chromatophore covering the internal side of the total membrane and they contain numerous pyrenoids, i.e. small refractive protein globules concerned in the formation of starch; they will stain blue on addition of iodine. *Chlorochytrium* reproduces by the formation of morphologically identical spores of oval shape. These possess two flagella. They are released from the mature cell contained in a slimy capsule, in which copulation takes place. The resulting zoospores with four flagella swim around in the water for some time, till they settle on a fish and after having produced a membrane penetrate between the epidermis cells, where they develop into new vegetative forms. Asexual zoospores may also be

produced in some species of *Chlorochytrium*; these are released one
at a time and do not conjugate.

Chlorochytrium piscicolens has been observed on Carp (*Cyprinus carpio*),
Tench (*Tinca tinca*) and young Perch (*Perca fluviatilis*). Other species
of *Chlorochytrium* are parasites of aquatic plants.

The small wounds resulting when the parasites leave the fish for
reproduction may easily become infected by bacteria or fungus.
Specific cures are not known.

KNOT OR PIMPLE INFECTIONS

Morbus nodulosus or *Sporozoasis tuberosa*, commonly known as knot or
pimple disease, is a collective name for several diseases, caused by
sporozoans. Symptoms are the formation of little 'knots' in the
skin, often closely resembling those caused by *Ichthyophthirius*, or
larger pimples or bumps. If there are only little knots in the skin, as
is usually the case in Carps and related groups, it is difficult to
distinguish between this disease and white spot. But, since the
disease cannot be cured either by quinine or methylene blue, the
difference will show on treatment.

Sporozoans are a group of the protozoans, characterised by the
production of spores. The normal form of the parasite is amoeboid
and for reproduction it encysts and produces hundreds or even
thousands of spores. All sporozoans are parasites. The life cycle of
several of them is more intricate, but to give further details here
would be beyond the scope of this chapter. A more detailed description of sporozoan infections is given on pages 125–147. The spores
have a size of 0.004–0.020 mm (4–20 µm). The germ (sporozoite)
lies inside together with one or two polar cells with a spirally rolled
nettle thread which can be pushed out. This thread generally has a
length of 2, 5 or 25 times that of the diameter of the spore. Under
good conditions the sporozoite leaves the spore and lives for a time
in the amoeboid stage. After some time a new cyst is produced and
the cycle starts anew. Sporozoans may be found in all organs of
fishes but in the skin they are relatively rare, and these include
Myxobolus exiguus (spores with two polar capsules)in Carps (Fig.
2.39); *Myxobolus dispar* in Bleak (*Alburnus lucidus*); *Myxobolus oviformis*
in Roach (*Rutilus rutilus*); *Glugea anomala* (oval-shaped spores with
one polar capsule) in Sticklebacks and other fishes; *Henneguya* species
(spores with two polar capsules).

The little knots are formed when the parasites are situated in the
skin, while bumps and pimples originate from a process in the
muscles.

For exact diagnosis cysts may be opened by exerting slight pressure
or by piercing with a (disinfected) needle and collecting their
content in a drop of tap water on a slide for microscopical
examination (preferably with phase-contrast). Addition of some

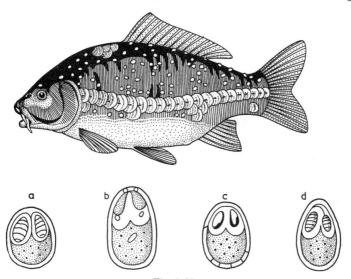

Fig. 2.39.
Top: CARP WITH KNOTS
*Carp attacked by knots (*Myxobolus *infection). It is possible for this disease to be confused with white spot.* Bottom: *Spores of* (a) Myxobolus dispar; (b) Myxobolus ellipsoideus; (c) Myxobolus exiguus; (d) Myxobolus oviformis

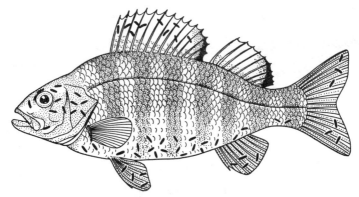

Fig. 2.40. Perch with cysts of Dermocystidium percæ
at the fins, belly and operculum

iodine solution improves visibility and allows discrimination between species containing a brownish-yellow staining vacuole in the sporozoite and others that have not. Dried smears may be fixed and stained by usual cytological techniques.

In Perch (*Perca fluviatilis*) oblong cysts, 1–2 mm long and 0.04–0.2 mm wide, may be produced by *Dermocystidium percæ* (Fig. 2.40), first described and named by Dr. Reichenbach-Klinke in 1950.[37] These cysts are found most often at the fins (especially the first dorsal), the head and the belly, further at the border of the operculum and under the cornea of the eye. The condition proved to be non-infectious from fish to fish, so it is presumed that the life cycle of the parasites includes some intermediate host, perhaps water fleas or cyclopids. The infection starts in the intestine of the fish, where from the ripe spores plasmodia are released, that are transported by the blood stream and finally settle in the tissue of the cutis (lower layer of the skin). There each plasmodium becomes polynuclear and divides into a number of globular sporoblasts, 2–7.8 μm in size. The cyst around the parasites is produced by the connective tissue of the fish. The ripe cysts filled with spores shove between the epithelial cells of the epidermis till they approach the surface, which is pressed upwards till the walls of the cysts burst open and release the spores into the water. The spores are globular or pear-shaped. Their size is 3.5–13 μm.

In 1962, Dr. E. Elkan investigated an until then unknown species occurring in Sticklebacks (*Gasterosteus aculeatus* and *Pygosteus pungitius*), which he named *Dermocystidium gasterostei*[38] (Fig. 2.41). The

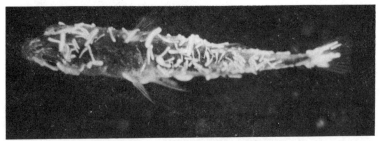

Fig. 2.41. Stickleback (Gasterosteus aculeatus) *with numerous cysts of* Dermocystidium gasterostei *(photograph Dr. E. Elkan)*

infected fish look at first sight to be covered with white worms, or bearing *Lernæa* parasites ('anchor worm', see page 14), but in reality the worm-like appendages are cysts, 2–3 mm long and 0.2–0.3 mm wide. On the tail fin their arrangement followed the direction of the tail bones. No cysts were encountered on the gills or in the internal organs, but in several of the attacked fish cysts also appeared in the cornea of the eye, some of them being deeply embedded between the skull bones, close to the brain capsule. As in the infections of

Perch by *Dermocystidium percæ* the cyst walls always consisted entirely of connective tissue of the host, but there was considerable variation as to the thickness of the cyst wall, without detectable relationship with the stage of development. Some cysts, containing mature spores, even lacked walls. The spores have a size of 3–5 μm. Morphologically, *D. gasterostei* appears to be rather similar to *D. percæ*, but it penetrates much deeper, even to the skull, whereas the latter is restricted to the surface or the cutis. Further, *D. gasterostei* was not found on any Perch inhabiting the same water in which the Sticklebacks were epidemically affected. The new parasite was found in the locality of Newdigate, Surrey, England.

Other species of *Dermocystidium* are typical parasites of the gills.

At present there are no known methods of curing infected fish. It is therefore important to remove infected fishes from a collection as soon as possible. Fortunately these diseases do not appear often in aquaria.

SLIMINESS OF THE SKIN (CYCLOCHÆTIASIS, CHILODONELLIASIS AND COSTIASIS)

A disease sometimes occurs in fish which is characterised by the formation of a slimy secretion on the skin. The colour of the infected fish is pale as the slime covers the whole skin like a thin, grey fog. The fins are usually folded up. The symptom of sliminess of the

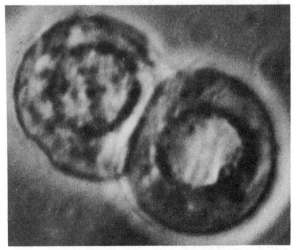

Fig. 2.42. Two globular slime cells in smear from slime of a fish suffering from sliminess of the skin. Photographed in the living state with a phase-contrast microscope. × 4000

skin may be observed very easily in dark-coloured fishes, while in others it does not show so clearly, since there is less contrast between the grey fog of the slime and the parts of the body that are not affected. On inspection under the microscope (Figs 2.42–2.47) unicellular parasites may be found in the slime. Three main species are known which may give the symptoms described.

CYCLOCHÆTIASIS

The most common of these in aquaria is probably *Cyclochæta* (*Trichodina*) *domerguei** (Figs 2.43, 2.44). This is a beautiful, symmetrically shaped micro-organism, which generally measures from 40–50 μm (0.04–0.05 mm), although sometimes specimens as small as 9 μm may be found. These may be of a different species. *Cyclochæta*

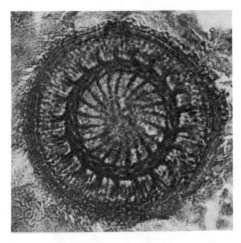

Fig. 2.43. Cyclochæta domerguei (Wallengren), from a smear of the slime of a diseased fish (photomicrograph by the author. × 1000)

domerguei belongs to the Order of the *Peritricha* in the *Ciliata*, Family *Urceolariidæ*. Members of this Family are characterised by the possession of an attaching disc with a horny corona of teeth. Seen from above, the micro-organism shows a ring of relatively large hooks, 20–32 in number, with which the parasite attacks the skin

* Some confusion has arisen as to the taxonomy of the *Urceolariidæ*, to which Family this parasite belongs, especially with respect to the definitions of the Genera *Cyclochæta* and *Trichodina*. It has even been suggested that the parasite of *Hydra*, *Trichodina pediculus*, might be identical with *Cyclochæta domerguei*. In agreement with Schäperclaus, I see no necessity at present to accept changes of nomenclature suggested by Zick. For a complete discussion, see Schäperclaus, *Fischkrankheiten*, 3rd ed. Berlin 327–33 (1954) and, further, Reichenbach-Klinke, *Krankheiten und Schädigungen der Fische*, Stuttgart 137–41 (1966).

of the victim. This ring of hooks is part of a kind of sucker. In side view the parasites look like a bell if they are swimming freely in the water, but on the fish they often suck so strongly that their bodies become flattened. As a result of this suction the cells of the epidermis are irritated and the slime cells secrete a large quantity of slime and die. The parasites then proceed to feed on these dead cell particles.

Cyclochæta domerguei may be found on all kinds of fish, but the parasite most frequently attacks Goldfish and other members of the Carp Family, Trout and other *Salmonidæ*, and Eels, while according

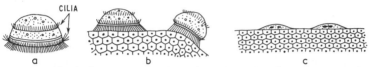

Fig. 2.44. Cyclochæta domerguei, *as it appears when free-swimming (after Moroff). Specimens of the same organism on the skin of a fish (after Roth).* (c) *Section through the skin of a fish showing two* Cyclochæta *organisms flattened by strong suction (after Doflein) (all schematised)*

to statements of Dr. W. Roth, in tropical tanks Paradise Fish, Guppies and *Brachydanio* species are the most common victims. The infection can remain in a latent stage if the fishes are in good condition and this may explain the higher resistance of fishes when living in completely natural conditions.

Nowadays quite a lot of different species have been described and distinguished by taxonomists, divided among the Genera *Trichodina, Trichodinella, Tripartiella, Dipartiella* and *Foliella*.[39] For practical purposes (treatment of disease rather than studying the biology of parasites) it does not make any difference which species is encountered. Morphological differentiation depends on the structure of the ring of hooks, the implantation of the cilia, and size and shape of the nucleus. There is further difference with respect to the preferred host species. Members of the Genus *Tripartiella* are typical parasites of the gills.

The related species *Trichodina urinaria* Dogel and *T. polycirra* Lom have been found in the urinary bladder and the ureters of Roach, and *T. alburni* in those of Bleak (*Alburnus alburnus*).[40] Still others occur in the urinary system of male newts, and in bitterling mussels (*Unio*).

TREATMENTS

Affected fishes can be cured by immersion in salt or quinine hydrochloride solution. If salt is used the fishes are bathed in a one per cent solution of salt for a quarter to half an hour. Since it is possible that the parasites produce cysts with a higher resistance, treatment must be repeated after two days; during this period encysted specimens will have left their cysts and then they will be killed, too.

Alternatively, a permanent salt treatment may be applied, as described on page 348, but going no further than the third addition and then, starting at the fourth day, gradually changing the water. Investigations by Schäperclaus have shown that for a sure cure of this infection much lower salt concentrations are sufficient than was thought necessary in the past. Therefore it is better for the condition of the fishes to reduce the strength of the medication accordingly; that is why the present treatment indicates a lower concentration of the bath than was given in the first edition of this book.

Quinine hydrochloride may be used at a strength of one part in 50 000 (about $1\frac{1}{2}$ gr to 1 Imp. gal, 1.3 gr/U.S. gal). The quinine must be dissolved in water before putting in the tank. The diseased fishes should be kept in the quinine solution until they are cured. It takes only 6 h to kill the parasites on the skin; generally, however, prolonging treatment to 24–48 h is recommended. Prussian Carp (*Carassius carassius*) seem to be hypersensitive to quinine treatment and should not be subjected to it.

D. Bailösoff found Neguvon (Bayer) highly effective. Fishes are bathed for 2–3 min in a 2–3.5% solution, which kills the free parasites within 10–30 sec. This is also true with respect to infections by *Chilodonella*, see further page 336.

According to Tsutsumi and Murata an alternative treatment consisting of a permanent bath 1 : 250 000 kills all parasites of the *Urceolariidæ* Group in 35 h. This will be the method of choice for fully planted tanks with a crowded population, and in all cases of delicate fishes. After treatment the water is changed.

Other treatments that have been reported to be effective are malachite green 1 : 200 000–1 : 400 000 for 30 min (not recommended for aquarium fishes, see discussion on pages 86–87 and pyridyl-mercuric acetate 1 : 500 000 for 1 h, which is not recommended for aquarium fishes either.

Potassium permanganate 1 : 500 000 for about half an hour should be effective, too, but is not recommended for reasons given at pages 344–345.

Benzalkonium chloride 1 : 40 000 up to 1 : 20 000 for 30 min only has also been advocated (see p. 320).

CHILODONELLIASIS

The same symptoms of disease may be caused by *Chilodonella cyprini* (Moroff) (Fig. 2.45a–b), or the closely related Species *Chilodonella hexastichus* (Kiernik) (Fig. 2.45c–d), belonging to the Order *Heterotricha* of the *Ciliata*. The genus has been known for more than a century under the name of *Chilodon*, but the name had to be changed after it had been discovered that a few years prior to its use for a genus of protozoans, it had already been reserved for a mollusc.

These organisms are heart or leaf shaped. The body is flattened from the dorsal to the ventral side. The dorsal side is vaulted, bare and has no stripes, while the ventral side is completely flat, striped and covered with cilia. At the front side the cilia are a little larger.

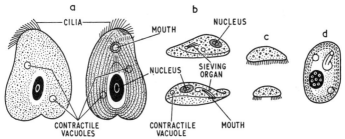

Fig. 2.45. (a) Chilodonella cyprini. Left: *dorsal view*. Right: *ventral (re-drawn after Hofer)*. (b) *side view of* Ch. cyprini *(redrawn after Roth)*. (c) upper illustration, *section of* Ch. cyprini*; lower, *section of* Ch. hexastichus *with cilia variation (redrawn after Roth)*. (d) *ventral view of* Ch. hexastichus *(redrawn after Roth)*

Inside are a nucleus and two contractile vacuoles (in the living parasite the nucleus is often not showing, but it can be made visible in a microscopical preparation by staining with suitable dyes, such as methylene blue, aniline blue, methyl violet or fuchsine). *Chilodonella cyprini* has a length of 40–70 μm and a breadth of 30–50 μm, whereas *Chilodonella hexastichus* has a length of 42–54 μm and a width of 34–42 μm.

Reproduction takes place by simple division in two parts after division of the nucleus and preparatory processes. Division takes place perpendicularly on the longitudinal axis of the body. From time to time two individuals unite and exchange parts of nuclear matter (conjugation).

Under good conditions, an infection may remain latent for weeks, even months. If the fishes are weakened by bad conditions, however, the parasites may multiply in rapid tempo and, if the gills are affected too, they can do considerable harm. In such cases, an epidemic may occur.

The parasites can only be detected in the slime collected from living fishes, since they leave their host very soon after it has died. Killed and preserved fishes are unsuited for diagnosis.

In big Carp-breeding ponds in Northern Russia heavy losses have regularly occurred in the winter season, due to *Chilodonella* infections (Golovkow and Abrosow[41]). In a period of 11 years, some 14 millions of one-summer-old Carp were lost in this way. In

Germany, Schäperclaus observed large epidemics in young Carp and Trout. Treatment is the same as for fishes that are infected by *Cyclochæta*. Very good results are obtained with salt. *Chilodonella* can be killed with quinine, too, but instead of 6 h, as in *Cyclochæta*, it takes 18 h to eradicate the parasites on the fish. Acriflavine was found much more effective than quinine, however. Schäperclaus recommends treatment with a solution of 1 g of acriflavine (indicated by the trade mark 'Trypaflavin' by him) per 100 l of water (equivalent to 0.7 gr/Imp. gal or 0.58 gr/U.S. gal). At this strength *Chilodonella* is killed within a period of 2–10 h; thus treatment does not need to be continued for much more than half a natural day.

Methylene blue has also proved effective, but at a much slower rate; it takes several days before the infection is eradicated. It should be applied in the same way as indicated for treatment of white spot (see pages 45–47).

Chilodonella is not susceptible to changes of temperature or to the oxygen content of the water within the range in which fish can live. Therefore, during any treatment the temperature should be kept at the normal level.

COSTIASIS

The third micro-organism that may cause sliminess of the skin is *Costia necatrix* (Figs 2.46, 2.47). This is the most dangerous of the three parasites. It may reach a length of 12–20 μm and a breadth of

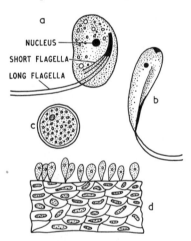

a

NUCLEUS

SHORT FLAGELLA

LONG FLAGELLA

c

b

d

Fig. 2.46. (a) *ventral view of* Costia necatrix. (b) *side view.* (c) *cyst.* (d) *section through skin of young Trout showing numerous specimens of* Costia *parasites (all redrawn after Moroff)*

6–10 μm. I have also found numerous specimens which were only about half this size. It belongs to the Class *Mastigophora*, Sub-class *Zoomastigina*, which are protozoans having large flagella by means of which they can swim through the water. *Costia* has two long and two short flagella. According to Hofer,[42] they stick to the skin of the fish by means of the long flagella, while the short ones are used for bringing food (consisting of epithelial cells) to the mouth. However, this is denied by Schäperclaus,[43] who states that attachment on to the skin of the fish should take place by tucking up part of the thinner

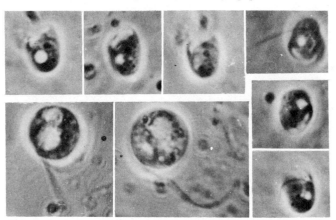

Fig. 2.47. Living Costia *necatrix. Phase-contrast photomicrographs (× 1000 and × 2000 approx.) of slime from a diseased fish. The pictures were taken at 1/10th second exposure and give an impression of the parasite swimming*

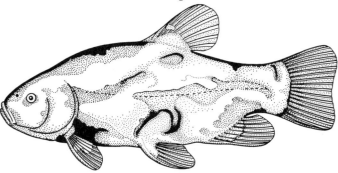

Fig. 2.48. Tench (Tinca tinca) *afflicted with sliminess of the skin* (Costiasis). *Infections caused by* Costia *are particularly dangerous*

lower side of the body, thus forming a kind of little gutter, enabling them to hold fast by suction. The present writer fails to understand the mechanics of this presumed process, and Schäperclaus himself does not seem to be completely convinced, either, since he adds that perhaps the parasites may have some stickiness from themselves aiding their adhesion. The activity of the parasites irritates the fish's skin and the slime cells secrete a large quantity of slime (Figs 2.48, 2.49), as is also the case with *Cyclochæta* and *Chilodonella* infections. Reproduction of *Costia* takes place by simple transverse division. The tempo of subsequent divisions may be very rapid so that in from one to two weeks a fish of great size may be covered over its whole skin with specimens of this parasite, which can encyst. When

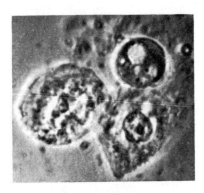

Fig. 2.49. Smear from the slime of a fish infected by Costia necatrix. *Left: slime cell. Right: a C.* necatrix *and epithelial cell with nucleus and nucleolus (photomicrograph taken in living state by phase contrast (× 1170))*

it leaves the fish and reaches the tank or pool bottom it thrusts out part of its protoplasm, after which it produces a membrane around itself. This cyst is spherical and has a diameter of 7–10 μm. Such cysts can also be found on the skin of the fish. Generally, the parasite attacks the gills as well. Infection of the gills is favoured at low pH values (4.5–5.8), at which the gills are affected chemically by the acid reaction of the water. In small fishes, death may occur in a few days, while large ones can stand the infection for a longer period. If no suitable treatment is used, all infected fishes will eventually die

Costia pyriformis is a smaller species, measuring only 9–14 μm × 5–8 μm, which has been found on North American Trout.[44]

TREATMENT FOR COSTIA

Costia necatrix infections require more drastic treatment than the other parasites which cause sliminess of the skin, due to the higher resistance of this organism. The free parasite may be killed by bathing the infected fishes in a 1% solution of salt for half an hour. In this solution *Costia* is killed in 15 min; a longer period of treatment is required to make sure that any specimen with an exceptionally high resistance, or that is protected by a more hidden site at the body of the fish, should be killed, too.

When separated from the fish, *Costia* will not survive for much more than one hour. Consequently, if all fish are removed from the infected tank for separate treatment, this tank will be safe again after having stood unoccupied for several hours. No further treatment would then be required.

Before this short survival of the parasite when separated from the fish was known, treated fishes were put back in the tank immediately and would be reinfected, so that treatment had to be repeated two, three or, in very bad cases, even four times every two days. This was thought to be due to survival of part of the specimens on the fish, and of survival of cysts. With the present better understanding of the physiology of the parasite, reliable results can be obtained more easily and with less drastic medication than formerly.

Instead of salt a formalin bath may be applied. This is used in a strength of $\frac{1}{4}$: 1000, i.e. 2–5 cm^3 of common formalin solution per 10 l of water or 1–2.5 cm^3/Imp. gal (0.85–2.2 cm^3/U.S. gal). The fish should be bathed in this solution for a quarter of an hour. The tank should be kept unoccupied for several hours before the fish may be reintroduced. Permanent treatment with low concentrations of formalin, as are successfully employed against skin flukes (see page 29), has been proved to be ineffective against *Costia*.

A short bath (30 min only) in a solution of benzalkonium chloride 1 : 40 000 up to 1 : 20 000 has also been recommended.

Quinine hydrochloride at a strength of 1 : 50 000 (1 g in 50 l, or $1\frac{1}{2}$ gr to 1 Imp. gal, 1.3 gr/U.S. gal) kills *Costia necatrix* after 24–26 h. Add the separately dissolved drug in two equal portions at half a day's interval and prolong treatment for 36–48 h after the first addition. Do not apply this cure to Prussian Carp.

Methylene blue (3 g/100 l) has been found efficacious in 3–5 days, as mentioned by Amlacher.

Results with acriflavine are not yet available, but considering the experience with this drug for treatment of *Cyclochæta* and *Chilodonella* infections and the relative drug resistance of these three parasites, Schäperclaus recommends acriflavine at a strength of 1 g/100 l (0.7 gr/Imp. gal, 0.58 gr/U.S. gal), but prolonged for two days.

Since both quinine salts and acriflavine (particularly in such a strong concentration) have a very bad effect on plant growth and are not completely harmless to fish, either, personally I prefer separate treatment with salt or formalin, keeping the aquarium or pond unoccupied for several hours, or a permanent salt or methylene blue bath as mentioned for curing *Cyclochæta* infection.

Up to 25°C (77°F) the viability of *Costia* does not show any observable dependence on temperature. At higher temperatures, however, viability apparently decreases till above 30°C (86°F) the parasites gradually disappear from the skin of the fish. This explains why *Costia* infections rarely occur in tropical aquaria. In case the infection should occur in Labyrinth Fishes, a cure could then be effected by simply raising the temperature of the water to 30–33°C (86–91.5°F) and keeping it at this level till every symptom of the disease has disappeared completely. For other fishes, however, such prolonged heat treatment is not to be advised because it weakens them.

Without the aid of a microscope it is impossible to distinguish *Cyclochætiasis*, *Chilodonelliasis* and *Costiasis*. Therefore one might ask, what course should be taken if symptoms of sliminess of the skin are observed and a microscope is not available for ascertaining an exact diagnosis. Since *Costia* is the only one of the three parasites which dies soon when separated from the fish, whereas the other two may survive for long periods, permanent treatment is to be preferred, of such duration as would be required in case of *Costiasis*.

As set forth in the description of diseases caused by skin flukes, a sliminess of the skin may occur also in cases of *Gyrodactylus* infection. Since treatment in this case is not the same, it is important to notice differences in the symptoms; in *Gyrodactyliasis* small blood spots may be showing in the skin; these do not occur with the three unicellular parasites (*Cyclochæta, Costia, Chilodonella*). In *Gyrodactyliasis* breathing is always increased in frequency, while in the others this is rare, occurring only at the end of the course of the disease, shortly before the death of the victims. If it is possible to make a microscopical examination of the slime from the skin, diagnosis is easy, since the parasites may be recognised from the illustrations on pages 68, 71–73. *Gyrodactylus* may be recognised even with the aid of a good magnifying glass (about × 10). (See Fig. 2.18, page 30.)

ULTRAVIOLET IRRADIATION

Recent investigations in Russia seem to indicate that irradiation of fish larvae and fry with ultraviolet rays may be successfully applied for combating infections by *Costia*, *Cyclochæta* or *Trichodina*, *Chilodonella* and *Ichthyophthirius*.[45] Since glass absorbs ultraviolet rays, the source should be placed over the water surface and the water depth should be low.

It must be emphasised, however, that eggs and embryos are damaged by irradiation, even with visible light;[46] therefore these should not be present if one wishes to try this treatment. Further, prolonged ultraviolet irradiation may induce tumours and skin lesions, so anyhow the method should be used with caution.

GLOSSATELLA (APIOSOMA) INFECTIONS

Members of the Genus *Glossatella* Bütschli (formerly *Apiosoma*) are Infusorians, belonging to the Order of the *Peritricha* in the *Ciliata*. Some of them occur occasionally on the skin and the gills of fish, where they may produce whitish spots. Diagnosis of the infection is only possible when the causative organisms are found in smear preparations from the slime of the skin or the gills. They are characterised by a more or less cylindrical shape and a definite stem with which they adhere to the fish skin.

Glossatella piscicola (Blanchard) possesses two rings of cilia, one round the mouth and the other about half-way along the body. Its length is from 62 to 86 μm and it is from 23 to 27 μm wide at the broader part of the body. Related species are *Glossatella glabra*

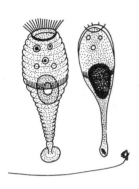
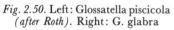
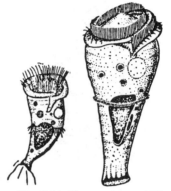

Fig. 2.50. Left: Glossatella piscicola   *Fig. 2.51. Two specimens of* Glossa-
(after Roth). Right: G. glabra   tella amœba *(after Bychovsky)*

(Roth), with a length of 75 μm and *G. amœba* (Grenfell) (see Figs 2.50, 2.51).

Infected fishes can be cured by bathing them in a 1% solution of ordinary salt (sodium chloride) for a quarter to half an hour, or by a formalin bath as described for treatment of *Costiasis* (page 75).

SCYPHIDIA AND *CALLIPERIA* INFECTIONS

These are organisms closely related to *Glossatella*, from which they differ by their very short stem that may have developed into a definite sucking disc (*Scyphidia*) or even a special attachment organ (*Calliperia*)—see Fig. 2.52. *Scyphidia macropodia* Davis, *S. micropteri* Surber and *S. tholoformis* Surber have been found on North American fishes; *S. pyriformis* Tripathi on species from India. *Calliperia brevipes* Laird and *C. longipes* Laird are parasites of marine fishes.

Treatment consists of bathing infected fishes in a 1.5% salt solution for 1 h, or by a formalin bath, as indicated for *Costia* (p. 75), but extended to 1 h.[47]

HARMLESS ORGANISMS ON THE SKIN

Sometimes completely harmless microscopical organisms can be found on the skin of a fish, e.g. bell animalcules (*Vorticella, Carchesium* and *Epistylis* species). These are Infusorians which are highly

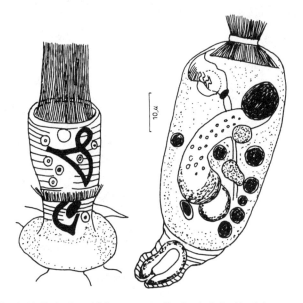

Fig. 2.52. Left: Scyphidia macropodia *Davis (after Davis).*
Right: Calliperia brevipes *Laird (after Laird)*

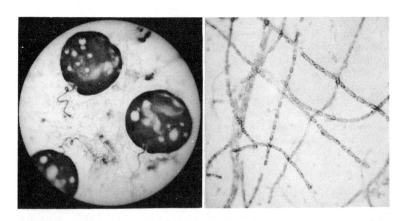

Fig. 2.53. Left: *Bell animalcules* (Vorticella globularis), × *150.* Right: Desmobacteria, × *950. Both were found in Siamese Fighters*, Betta splendens

appreciated as a food by small fry. They will settle only on fishes that are slow swimmers, such as *Bettas*. They do not penetrate into the skin, nor do they irritate the epidermal cells and these organisms are consequently only commensals, profiting by the good supply of fresh water, containing oxygen and food, given to them by the movement of the fish.

Obviously such moving life has great advantages for the organisms over settling on immovable objects, such as plants, stones, or glass

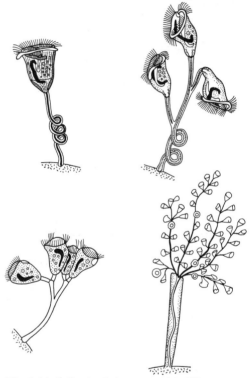

Fig. 2.54. *Bell animalcules representing different genera.*
Upper left: Vorticella nebulifera. Upper right:
Carchesium polypinum. Lower left: Epistylis leucos.
Lower right: Zoothamnium arbuscula. *All are harmless organisms*

tank sides. Settling on a fish, however, can only take place under very favourable conditions, so that bell animalcules are not very often found on fishes. If there is some fungus growth or development of bacteria on the skin, the latter will give a better hold to these Infusorians and they may therefore occasionally be found with real parasites. Then care should be taken not to confuse these harmless micro-organisms with the real cause of the disease.

Under the microscope the bell animalcule (Figs 2.53, 2.54) is easily recognisable by the bell-like body, situated on a long flexible stem, which may contract to a rolled-up spiral. The organisms are clearly visible at such low magnifications as $\times 20$, although at higher magnifications greater details of their structure will be seen. Without the aid of a microscope it is difficult to recognise a growth of these organisms. If they form large colonies, a thin veil may be seen. Some species, however, particularly those of the Genus *Carchesium*, may form such large colonies that they can be recognised with the aid of a simple magnifying glass. If no microscope is available, the easiest method of observing the tiny creatures is to introduce them (in a drop of water) on the surface of a small plane mirror. Now let the light (from a window, or from an electric bulb) fall on one side, and observe the drop with the aid of a magnifying glass from the opposite side, thereby looking at an angle that is approximately the same as that at which the light is reflected by the mirror, but preventing the directly reflected rays from entering the eye. Then only the light scattered by the organisms will reach the eye and they will become visible as tiny illuminated specks against a dark background. By this arrangement it is possible to see particles that in other circumstances are completely invisible at the same magnification. This phenomenon is known in physics as the 'Tyndall effect'.

According to Reichenbach-Klinke, accumulations of *Carchesium* and *Epistylis* can be killed by bathing the fishes in a 3% sodium chloride (salt) solution, a solution of malachite green 1 : 15 000 or pyridylmercuric acetate 1 : 500 000. These concentrations are all rather strong and risky for small fishes (see particulars given in Chapter 10), so I am opposed to their use, especially as these organisms do not impair general health of the fish.

On the skin of Carp local overgrowth with different kinds of algae has been observed by Van Bergeijk.[48] Among them were the green alga *Stigeoclonium tenue* Ktzg., the blue-green alga *Lyngbia diguetti* Gom. and a small amount of *Oscillatoria*, as well as a fairly large amount of diatoms. No harmful effects could be observed.

Other harmless micro-organisms that may sometimes be found on the skin of a fish are *Desmobacteria* (see Fig. 2.53 right), a group of bacteria that form long thread-like vegetations, so that the layman could confuse them with fungus when he sees them under the microscope. Actually the threads of *Desmobacteria* are much thinner than those of fungus, and show other structures, whilst on fishes they have a totally different appearance. There is no tuft (resembling cotton-wool) formed, but only a very thin veil. These organisms may be found mostly in water that contains a large amount of iron.

FUNGUS INFECTION

Dermatomycosis or fungus is one of the commonest diseases affecting fresh-water fishes. It is characterised by the growth of thin threads of a more or less dirty white or grey colour (Fig. 2.55) on the skin or fins. If fungus growth is abundant it may resemble tufts of

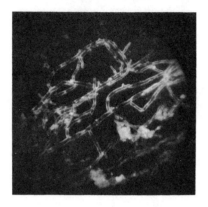

Fig. 2.55. Threads of fungus taken from an affected fish—photomicrograph (dark-ground illumination, × 500)

cotton-wool. Fungus is due to a mould which attacks only fishes that have been wounded or whose resistance has been weakened by other parasites or bad conditions. Thus, fishes which are suffering from white spot, flukes or other parasites which cause heavy injury to the skin, often develop fungus in addition, and this always means a serious complication. Fishes which are completely healthy and

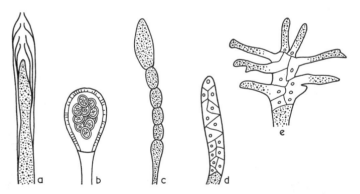

Fig. 2.56. (a) *Sporangia of* Saprolegnia Thureti *(after Thuret).* (b) *Oogonium of* Saprolegnia Thureti *(after Thuret).* (c) *Conidia of* Saprolegnia *spec. (after Maurizio).* (d) *Oogonium of* Saprolegnia *spec.* (e) *The same three hours later, completely germinated (after Roth)*

undamaged cannot get fungus, although the spores of these parasites are present in the water in large numbers.

Fungus is caused by a great many kinds of moulds of the Family *Saprolegniaceæ*. The most common members of this Family are the species of the Genera *Saprolegnia* (Fig. 2.56) and *Achlya* (Fig. 2.57). Correct determination of species is difficult, since this is only possible if they are in the stage of sexual reproduction. In practice it is not

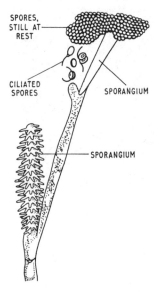

SPORES, STILL AT REST

CILIATED SPORES

SPORANGIUM

SPORANGIUM

Fig. 2.57. Achlya prolifera, *the lower sporangium with spores germinating and the upper one after spore dispersal (after Maurizio)*

very important, although probably different types may cause different forms of disease (all more or less serious).

Moulds consist of threads, called hyphae, which are often branched. The lower parts of the hyphae are thinner and grow into the sub-stratum (in this case the skin of the fish) like roots. This part of a fungus is called the mycelium. To kill the hyphae is relatively easy, but to kill the mycelium is more difficult, as it is protected by the skin of the victim. The length of the hyphae may vary between a few millimetres to 3 cm (about 1.2 in).

The tempo of development of fungus depends on conditions. On dead fishes growth is very rapid, whilst on living fishes it may take days or even weeks before larger areas of the skin are covered. At pairing time most fishes are more susceptible to fungus infections. This is partly due to greater chances of injuries during mating, or in fights with rivals, and partly to a weakening through exhaustion.

After a vegetative period in which the mycelium grows progressively through the skin of the fish, and the hyphae grow until a more or less large tuft has been formed, reproduction of the fungus will take place. For this purpose sporangia are usually formed at the end of the hyphae, and in these a large number of spores (up to 800) are produced. Each spore has two cilia (thin thread-like processes) with which it can move through the water like a little animal; therefore this form of spore is called the zoospore (from Greek: ζωός living, moving, and σπορά, what is sown). Each zoospore can produce a new mycelium, which forms new hyphae. When the first sporangium at the end of a fungus thread has been emptied, a second sporangium is formed, growing through the space that was at first occupied by the primary one. In this way two to eight empty sporangia walls may be enveloping each other.

A second form of reproduction consists of the formation of so-called conidia, which are club-shaped swellings at the end of the hyphae. These divide themselves into several parts, which may produce new fungus plants just like the zoospores, if they reach a suitable substratum.

These reproduction methods are all asexual, but a true sexual reproduction may appear, too. For this purpose, oospores (a kind of ova) are formed in oogonia ('ova-producers'), which may, or may not, be fertilised by spermatozoids. The oospores are the most resistant forms in the life cycle of a fungus. After a period of rest they may produce a new fungus thread directly, or a large number of zoospores. Which process will actually take place depends on conditions.

Fungus is not an obligatory parasite. It can live very well without the presence of fishes provided there is sufficient organic material present (decaying plants). Fishes are attacked only if their resistance has been weakened by other diseases, wounds, or bad conditions.

If infection of the fish's skin has occurred, at first a mycelium will be formed, growing between the cells of the epidermis and penetrating from there into the cutis and even to the underlying muscles. Meanwhile, hyphae are formed which grow not only upon the skin, but also through the skin and into the muscles, too. By their action the cells of the skin and the muscles begin to degenerate and eventually die. In very bad cases, the fungus may even penetrate to the skeleton.

TREATMENTS OF FUNGUS

Since fungus is not dangerous to healthy and undamaged fishes, it is not strictly necessary to remove a fish with fungus from a community tank, although it is advisable to do so for treatment of the victim. Precautions against fungus infections, following fishes becoming wounded, can never be absolute, but the chances can be diminished by keeping the aquarium or the pond in which the fishes are living, very clean. Aeration of the water is also helpful. The condition of the water is important. Very alkaline waters, such as are often found in ponds where the concrete has not properly matured, have a bad effect on the protecting mucous coat of fishes, and this increases their susceptibility to fungus infections. Sudden changes of water may have a bad effect, e.g. when fishes which have been living in slightly acid water are suddenly transferred into alkaline water. If the change is gradual, fishes will adapt themselves to the new conditions and no harm will be done. Water which is very acid has a bad effect, too. Experience has shown that for most fishes the best conditions obtain when the reaction of the water lies between the pH range of 6.8–7.2 (in sea-water a suitable pH range is from 7.6 to 8.0).

If only a small part of the skin is covered by fungus, the best way to treat it is by taking the fish from the water and touching the affected places with a solution of a good disinfectant, e.g. a solution of iodine, 1 : 10; or Mercurochrome^R 1 : 10 (one part by volume of commercial 2% solution with nine parts of water, making the final strength 0.1%); or merthiolate 1 : 1000; or 1% solution of potassium dichromate. The first three of these chemicals have the strongest activity but for very delicate, or very small, fishes it is better to use the last-named. A pencil or brush is dipped into one of the solutions and the mouldy places are touched with this, holding the fish in your left hand in such a way that its head and gills remain in the water, if possible, and only the body and fins are out. Take care to avoid touching healthy parts of the skin of the fish, since this would have a bad effect.

After this treatment the fish may be put into a tank containing potassium dichromate in a strength of 1 : 25 000 to 1 : 20 000, that is, 1 g in 5 or 6 Imp. gal (6–7 U.S. gal) of water, or $2\frac{1}{2}$–3 gr/Imp. gal (2–$2\frac{1}{2}$ gr/U.S. gal). This treatment should continue for about a week to 10 days, unless complete recovery has occurred before that time. Longer treatment is not advisable, since this could have a bad effect on the fishes. If necessary, primary treatment, by touching the fungus with the stronger chemicals, may be repeated. The water must be well aerated, while in tropicals it is advisable to raise the temperature several degrees to a maximum of about 27–28°C (about 80–82°F). Potassium dichromate may be used in fully planted tanks; its activity will not suffer and the plants will not be affected. After the period of treatment, the water must be changed. In ponds this chemical may be used only if it is possible to change at least two-thirds of the water after the cure.

It has been stated that ozone treatment for 1 h, repeated three to four times a day, will effect a cure in 10 days.[49]

In Russia, good results in preventing fungus growth on Sturgeon eggs have been obtained by disinfection of the water with ultraviolet irradiation,[50] as did periodical treatment of the eggs with malachite green 1 : 200000. Sodium chloride and formalin proved inadvisable. Also see pages 86–87.

DISADVANTAGES OF PERMANGANATE

According to my experience, the above-mentioned methods are very effective treatments for fungus. Potassium permanganate, often recommended, has several disadvantages, one of the most important being its dependence on the quantity of organic matter in the tank, so that it is often not easy to estimate the correct amount of permanganate that has to be added. An excessive dose of permanganate will kill fishes, while a perfectly safe dose is frequently not strong enough to guarantee a cure. Further, the activity of permanganate depends on the reaction of the water. This activity is relatively good in acid waters, while in neutral or alkaline water it is much less. If there is not enough acid present in the water, a precipitate of manganese is formed, which may accumulate on the body and gills of the fishes and damage them. This risk can be lessened by the use of artificial aeration. On the other hand, potassium dichromate shows no great dependency on the presence of organic matter in the water, nor on the reaction of the water, and no precipitates are formed. While a strength of 1 : 100 000 of permanganate is much too strong for use as a permanent treatment, a solution of 1 : 20 000 of dichromate is safe if it is not used for more than 10 days. Gosh and Pal also found dichromate preferable to permanganate.[51]

Potassium dichromate has a hardening effect on the skin of the fish (in tanning it is used for producing fine qualities of leather) which will increase the resistance to further outbreaks of infection. In ponds that cannot be streamed through with fresh water it is, unfortunately, impossible to use potassium dichromate. In such cases, one depends solely on potassium permanganate in a strength of 4–5 mg/l (0.25–0.3 gr/Imp. gal or 0.2–0.25 gr/U.S. gal). It is, therefore, better to catch diseased fishes in the pond and to treat them separately in an aquarium. Disinfection of the pond is not necessary since healthy fishes cannot be infected.

Although the potassium dichromate treatment has been used successfully during the many years since I first introduced it in 1935 in Holland (1938 in Britain[52]), it might become obsolete in the near future now that a very effective new cure has been found.

PHENOXETHOL

This is the phenoxethol treatment found by Ian M. Rankin. Phenoxethol (2-phenoxyethanol; spelt without the 'h'—Phenoxetol —it is a registered trade name) is an oily liquid with faint aromatic odour and burning taste. It is slightly soluble in water. For use, a stock solution of 1 cm^3 of phenoxethol in 99 cm^3 of distilled water is prepared. From this stock solution 10–20 cm^3 are added per litre of aquarium water. It is advisable to use the lowest concentration wherever possible. The maximum tolerance is 30 cm^3/l, while there is but a small margin between this maximum and a generalised lethal dose for some fish, the latter being 40 cm^3 of stock solution per litre. The lowest dosage of 10 cm^3/l, however, has proved safe even for Veiltail fry, two months old, and for tropicals. The dosage of 10 cm^3/l is equivalent to 45 cm^3/Imp. gal (or 38 cm^3/U.S. gal). Phenoxethol destroys fungus very rapidly; Rankin states: 'The fungus disappears literally overnight.'

OTHER TREATMENTS

Several other chemicals have been recommended for the treatment of fungus, but in my experience they seem less useful than the methods described. Mainly for completeness I will mention Collargol^R (colloidal silver). A stock solution is made by dissolving 0.1 g of Collargol in 100 cm^3 of hot, distilled water. From this solution 1–3 cm^3 are added to 1 l of water, or $4\frac{1}{2}$–$13\frac{1}{2}$ cm^3/Imp. gal ($3\frac{1}{2}$–$11\frac{1}{2}$ cm^3/U.S. gal). The fishes should remain in this bath for from one to three hours. Affected places may be treated with the stock solution in the same way as described for the iodine or Mercurochrome treatment. Collargol should not be used as a permanent bath.

Salt has been suggested, but to ensure success, a salt solution has to be made too strong for the fishes and this chemical cannot, therefore, be recommended.

Malachite green was tried by the U.S. Fish and Wildlife Service for treatment of eggs of Pike in hatcheries to prevent fungus development.[53] The eggs were treated with a 1 : 200 000 solution of the dye for 1 h. They were stained green, but this adsorption of dye is obviously harmless, since the percentage of hatches amounted to double that obtained from the untreated ones. This same treatment was used on Trout eggs by Burrows[54] who also concluded that the eggs had a wide tolerance to malachite green.

Merriner incubated Pumpkinseed (*Lepomis gibbosus*) and Bluegill (*L. macrochirus*) eggs with malachite green oxalate and found that the prolonged concentration for watchglass incubation coincided with the lower fungistatic limits of between 0.01 and 0.05 p.p.m. (0.1–0.5 mg/l).[55]

O'Donnell[56] successfully employed malachite green for eliminating fungus from 18 species of fish, including Brook Trout (*Salvelinus fontinalis*), Brown Trout (*Salmo trutta*) and Rainbow Trout (*Salmo iridaeus*), by dipping them for 10–30 sec only in a 1 : 15 000 solution. Allison[57] has reported that in Michigan (U.S.A.) malachite green is often used in pond treatment. At most fish-breeding stations, ponds are treated regularly with a dilution of 1 : 180 000 for 45 min. Where other external parasites, such as *Gyrodactylus*, are also present, malachite green would be combined with formalin in one treatment, which, however, increases toxicity to fish. As a method for disinfecting ponds or tanks without fish it might be a good policy.

All treatments should be performed in subdued light, because malachite green acts as a photosensitiser, i.e. toxic effects are highly increased by illumination.

For use in aquaria a lower concentration has been recommended, namely, 1 : 450 000 (0.22 mg/l). However, very bad results have been experienced with this prescription. Mr. Donald Speigal, Aquarium Sales Service, Vancouver, Canada, tried this treatment at an exact concentration of 2 gr for 15 U.S. gal in a bare aquarium with very soft water at pH 7 and temperature 24°C (75°F) and reported that it seemed to be very poisonous to live fish (personal communication 1958). Gills became inflamed and fish were near death in about 20 min. The reason for the apparent discrepancy between the experience in Pike and Trout hatcheries and this one could not be ascertained. However, later on great differences in susceptibility to this dye between different kinds of fish have been demonstrated. Amlacher has reported that Trout may die at 0.3 mg/l, but that they may stand up to 4 mg/l, if they get accustomed, with a slowly increasing concentration, whereas small aquarium fishes, especially members of the Genus *Hyphessobrycon* and its near relatives, could not even stand 0.1 mg/l. This same concentration was found to be the highest that was tolerated without casualties for 96 h by North American young *Siluriformes*, whereas at 0.19 mg/l all were killed.[58]

Therefore, application of malachite green in aquaria must be condemned as too risky, and the same may apply to the chemically closely related dye brilliant green. Also see pages 331–333.

COMBINED TREATMENT TRIED

A combined treatment with merthiolate, acriflavine and methylene blue was advocated by Dr. Aaron Wold.[59] According to Wold the effectiveness of merthiolate and other mercury compounds should be increased by the addition of acriflavine and methylene blue. He stated that the combination is quite effective. The dosage is given as two drops of 1 : 1000 aqueous merthiolate solution and two drops of 1 : 500 aqueous solution of acriflavine-methylene blue mixture (0.8 g of acriflavine neutral and 0.2 g of methylene blue, medical quality, in 500 cm³ of water) per U.S. gal, which should be equivalent to five drops of each solution to every 2 Imp. gal. During treatment artificial aeration must be employed. If the fish come to the surface of the water, gasping for air, one-third of the water must be changed immediately.

In the present writer's opinion, this treatment cannot be recommended. All mercury compounds are bound to give intoxication effects if the fish has to be in contact with them for some period, and merthiolate should make no exception. Further, acriflavine may cause a temporary sterility in fish. It would have been more satisfactory had a more exact prescription been stated; one should use an exact volume unit, since the actual volume of a drop will depend on the dimensions of the pipette used to measure it. Wold states 'acriflavine hydrochloride (neutral salt)' is to be used, but acriflavine hydrochloride is not a neutral salt but an acid one, known to be more toxic to fish.

Metaphen is mentioned as an alternative to merthiolate in this description, but metaphen is insoluble in water and has to be made soluble by adding alkali or ammonia. Apart from the toxicity due to its mercury content, it is also a blood poison, which does not seem to be desirable, either.

METHYLENE BLUE FOR MILD CASES ONLY

Methylene blue shows some slight fungicide activity, but it cannot be expected to cure advanced cases where the mycelium of the fungus has already penetrated deep into the body.

SULPHA DRUGS AND ANTIBIOTICS

Sulpha drugs and antibiotics have been reported to be effective in treatment of fish infected by fungus, but it seems that they do not attack the fungus itself. If the fungus is secondary to some bacterial infection, as is often the case, these drugs will act on the primary infection and by doing this, the resistance of the fish will be increased so that it may overcome the secondary fungus growth by virtue of its own defences. Apart from the regulations which may make it difficult to obtain antibiotics and sulpha drugs to treat diseased fishes, the cost may be prohibitive. These drugs should not be used indiscriminately, but only if there is no good alternative. A further discussion on sulpha drugs and antibiotics is given in the chapter on bacterial diseases (pages 152–156).

Recent new developments are types of antibiotics with specific activity against funguses only. As such griseofulvin (Fulvicin; Fulcin) has already been applied at 10 mg/l. A drawback of these types of substances (Nystatin = Mycostatin is another example) is that they are nearly insoluble in pure water, which makes treatment more difficult. The best way of application seems to be to use them locally in ointments, such as are commercially available for use in human and veterinary medicine.

FUNGUS AS SECONDARY INFECTION

In cases where fungus is only a secondary infection of fishes that have been weakened, or whose skin has been injured by other microscopical parasites, such as *Ichthyophthirius* or *Gyrodactylus*, or bacteria, treatment must first be directed at the primary disease. In such cases, it will often be best to give the fishes an initial treatment by touching the affected places of the skin with a suitable disinfectant, as mentioned previously, and immediately afterwards they can be treated with methods suitable for curing the primary disease. There are some other forms of fungus, needing special treatment. These are 'eye fungus', 'mouth fungus', and tail- or fin-rot. The first is a true fungus disease, which is dealt with in the chapter on diseases of the eye, while the latter two are primarily bacterial infections, although true fungus may appear as a secondary parasite. These afflictions are dealt with in the chapter on bacterial infections.

REFERENCES

1 STAMMER, J., 'Beiträge zur Morphologie, Biologie und Bekämpfung der Karpfenläuse', χ. *Parasitenkunde* **19**, 135–208
2 HOFER, B., *Handbuch der Fischkrankheiten*, Munich (1904)
3 CAMPBELL, A. S., *Aquarium Journal* (U.S.A.) **XXI**, 194 (1950)
4 KOLIPINSKI, M. C., 'Gar infested by *Argulus* in the Everglades', *Quart. J. Fla. Acad. Sci.* **32**, 39–49 (1969)
5 BAILÖSOFF, D., 'Neguvon—ein wirksames Mittel zur Bekämpfung der Karpfenlaus und sonstiger parasitärer Fischkrankheiten', *Deutsche Fischerei-Zeitung* **10**, 181 (1963)
6 HANSON, G. F., 'Effective parasitic worm treatment', *The Aquarium* (U.S.A.) **XVIII**, 275 (Nov. 1949)
7 WITENBERG, G., 'What is the cause of parasitic Laryngopharingitis in Near East ("Halzoun")?', *Acta Medica Orient.* **3**, 13–14 (1944)
8 DAWES, B., *The Trematoda*, Cambridge University Press (1946). *Also see:* MALMBERG, G., 'Om Förekomsten ow *Gyrodactylus* pa svenska fiskar', *Skrift. Sver. Fiskeriför*, 19–76 (1956)
9 PUTZ, R. E. and HOFFMAN, G. L., 'Two new *Gyrodactylus* (Trematoda: Monogenea) from Cyprinid fishes with synopsis of those found on North American fishes', *J. Parasit.* **49**, 559–66 (1963)
10 BOSHART, G., '*Gyrodactylus*-ziekte in mijn aquarium', *Het Aquarium* (Holland) **XI**, 320–22 (1940–41)
11 RANKIN, I. M., 'Treating fish affected by gill flukes', *Water Life* **VII**, 297–98 (Dec. 1952)
12 DOLLFUS, R. P., 'Sur un Trematode (Genre *Isoparorchis*) agent pathogene de la maladie de la *tache d'encre* chez des poissons du Vietnam', *Bull. Soc. Pathol. Exot.* **52**, 791–803 [1959 (1960)]
13 BUSCHKIEL, A. L., 'Neue Beiträge zur Kenntnis des *Ichthyophthirius multifiliis* Fouquet', *Archives Nederlandaises Zool.* **II**, 178–224 (21 Dec. 1936)
14 JUNG, W., 'Eine neue Behandlungsart der *Ichthyophthiriasis*', *Blätter f. Aquarien- und Terrarienkunde* **42**, 245 (1931)
15 SCHÄPERCLAUS, W., *Fischkrankheiten*, 3rd ed., 165 (1954)
16 VAN DUIJN, Jnr., C., 'Genezing van *Ichthyophthiriasis* met methyleenblauw', *Het Aquarium* **VII**, 205–07 (1936); '*Diseases of Fishes*—5. White Spot', *Water Life* **4** (new series), 273–74 (1949)

17 GODFREY, P. W., 'Methylene blue efficacious', *Water Life* **VI**, 83 (April 1951)
18 JOHNSON, D. W., *The Aquarium* (U.S.A.) **XVIII**, 232 (Oct. 1949)
19 VAN DER KROON, A. A., 'Een nooddeeling van *Ichthyophthirius* onder den microscoop', *Het Aquarium* (Holland) **5**, 58–59 (1934)
20 DEUFEL, J., 'Malachitgrün zur Bekämpfung von *Ichthyophthirius* bei Forellen', *Fischwirt* **1** (1960)
21 AMLACHER, E., *Taschenbuch der Fischkrankheiten*, pp. 179–80, VEB Fischer Verlag, Jena (1961)
22 SLATER, D. C., 'New treatment for white spot', *Water Life* **VII**, 122 (June 1952)
23 WADEMAN, L. C., *The Aquarium* (U.S.A.) **XVIII**, 237–38 (Oct. 1949)
24 VAN HENGEL, Jnr., J. F., 'Iets over *Ichthyophthirius multifiliis*', *Het Aquarium* **25**, 215 (1954–55); KRISTENSEN, I., '*Psettus* als witte-stip verdelger', *Het Aquarium* **25**, 279 (1954–55)
25 DE GRAAF, F., 'A new parasite causing epidemic infection in captive coral fishes', *Bull. Inst. Oceanog. Monaco, Num. Special 1A, Premier Congr. Inst. Aquariol. A.*, 93 (1962)
26 NIGRELLI, R. F. and RUGGIERI, G. D., 'Enzootics in the New York Aquarium caused by *Cryptocaryon irritans* Brown, 1951 (= *Ichthyophthirius marinus* Sikama, 1961), a histophagous ciliate in the skin, eyes and gills of marine fishes', *Zoologica* **51**, 97 (1966)
27 KOZLOFF, E. N., 'Velvet: a common protozoan infection of aquarium fish', *All-Pets Magazine* (U.S.A.), 43–44 (May 1948); *Oregon Aquatic News* (U.S.A.) **X**, No. 9 (Dec. 1949); PATTERSON, E. E., 'Velvet—a sure cure', *Oregon Aquatic News* (U.S.A.) **X**, No. 9 (Dec. 1949)
28 PATTERSON, E. E., 'Effects of acriflavine on birth rate', *Aquarium Journal* (U.S.A.) **XXI**, 36 (1950)
29 REICHENBACH-KLINKE, H., *Krankheiten und Schädigungen der Fische*, Stuttgart (1966)
30 WOLD, A., *The Aquarium* (U.S.A.) **XX**, 13 (Jan. 1951)
31 McKAY, R. J. and WORTHINGTON, R., *Corrosion Resistance of Metals and Alloys*, New York (1936)
32 SCHÄPERCLAUS, W., 'Der Colisa-Parasit, ein neuer Krankheitserreger bei Aquarienfischen', *Die Aquarien- und Terrarienzeitschrift* **4**, 169–71 (1951)
33 HIRSCHMANN, H. and PARTSCH, K., 'Der Colisa-Parasit—ein Dinoflagellat aus der Oodiniumgruppe', *Die Aquarien- und Terrarienzeitschrift* **6**, 229–34 (1953)
34 REICHENBACH-KLINKE, H., 'Untersuchungen über die bei Fischen durch Parasiten hervorgerufenen Zysten und deren Wirkung auf den Wirtskorper', *Zeitschrift für Fischerei N.F.* **3**, 565–636 (1954); (*see also* pp. 585–88)
35 BROWN, E. M., 'On *Oodinium ocellatum* Brown, a parasitic Dinoflagellate causing epidemic disease in marine fish', *Proc. Zoo. Soc.*, London **3**, 583–607 (1934); NIGRELLI, R. F., 'The morphology, cytology and life history of *Oodinium ocellatum* Brown, a Dinoflagellate parasite on marine fishes', *Zoologica, N.Y. Zoo. Soc.* **321**, 12–164 (1936)
36 RISELEY, R. A., *Tropical Marine Aquaria—the Natural System*, Allen & Unwin (1971)
37 REICHENBACH-KLINKE, H., *Verh. deutsch. Zool. Mainz* (Aug. 1949); *Publ. Zool. Anzeiger*, Supp. 14, 126 (1950); 'Beobachtungen an einer Barschseuche (Dermocystidiose)'; *Deutsche Aquarien- und Terrarienzeitschrift* **4**, 213–14 (1951); also in: 'Untersuchungen über die bei Fischen durch Parasiten hervorgerufenen Zysten und deren Wirkung auf den Wirtskörper, *Zeitschr.f. Fischerei N.F.* **3**, 602–04 (1954)
38 ELKAN, E., '*Dermocystidium gasterostei* n. sp., a parasite of *Gasterosteus aculeatus* L. and *Gasterosteus pungitius* L.', *Nature* **196**, 958–60 (1962)

39 LOM, J., 'The Ciliates of the Family *Urceolariidae*', *Vestn. Českosl. Zool. Spol.* **27**, 7–19 (1963)
40 VOJTEK, J., 'Zur Kenntnis der Gattung *Trichodina* Ehrenberg 1830', *Vestn. Českosl. Zool. Spol.* **21**, 173–80 (1957)
41 GOLOVKOW, G. A. and ABROSOW, W. W., *Zool. J.* **XXXI, A.**, 128 (1952) (in Russian)
42 HOFER, B., *Handbuch der Fischkrankheiten*, Munich (1904)
43 SCHÄPERCLAUS, W., *Fischkrankheiten*, 3rd ed., Berlin (1954)
44 DAVIS, H. S., 'Studies of the protozoan parasites of freshwater fishes', *Fish. Bull.* **51**, 1–29 (1947); *Culture and Diseases of Game Fishes*, Berkeley and Los Angeles (1953)
45 VLASENKO, M. J., 'Ul'trafioletovye luchi kak metod bor'by s boleznyami ikry i molodi ryb', *Vop. Ikthiol.* **9**, 917–27 (1970)
46 PAINLEVÉ, J., 'Inluence de la lumière visible sur les structures vivantes en microcinématographie', *Research Film* **3**, 1313 (1958); MacCRIMMON, H. R., 'Influence on early development and meristic characters in the rainbow trout, *Salmo gairdneri* Richardson', *Can. J. Zool.* **47**, 631–37 (1969)
47 DAVIS, H. S., *Culture and Diseases of Game Fishes*, Berkeley and Los Angeles (1953)
48 VAN BERGEIJK, W. A. M., 'Merkwaardige begroeiing bij vissen', *Het Aquarium* **24**, 35 (1953–54)
49 SANDER, E., 'Ozone—its application to aquarium-keeping', *Pet Fish Monthly* **I**, 9–10 (1966)
50 ASTAKHOVA, T. V. and MARTINO, K. V., 'Mery bor'by s gribkovyn zabolevaniem ikry osetrovykh na rybovodnykh zavodakh', *Vop. Ikthiol.* **8**, 332–41 (1968)
51 GOSH, A. K. and PAL, R. N., 'The toxicity of four therapeutic compounds to Indian Major Carp', *Fish. Technol. (India)* **6**, 120–23 (1969)
52 VAN DUIJN, Jnr., C., 'Bichromate of potash', *Water Life* **IV** (old series), 108 (1 Mar. 1938)
53 *The Fish Culturist*, Pennsylvania (U.S.A.) (Jan. 1952)
54 BURROWS, R. E., 'Prophylactic treatment for control of fungus (*Saprolegnia parasitica*) on Salmon eggs', *Progr. Fish-Cult.* **II**, 97–103 (1949)
55 MERRINER, J. V., 'Constant-bath malachite green solution for incubating sunfish eggs', *Progr. Fish-Cult.* **31**, 223–25 (1969)
56 O'DONNELL, J., 'A method of combating fungus infections', *Progr. Fish-Cult.* No. 56, 18–20 (1941)
57 ALLISON, L. N., 'Advancements in prevention and treatment of parasitic diseases of fish', *Trans. Am. Fisheries Soc.* **83**, 221–28 (1953)
58 CLEMENS, H. P. and SNEED, K. E., 'The chemical control of some diseases and parasites of Channel Catfish', *Progr. Fish-Cult.* **20**, 8–15 (1958)
59 WOLD, A., *The Aquarium* (U.S.A.) **XIX**, 86–97 (April 1950)

3

RESPIRATION AND DISEASES OF THE GILLS

The gills of a fish each consist of four hard bones (gill arches) on which the gill sheets are attached (Fig. 3.1). They are situated in two alternating rows. Each gill sheet is more or less lancet shaped and has a great number of fine transverse folds on the broad sides; these are called respiratory folds (Figs 3.2, 3.3). They contain a net of fine capillaries lying near the surface and this enables oxygen to diffuse from the water into the blood and carbon dioxide (carbonic acid) from the blood into the water.

Hence the gills of healthy fishes have a reddish colour, unless they are pigmented as in the case of Bettas and some other species

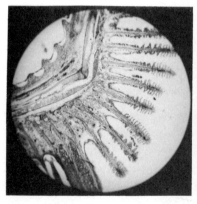 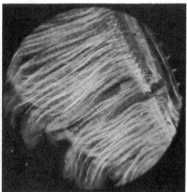

Fig. 3.1. Photomicrograph of a section through gill of a fish showing the bone (left) and the gill sheets with respiratory folds (right)

Fig. 3.2. Part of the gill of a Platyfish under dark ground illumination. Photomicrograph of magnification × 15

when the colour is dark. Pale gills are always a sign of disease in living fish. When the fish dies, the gills will always become pale, but this process takes some time, the exact period depending on conditions. In water it will take place more quickly than if the fish is brought into the air while, at low temperatures, the rate of fading

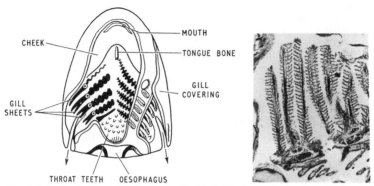

CHEEK

MOUTH

TONGUE BONE

GILL COVERING

GILL SHEETS

THROAT TEETH   OESOPHAGUS

Fig. 3.3. Left: *Section of the head of a Haddock* (Gadus æglefinus) *indicating the situation of the gills (after Hertwig).* Right: *Transverse section of the gill sheets showing the situation of the respiratory folds (photomicrograph by the author)*

is much slower. It will be understood from this why it is that housewives, buying fish to cook, look at the colour of the gills to see if the fish is fresh.

On the sides of the gill sheets that have no respiratory folds, a thick, mucous epithelium is present. The slime cells in this tissue secrete a slimy liquid that forms a protective layer, like the action of the slime cells of the skin. Thus, if parasites are present that cause an irritation of the epithelium, the slime cells will secrete a larger quantity of slime, which covers the gill sheets to some extent and gives the impression of a fading of the colour of the gills— although they may be filled with blood in the normal way. Such a slime-covering hinders the diffusion process of oxygen and carbon dioxide to and from the blood and, consequently, respiration becomes difficult. The fish tries to overcome this handicap by a wider opening of its gill coverings and by increasing the frequency of breathing. These symptoms are common features of all diseases of the gills, but since they depend ultimately on lack of oxygen they are also shown by fishes that are healthy, but are in situations where there is too low an oxygen content in the water. Increased frequency of breathing will also occur when fishes are taken from colder water and put directly in water that is warmer. Breathing frequency is always dependent on the oxygen content of the water, but since, even in epidemics, not all fishes will be infected at once, it is always possible to observe the symptom of increased breathing frequency by comparing with that of other fishes of the same, or closely related, species in the same tank.

OXYGEN REQUIREMENTS OF FISH

There are not many data available on the concentration of oxygen that is needed to keep fish in good health, although it is a well-established fact that there are considerable variations between different groups of fish.

The following figures have been calculated from investigations by Bruno Hofer.[1] The normal oxygen content of natural waters is 8.6–11.5 mg/l; 4.3–5.75 mg/l is sufficient in winter, even for *Salmonidæ*, such as Salmon and Trout. *Salmonidæ* die when the oxygen content has fallen to 2.16 mg/l, whilst *Cyprinidæ* (Carp and relatives) die at a concentration of 0.72 mg/l. Trout showed a breathing frequency of 60–70 respirations per minute with 10.8 mg/l and this was increased to 140–150 respirations per minute when the oxygen content had fallen to 2.88 mg/l.

Schäperclaus[2] states that at summer temperatures *Salmonidæ* already show signs of distress at an oxygen content of 5–5.5 mg/l, and increased breathing frequency and gasping at 4 mg/l. 3 mg/l is insufficient when persisting for any longer period of time, whereas 1.5–2 mg/l proves fatal within a short time.

Carps in fish ponds apparently do not feel happy at 3–3.5 mg/l and at 0.5 mg/l they are gasping for breath, snapping air at the surface of the water until eventually they die. The same limit holds for Tench.[2]

Dr. E. Fink[3] gave the minimum oxygen content of water for European wild fishes as 6.5 mg/l (which does not agree very well with the values given by Hofer and Schäperclaus) and approximately 1.3 mg/l only for tropicals. This latter value is extremely low and, in my opinion, it should be a lethal limit rather than a concentration which allows fish to keep in good health.

In my own investigations I found no signs of lack of oxygen in Goldfish of 2-in length at an oxygen content of 1.8 mg/l (temperature 17.5°C), but, when there was not more than 1.63 mg/l, the fish came gaping at the surface. The carbon dioxide content of the water in the latter case was 101 mg/l (pH 6.8; temperature 15°C).

Dr. Kurt Smolian gave values of oxygen requirements for large fish cultured in ponds for food purposes; this is done to a large extent in Germany.[4] He gave the oxygen requirements as a function of both the weight of the fish and the temperature, while he also pointed out that the nutritive condition and the motility of the fish influenced the figures he obtained.

The following table has been derived from the figures given by Smolian (after Maier and Hofer). His values in volume units have been recalculated in weight units by the author:

| Temperature of the water | | Oxygen consumed by 1 kg of various fish in mg/h | | |
°C	°F	Carp, Eel, Tench	Salmonidæ, Coregonidæ, Pike, Perch	Prussian Carp, Goldfish, Weatherfish
2	35.6	7.2	100	14.4
5	41	14.4	130	26
10	50	36	160	53
12.5	54.5	68.5	175	68
15	59	58–72	173–216	83.5
30	86	200	432	216

At 5°C numbness caused by cold occurs in the *Cyprinidæ*, while *Salmonidæ* fish just stop eating. 30°C is the highest temperature that can be stood by *Salmonidæ* and then only for a short time.

Although the figures given in this table are of little value to persons keeping fish in aquaria, they have been stated because they furnish a good comparison between the relative oxygen requirements of different kinds of fish.

More recent data are represented in the graph on page 96.

For several kinds of fish the partial pressure of oxygen in the blood, required for keeping 95% of the blood haemoglobin in the oxidised state (oxyhaemoglobin), has been determined. Results were:

Fish	Partial pressure of oxygen maintaining 95% oxyhaemoglobin[6] mm of mercury	Corresponding oxygen content of water at 15°C and 1 atm total pressure[7] mg/l
Carp, Eel, Pike	10	0.6
Trout	30–40	1.8–2.4
Plaice	40	2.4
Cod	70	4.2

Winterstein[8] has found that a partial pressure of oxygen in the water of 9.5–11.5 mm of mercury is insufficient for Roach (*Rutilus rutilus*) and Rudd (*Scardinius erythrophthalmus*), but a partial pressure of 16.6 mm of mercury will do. These amounts correspond to 0.57–0.69 and 1.0 mg/l at 15°C and 1 atm total air pressure.

Fishes that are suffering from lack of oxygen will swim near the surface of the water. Often they swim more rapidly than normally, sometimes even jumping out of the water; this is the reaction of fishes that are lively swimmers. Slower-swimming species often swim near the surface, put their mouths above the water and swallow air that is distributed in small bubbles in the mouth and after that mixes with the water that flows to the gills. In doing so, they can stand a low oxygen content of the water, that would otherwise be fatal, for some time, but if conditions do not improve this is insufficient to satisfy the oxygen requirements and they will die from suffocation. Fishes that have died in this way show a widely gaping mouth, while the coverings of the gills stand out, showing the gill sheets which are pale and swollen. The heart of such fishes is expanded, too, and shows excessive filling with blood.

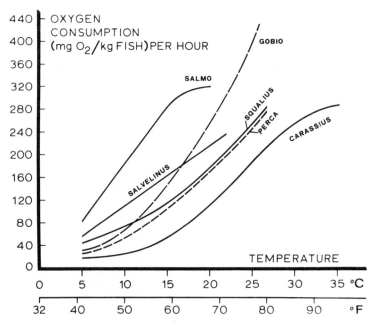

Oxygen consumption of different fishes in relation to temperature. Redrawn with linear co-ordinates after data by M. Flörke, G. Keiz and G. Wangorsch, Z. Fisch. 3, N.F. (1954)

In young fishes deformities of the head may be produced if they are growing in an environment with low oxygen content (see page 309).

Lack of oxygen will occur in tanks or ponds that are overcrowded, or contain too few plants, or receive insufficient light to allow good assimilation by the plants. Lack of oxygen can also occur on very hot days, when the temperature of the water rises rapidly so that much of the oxygen in the water is driven out (gases are less soluble in warm than cold water), while at higher temperatures fishes will often be more lively and consequently will want more oxygen than at lower temperatures. In fully planted tanks this is compensated by increased oxygen production by the plants. Thus, lack of oxygen will not manifest itself immediately in tropical tanks during the summer but in autumn and winter, when the temperature of the water is kept relatively high, while oxygen production is lower, it can often occur. In cold-water tanks, however, conditions are different. Here, lack of oxygen may occur more often in summer than in winter, since in winter the water is colder and can hold more oxygen, while the fishes need less oxygen due to decreased activity at this time.

Another important factor is the presence of much organic matter that is used by bacteria. Abundant growth of bacteria in the water causes a high oxygen consumption and, as this is stimulated by lack of light, it is important to keep the aquarium clean. From the data given above, measures to be taken to avoid distress due to lack of oxygen can easily be deduced. Keep the aquarium clean and take care that it receives enough light, but prevent direct sunlight shining on cold-water tanks in summer. Take care that the tanks are not overcrowded and use artificial aeration if necessary.

According to experiments by Dr. Kurt Kramer (Mulheim-Ruhr, Germany) coarse-bubble aeration should provide an air displacement of 47 l/h, medium-coarse 29 l/h and fine 6 l/h. The efficiency of fine-bubble aeration is much greater than of the other two, however. Kramer found that at the same rate of air displacement (10 l/h per 100 l of oxygen-free water) the following oxygen contents were obtained:

	mg/l
Coarse-bubble aeration	1.15
Medium	2.20
Fine	3.30

There are fishes which can stand a low oxygen content of the water. Loaches and Catfishes are able to swallow air at the surface of the water, which passes through the gullet and the stomach and comes into the intestine, where the oxygen is absorbed by the capillaries. This 'intestinal respiration' is a very great help to these animals. After being deprived of its oxygen, the air escapes through the anal opening.

In Labyrinth Fishes there is a special organ (the so-called labyrinth, after which they are named) for using atmospheric oxygen. While in Loaches and Catfishes respiration of air from the atmosphere is only a help to normal respiration, if this is required by conditions, in Labyrinth Fishes it is an absolute necessity. It may sound unusual, but these fishes can be drowned. If one of them is prevented from taking in fresh air (e.g. by stretching a net under the surface of the water) then, after ejection of the spent air, water is taken in and fills the swim bladder, drowning the fish. Newly hatched Labyrinth Fishes lack this labyrinth organ and breathe with their gills only until the labyrinth has developed. Too great a water depth will give trouble to such youngsters but 25–30 cm (10–12 in) may be considered safe.

OXYGEN REQUIREMENTS OF FISH EGGS

Oxygen requirements of developing fish eggs may be even higher than those of adult fish. Lindroth[9] studied oxygen consumption and required levels of oxygen concentration in the water in eggs of Pike (*Perca fluviatilis*). Both are significantly correlated and increase rapidly with increasing degree of embryological development, as shown by the graph in Fig. 3.4. For hatching, the water should be nearly saturated with oxygen, the actual oxygen concentration depending on temperature (see Fig. 3.5).

On the other hand, a lack of oxygen of short duration may be tolerated. At the beginning of development about 12 h of absolute lack of oxygen can be survived, but in later stages this period is a few hours only. Newly hatched fry may survive 1–2 h of complete lack of oxygen, but youngsters that are already able to swim and seek food will only stand this unfortunate condition for 5–10 min. Schäperclaus points out that the possibility must be considered that severe lack of oxygen during development of the eggs may lead to deformities in the hatching fry (compare page 309).

From these data it may be concluded that it is very important to keep breeding tanks for egg-laying fish in good condition with respect to oxygen content of the water. In order to prevent undue oxygen consumption by bacteria and other micro-organisms, the bottom should be kept clean. Excessive dirt on the bottom and lack of oxygen increase the risk of infection of the eggs by fungus, too.

GAS EMBOLISM IN FISH ('BUBBLE DISEASE')

Whilst lack of oxygen is dangerous to the health of fishes, there can be conditions in which oxygen is supplied so abundantly that this, too, is dangerous. A disease may then be caused which is known as gas embolism.

In fully planted tanks, receiving direct sunlight, so much oxygen may be produced on a hot day that the oxygen content of the water increases to 20–30 mg/l instead of the normal amount of 5–10 mg/l.[10] Leaves of *Vallisneria spiralis* of 30 cm length may produce 0.63 mg of oxygen per leaf per hour during daylight.[11] For other aquatic plants an oxygen production in the range of 0.013–0.07 mg/cm^2/h has been observed by Rabinovitch.[12] The value given for *Vallisneria* falls in this same range. The rate of respiration of plants amounts to about

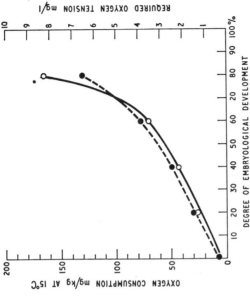

REQUIRED OXYGEN TENSION mg/l

OXYGEN CONSUMPTION mg/kg AT 15°C

DEGREE OF EMBRYOLOGICAL DEVELOPMENT

Fig. 3.4. Right: *Oxygen consumption (dashed line; left-hand scale) and required oxygen content of the water (solid line; right-hand scale) by Pike eggs during progressing embryological development (after numerical data by Lindroth)*

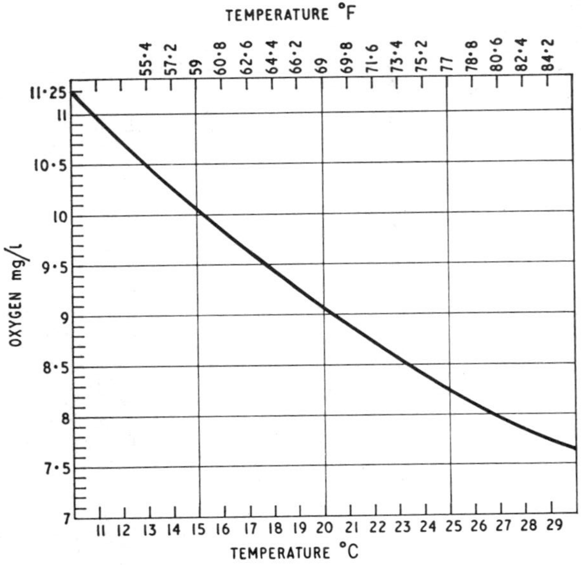

TEMPERATURE °F

TEMPERATURE °C

OXYGEN mg/l

Fig. 3.5.
SOLUBILITY OF OXYGEN
Left: *Graph showing the solubility of oxygen at different temperatures. Atmospheric pressure is 1 atm. (760 mm of mercury) and partial pressure of oxygen is 0.2075 atm. Temperatures are given in Fahrenheit and Centigrade for comparison*

5–15% of photosynthesis, so the net oxygen production available for the fish amply exceeds that of oxygen consumption by the plants themselves during the night.

If the temperature of the water is high, it can become over-saturated with oxygen which may cause an oversaturation in the blood of the fishes. So long as there is equilibrium between the partial pressure of oxygen in the blood and in the water no harm is done, but if the external pressure decreases suddenly or more rapidly than the rate of diffusion of oxygen from the blood vessels to the outside can cope with to maintain equilibrium, dissolved gas will escape from the solution in the form of bubbles that can obstruct the blood vessels and, if they reach the main vessels, so much hindrance is given to the normal circulation of the blood that the victim dies from gas embolism.

In this condition, the gas bubbles consist mostly of nitrogen instead of oxygen. The reason for this is as follows. In the gill sheets there is a direct exchange of dissolved gases between the water and the blood vessels of the fish, the gases including all that are present in atmospheric air, although in different relative amounts owing to the differences in solubility. Now of these gases, oxygen is removed from the dissolved state in the blood by combining chemically with haemoglobin so that the total gas pressure in the blood is lowered. This means an increase of the partial pressure of the other gases in the blood, mainly nitrogen and carbon dioxide. The latter is of minor importance in this respect because it is highly soluble in water and in blood it will not escape in a gaseous form, because it is held back by combination with calcium salts and other blood constituents. Nitrogen, on the other hand, is chemically inert under atmospheric conditions and in the blood, whereas its solubility is very low, so that supersaturation with this gas is reached much sooner. High gas tension in the water in itself does not cause gas embolism, but it is a rapid change in this tension which may produce it, the essential cause being that the gas exchange by diffusion cannot maintain the internal and external pressures near equilibrium. The condition is analogous to caisson disease occurring in workers in compressed air, who are too suddenly returned to atmospheric pressure.

When the plants are assimilating very rapidly, they take so much carbon dioxide from the water that bicarbonates are converted into carbonates, while the process may even go so far as to take carbon dioxide from the carbonates. As a result of this process, the water becomes more and more alkaline and ultimately its pH may reach a value which is dangerous to the health of the fishes. Water which is too alkaline (about pH 9 or more) has the effect of corroding the skin of the fish and normal respiration is hindered. Fins may become ragged, the pupils of the eyes appear enlarged and the lens of the eye may lose its transparency.

Gas embolism may show externally by the presence of small

bubbles in the body of the fish, to be seen when looking through the animal against the light. Of course, only more or less transparent fishes can show such signs. Gas bubbles can also accumulate under the skin of the head and the eyes, where they can be observed easily, even in big fish. If gas bubbles occur between the cornea and the lens of the eye, the eye may swell and protrude, producing the symptom of *exophthalmus* (see also page 214). Fishes suffering from gas embolism generally swim restlessly near the surface of the water and they are very easily frightened. Later on, when the number of gas bubbles increases, they become apathetic and will die in the end if no suitable measures are taken.

Symptoms may vary to some extent in different species of fish. In Carp and Prussian Carp the first indication is given by the formation of vesicles of gas in their fin membrane or by protrusion of the eyeballs, whereas in the Japanese Bitterling (*Rhodeus ocellatus*) the first symptom is appearance of gas blisters on the fins.[13] In Killifish (*Oryzias latipes*) it is distention of the belly owing to accumulation of gas in the swim bladder, the intestine and/or the abdominal cavity, producing considerable buoyancy so as to lift the body of the fish up to the surface. In the Japanese Eel (*Anguilla japonica*) at first several small swellings filled with gas appear on the head. In Killifish, especially fry and youngsters, death results from the laceration of the belly wall, caused by the expansive pressure of the gas accumulated in the swim bladder, intestine and belly cavity, but in other fishes death is generally caused by asphyxiation resulting from gas embolism in the circulatory system.[13] Up to the last moment before death fishes will show full colours. Post-mortem examination may reveal dilation of the heart, accumulation of gas bubbles under the peritoneal covering of the kidneys, in the intestine and in the descending part of the aorta; further, small haemorrhages may be found in the brain, caused by bursting of the smaller capillaries that could not stand the excessive gas pressure.[14] In Carp, external symptoms of gas embolism are rarely observed, but the internal blood vessels are filled with bubbles just as well as in other fishes. Engelhorn supposes that jumping above the water surface sometimes exhibited by Carp on hot summer days may be due to a concealed condition of gas embolism.

Generally, if fishes are likely to suffer from gas embolism, bubbles will settle on the skin, the fins or the gills, where they can easily be seen. In such cases, it is advisable to change the water to avoid distress. Fishes that already show signs of gas embolism should be put direct in fresh water. If great damage has not already been caused they can be restored to normal completely.

If care is taken that the sun is not shining directly into the tank during the hottest part of a summer's day, you need have no fear that gas embolism will occur.

Further, it is important not to use artificial aeration in small bubbles when there are reasons to expect a high oxygen production

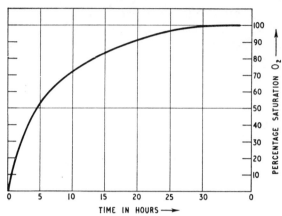

Fig. 3.6. Rate of oxygen saturation of stagnant water from experiments by the author. Water depth was 28 cm, in a cylinder filled with tap-water from which all dissolved gases were previously driven off by boiling. At regular intervals the oxygen content was determined by chemical analysis and the results expressed as percentage saturation. The graph shows that oxygen uptake by stagnant water by pure diffusion from the air above is a very slow process, incapable of coping with oxygen consumption by a good stock of fish

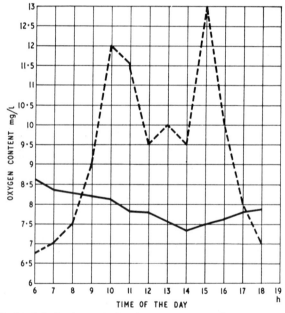

Fig. 3.7. Graph indicating variations in oxygen content of stagnant tropical water. Unbroken line shows normal equilibrium values at 100% saturation; broken line, the amounts of oxygen found (after Buschkiel)

by the plants alone. If you wish to continue artificial aeration, then use it in the form of large bubbles near the surface. The movement, given to the water by this form of aeration, has the effect of increasing the surface area, thus accelerating gas diffusion between the atmosphere and the water so that, if the water should become oversaturated with oxygen, this may escape easily into the air (Figs 3.6–3.8).

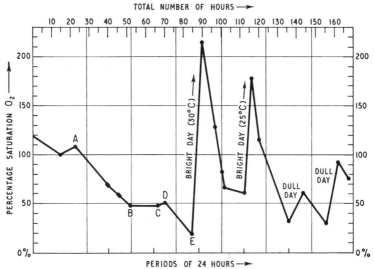

Fig. 3.8. Variations in percentage oxygen saturation in an experimental tank after investigations by the author. The tank contained a sand bottom but no plants or fish at the start. At A two Goldfish were introduced; at B some fresh water added and at D plants were introduced. The graph clearly shows the effect of oxygen production during the day and oxygen consumption by both plants and fish during the night, as well as the effect of light intensity on the efficiency of the process

Thus, if the water is oversaturated with oxygen, artificial aeration decreases the oxygen content, instead of increasing it.[15]

CARBON DIOXIDE POISONING

In water containing only small amounts of carbonates and bicarbonates and having an acid reaction (pH below 7.0), excess carbon dioxide ('carbonic acid') may be formed if there is insufficient photosynthetic activity of plants to remove this substance during the bright hours of day. Actually, some writers have tried to convince us that the symptoms of fish coming gasping to the surface of the water should be due to an excess of carbon dioxide and not to a deficiency of oxygen.[16] This theory has been refuted by the present author, based on specific experiments.[17]

The symptoms of carbon dioxide poisoning in fish are quite different from those of lack of oxygen whilst, if both conditions exist at the same time, symptoms of carbon dioxide intoxication are prevalent over those of lack of oxygen.

In carbon dioxide poisoning, at first the fish show signs of distress, namely equilibrium disturbance and slowing up of movement. This is followed by symptoms of numbness, tumbling and decreased breathing frequency, whilst lack of oxygen causes increased breathing frequency. They never show any tendency to come to the surface. A similar description of symptoms was already given by Steinmann as early as 1927.[18]

In an experiment with a Goldfish showing symptoms of lack of oxygen, staying at the surface and snapping air, pure carbon dioxide was bubbled through the water. Then the symptoms of lack of oxygen gradually vanished, symptoms of carbon dioxide poisoning occurring instead. The fish left the surface and breathing frequency gradually decreased, whilst after some time the same symptoms showed as described above. Finally the fish developed some kind of asphyxiation, breathing stopped almost completely and the fish hung in the water in an elevated position, the slope of the longitudinal axis of the body being about 45°. The head was held at the higher level but before this stage was reached the fish sometimes tumbled in a vertical position with its head down. However, the fish recovered completely after having been placed into fresh water, where normal breathing was restored immediately.

Such severe cases of carbon dioxide poisoning are not very likely to occur in aquaria, since it requires rather high amounts of that gas. In my experiments, concentrations of 430 and 558 mg/l were found to produce these severe symptoms in Goldfish. It might be expected, however, that in more susceptible species of fish extreme intoxication effects could be produced at much lower concentration. If any of the symptoms described should be observed in a tank, it would be wise to make a quick change of water.

Although the absolute solubility of carbon dioxide in pure (distilled) water is much greater than that of oxygen (at equal pressure) the concentration which will be in equilibrium with the atmosphere is much lower, owing to the very small amount of carbon dioxide present in the air. The normal carbon dioxide content of the air is about 0.03% by volume, and its partial pressure is 0.0003 atm. Solubility at 20°C (68°F) is only 0.77 mg/l. This figure is of little importance in fish-keeping, however, since the solubility of carbon dioxide is greatly increased by the presence of calcium bicarbonate in the water. If the water contains 297 mg/l of calcium bicarbonate the solubility of carbon dioxide is increased to 1.3 mg/l whilst, with an amount of bicarbonate four times greater (1188 mg/l), the normal solubility of carbon dioxide is increased super-proportionally to 63.6 mg/l. Consequently, it is not the partial pressure of carbon dioxide in the air that is the primary factor in solubility, as it is with oxygen, but the bicarbonate (and normal carbonate) content of the water.

There is a constant equilibrium according to the chemical equation:

$$CaCO_3 + CO_2 + H_2O \rightleftharpoons Ca(HCO_3)_2$$
(calcium carbonate) (carbon dioxide) (water) (calcium bicarbonate)

If carbon dioxide is removed from the water (e.g. by the action of plants) until the concentration falls below the equilibrium value, a certain amount of bicarbonate will be decomposed into carbonate and free carbon dioxide until a new equilibrium is reached. If more carbon dioxide is introduced into the water, normal carbonate is converted into bicarbonate. These conversions also affect the pH value of the water, since pH in natural water depends directly on the ratio of free carbon dioxide to bicarbonate. So true is this, in fact, that over the ordinary range of concentrations we can calculate the pH value from these concentrations.

An increased amount of free carbon dioxide will lower the pH, whilst decreasing the concentration of free carbon dioxide will increase the pH value. Increased carbon dioxide production in a crowded and fully planted tank during the night may even lower the pH to a critical value of 5.0, whilst a high photosynthetic activity of plants in a tank with low bicarbonate content may sometimes increase the pH value to 8.5 and even higher. pH values of 9–11 are dangerous to fish (higher values than 11 never occur in natural conditions; they could appear by introducing alkaline chemicals).

At extreme pH values the gills are the first organs that are affected. Characteristic symptoms are a brownish or red discoloration of the gill sheets, extensive slime secretion, corroding and fibrillar necrosis. The latter two symptoms are especially characteristic in case of very high pH values ('*alkali disease*').

Lethal pH values for some species of fish are:[19]

Species	Acid limit pH	Aklaline limit pH
Perch	4.0	9.2
Trout	4.8	9.2
Roach	—	10.4
Pike	4.9	10.7
Tench	4.9	10.8
Carp	5.0	10.8
Stickleback	5.6	11.0

Plants use free carbon dioxide in photosynthesis (1.375 mg for every milligram of oxygen produced), but if the available amount is consumed, they will draw CO_2 from the bicarbonates. The resulting calcium carbonate, which is only slightly soluble, will often precipitate on the leaves of the plants, thus encrusting them. In natural conditions we see this very often on *Potamogeton crispus*.

If only small quantities of bicarbonates are present, so that even these are insufficient for the photosynthetic activity of plants on bright days, further CO_2 is taken from the normal carbonate, according to the equation:

$$CaCO_3 \quad + \quad H_2O \rightleftharpoons \quad Ca(OH)_2 \quad + \quad CO_2$$
(calcium carbonate)   (water)   (calcium hydroxide)   (carbon dioxide)

Calcium hydroxide is a strongly alkaline substance and this causes a considerable rise in pH, even when it is produced in very small quantities. A remedy can be effected by adding sufficient calcium bicarbonate and, if necessary, a few drops of diluted phosphoric acid, to restore the pH to a value of 7.2–7.4 for European fishes, or 6.8–7.2 for tropicals. In cases where the pH falls too low, owing to increased free carbon dioxide content, this can be remedied by adding normal calcium carbonate.

The equilibrium values of free carbon dioxide in ordinary conditions over the pH range of 6.9–8.22 vary from 147–1.3 mg/l. Obviously the risk of exceedingly high CO_2 concentrations is much greater when the initial pH is kept low.

DIETARY GILL DISEASE

An affliction in which the gill sheets appear soft and swollen in absence of gross parasites or specific micro-organisms is probably due to a lack of pantothenic acid (vitamin B_5). The easiest remedy is to supply the vitamin by feeding chopped *raw* liver (the vitamin is destroyed by heat). Occasionally, *Myxobacteria* of the Genus *Cytophaga* are found, but these are only secondary invaders.

PARASITIC DISEASES OF THE GILLS

PARASITIC COPEPODA

There are a great number of species of parasitic *Copepoda* (*Siphonostomata* or *Parasitica*) that may attack the gills of fishes (Fig. 3.9). They are all related to the anchor worm (*Lernæa*) which attacks the skin (see page 14). The most common of these parasites is *Ergasilus sieboldi*, reaching a length (without the egg sacs) of 1.7 mm in the female, and the related species *E. gibbus* with a length of 1.5–2 mm. *E. sieboldi* is characterised by the presence of an intense blue pigment, which is showing when it is observed from the back. These parasites show a remarkable resemblance to the well-known cyclops, an organism that is extremely useful as a fish food. *Ergasilus* has two large hooks that are driven into the gill sheets, but, since it is necessary that the gills should be of a reasonable size to allow the parasite to take hold, it is only found on fishes of about 2 in or more in length. For this reason the parasites will not often be found in aquarium fish. The females of the parasite produce egg sacs (approx. 1 mm long) in March and these disappear in October. From the eggs nauplius larvae hatch, up to 200 from one female, and these

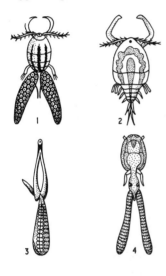
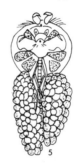

Fig. 3.9. Five parasitic Copepoda *known to attack the gills of fishes:* 1, Ergasilus sieboldi *(after Nordmann).* 2, Ergasilus trisetaceus *(after Nordmann).* 3, Tricheliastes maculatus *(after Kollar).* 4, Caligus lacustris *(after Lütken).* 5, Thersitina gasterostei *(after Thurbay)*

may be introduced into a pond or aquarium with live food. The eggs can only develop if the water temperature exceeds 14°C (57.2°F).

The incidence of infection with *Ergasilus* decreases with increasing mobility of the fish, so it is often found in Tench and Pike in natural waters, much less in Bream and Silver Bream and only occasionally in Carp.

On the gills of Sticklebacks *Thersitina gasterostei* may be found. The head of the ripe females appears heavily swollen and is much greater in size than the true thoracical part of the cephalothorax (as the region of the body formed by the fusion of the head and the thorax is called) and the abdomen. Seen from above the thorax is completely concealed. The parasite reaches a length of 0.8 mm.

The illustrations in Fig. 3.9 show some other species of parasitic *Copepoda*, that are found on the gills of fishes. If they are removed soon after their attack, fishes will recover completely but, if they have already done so much damage that a secondary fungus infection has occurred, the prospects of a cure are not so good.

For treatment of infected fishes potassium permanganate 1 : 10 000 (0.1 g/l) for 5–10 min only, or formalin 1 : 4000 for 1 h have been recommended. These are drastic treatments that should be applied with caution (see last chapter). The same holds true for treatments with DDT 1–2 : 100 000 000 or with lindane (same strength) for some days. If only a few parasites are present, it is recommended that they are touched with a pencil or brush dipped in a 1 : 1000 potassium permanganate solution and then removed mechanically by means of forceps. Formalin is ineffective against *Lernæa* and other *Copepoda*.

GILL FLUKES

These are closely related to skin flukes (*Gyrodactylus*) and will often appear together with them on the same fish. They are unsegmented flatworms of the Phylum *Platyhelminthes* and belong to the Class *Trematoda*, the Order *Monogenea* and the Super-Family *Gyrodactyloidea*. Skin flukes belong to the Family *Gyrodactylidæ*, members of which are viviparous, whereas most of the gill flukes belong to the Family *Dactylogyridæ* and produce eggs with *Dactylogyrus crassus* Kulwiéc

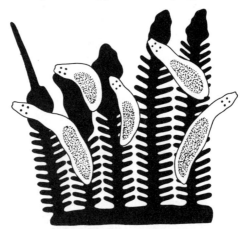

Fig. 3.10. Five specimens of Dactylogyrus *at the gill sheets. The pointed extension of the sheet at the extreme left is an abnormal tissue induced by the permeation (after Amlacher)*

as the only exception; this species has been described to be a live-bearing one just like *Gyrodactylus* (it has been found on Prussian Carp). The taxonomy of these organisms has been dealt with extensively by Dawes and by Bychovsky.[20]
There are many varieties of gill flukes to be found on fish, the more well known belonging to the Genus *Dactylogyrus* (Fig. 3.10).

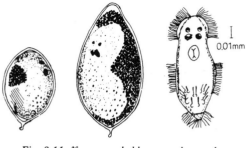 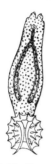

Fig. 3.11. *Younger and older egg and young larva of* Dactylogyrus vastator *Nybelin (after Bychovsky)*

Fig. 3.12. Dactylogyrus auriculatus *Diesing (after Roth)*

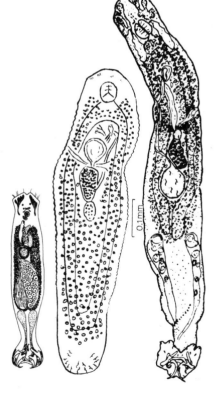

Fig. 3.13. *Gill flukes.* From left to right: Cichlidogyrus tilapiæ *Paperna (after Paperna)* ; Acolpenteron nephriticum *Gvosdev (after Bychovsky)* ; Ancyrocephalus balisticus *Hargis (after Hargis)*

They possess two pairs of head organs and have eyes, which skin flukes (*Gyrodactylus*) have not. The attachment organ has two strong and 14 small hooks (in *Gyrodactylus* there are 16). The pair of large hooks is supported by one clamp.

Some of the more important members of the Genus are: *Dactylogyrus vastator* Nybelin (Fig. 3.14), reaching a length of 1 mm. This is a typical parasite of young Carp and Prussian Carp up to 6–7 cm, causing epidemics among them in summer. *D. anchoratus* Dujardin, up to 0.6 mm, in Carp, Prussian Carp, Roach and Goldfish; *D. auriculatus* (Nordmann) (Fig. 3.12) and *D. wunderi* Bych, in Bream and aquarium fishes; *D. minutus* Kulwiéc, up to 0.5 mm,

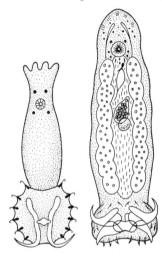

Fig. 3.14. Left: Dactylogyrus vastator *Nybelin (after Amlacher)*. Right: Tetraonchus (Monocœlium) monenteron *Wagener (after Reichenbach-Klinke)*

mainly in autumn on larger Carps; *D. macracanthus* Wegener, 1 × 0.2 mm, in Tench. In Germany 39 species of *Dactylogyrus* have been found.[21]

The Genus *Neodactylogyrus* is closely related, but the two large hooks are supported by two clamps, that may or may not be similar. Forty-five different species of this Genus are known, *N. megastoma* being one of them. Formerly, species of this Genus have been included in the Genus *Dactylogyrus*.

On the gills of *Cichlidæ*, especially of the Genera *Tilapia* and *Haplochromis*, heavy infestations with a different type of fluke, incorporated in the new Genus *Cichlidogyrus*, have been described by Paperna.[22]

Among the other related Genera are *Acolpenteron*, *Pseudocolpenteron*, *Bradactylogyrus*, *Dogiclus* and *Falciunguis* (see Fig. 3.13).

The Genus *Ancyrocephalus* (of the Sub-Family *Ancyrocephalinæ*), with two species, is characterised by the front of the body having three pairs of conical projections (head organs). The attachment organ has two pairs of large hooks supported by two large clamps, while the number of small hooks is the same as in *Gyrodactylus*, namely, 16. *Ancyrocephalus paradoxus* (Creplin) has been found on the gills of Perch (*Perca fluviatilis*) and Pike-Perch (*Lucioperca sandra*); *A. cruciatus* (Wedl.) on Weather Fish (*Misgurnus fossilis*).

Members of the Genus *Tetraonchus* (formerly placed in the Family *Dactylogyridæ*, now in a separate Family, *Tetraonchidæ*) possess two pairs or more conical projections at the front of the body. The attachment organ carries four large hooks supported by one clamp, and it has 16 small hooklets. *Tetraonchus unguiculatus* has been found on the gills of Perch and Pike-Perch; *T. monenteron* Wagener (Fig. 3.14) on the gills of Pike (*Esox lucius*), Angel Fish (*Pterophyllum*), Glass Fish (*Ambassis* or *Chanda lala*) and Puffer Fish (*Tetrodon fluviatilis*); and *T. cruciatus* on the gills of the Weather Fish (*Misgurnus (Cobitis) fossilis*).

Symptoms caused by gill flukes are increased breathing frequency, whilst the gill coverings are stretched open widely, the gills being expanded and very pale. Parts of the gills often become protuberant and show as a small pale fleece outside the covering. Parts of the gill sheets on which flukes have settled are covered with a cloudy film, consisting of slime and destroyed epithelial cells.

Apart from the exceptional *D. crassus*, gill flukes are not livebearing, as are skin flukes, but they produce eggs, which are deposited on the gills of the fish. These eggs have a higher resistance to chemicals than the adult parasites so that one treatment of the diseased fish is generally insufficient to obtain a complete cure. *Dactylogyrus* is an obligatory parasite and will not stand removal from the gills of a fish for more than a few hours. If fishes are removed from an infected tank for one day, the tank is safe again, provided that the temperature of the water is well above 15°C, otherwise the parasites may have produced highly resistant eggs, that will hatch after $2\frac{1}{2}$ days if the temperature rises to 23°C. However, the hatched youngsters of *D. vastator* can only live for 8–10 h without finding a host, whereas this period is 4–5 h in *D. macracanthus* Wegener. Development of the young parasites after hatching into the adult stage and dying after egg-production, takes 10–12 days in *D. vastator. D. macracanthus* produces eggs during the whole year; the eggs hatch after about 4 days and the youngsters grow into the adult stage in about $4\frac{1}{2}$ weeks at 13–14°C after having contacted a suitable host.

Overwintering of eggs of *Dactylogyrus* in a viable state at the bottom of ponds without water should be considered impossible,[23] although some eggs may survive in ponds filled with water in winter.

Eggs deposited by adult *Dactylogyrus* on the gills do not stay there, but fall off and settle at the bottom, which facilitates rapid spread of an infection to a large number of fish.

Young fry cannot be infected during the first days after hatching, because the gills are not yet fully developed, but in Carp the gills may become fully infected after about 13 days.[23]

There is also a relationship between the oxygen content of the water and the activity of these parasites.[24] When the oxygen content of the water decreases, *Dactylogyrus* parasites on the gills relocate themselves and then their egg-laying activity increases. If the oxygen content of the water increases again, the parasites change over again to their original positions.

TREATMENT OF GILL FLUKES

The same chemicals that have been recommended for treatment of fishes attacked by skin flukes may be used against gill flukes (see page 28). Treatments that may be used as a permanent bath are to be preferred, however, since the eggs are not destroyed in any treatment of short duration, thus necessitating several repetitions of such treatments at intervals of one or two days.

The formaldehyde treatment as advocated by Ian M. Rankin has proved to be highly effective against gill flukes as well as for curing fish infected by skin flukes. In my opinion, this is one of the best cures available at the present time.

Potassium antimonyl tartrate (Tartar Emetic) as described on page 342 may also constitute a good cure.

Good results have also been obtained by a combined treatment with ammonia and methylene blue. The diseased fishes are first given a treatment with a 1 : 2000 solution of ammonia for 15 min and then put in a tank containing 2–4 cm^3 of 1% stock solution of methylene blue per Imp. gal. Methylene blue will attack the adult parasites and the young hatching from the eggs, while it also has a palliative effect upon the breathing difficulties of the fish. Exact details for preparing the solution have been given previously (see pages 45 and 334–335).

Neguvon (Bayer) has been found highly effective for treatment of gill flukes by Bailösoff. Fishes are bathed for 2–3 min in a 2–3.5% solution, which kills *Dactylogyrus vastator* almost immediately and *Dactylogyrus anchoratus* (Dujardin) within 30 sec. See further page 336.

In very bad cases, a combined treatment with salicylic acid and methylene blue has been used with good results, but this should not be applied to the more delicate species of fish, since it is a rather drastic method. Salicylic acid should not be used unless other methods have failed. A bath is made up by dissolving 0.9–1 gr in 1 Imp. gal of water (0.75–0.85 gr/U.S. gal). The fishes may remain in this bath for a period not exceeding half an hour. During this time they should be watched carefully and if they show any sign of distress they must be removed from the bath immediately and put into clean, fresh water. One day later, methylene blue should be added as an after-treatment. Since fishes affected by gill flukes have a much greater need for oxygen than normal, owing to the decrease of gill capacity, it is advisable to aerate the water adequately by means of an air pump.

A further but risky treatment which has been suggested consists of dipping the diseased fish in a 0.2% solution of acetic acid for $2\frac{1}{2}$ min only, as a maximum. The acid coagulates the mucus of the gills and the skin and, with it, the worms. Nevertheless, only the adult parasites are destroyed, so that several repetitions are required to obtain a cure. The fish will develop a white colour as a result of the damage done to the mucous coat of its skin, which will gradually disappear after some time if no secondary infections should occur in the meantime, when the fish is susceptible to bacterial and fungal attack. In view of what happens I am opposed to its use.

TWIN WORMS (DIPLOZOON)

These parasites are also members of the *Trematoda* or sucking worm Class. The best-known species, *Diplozoon paradoxum* (Figs 3.15, 3.16), has a size of 4–5 mm (occasionally up to 11 mm) and thus it can easily be seen with the naked eye, although a magnifying glass is helpful. The animal has a typically X-shaped body with two heads and two hind parts. It settles between the gill sheets and, although it does little harm, its presence does hinder breathing.

The life history of *Diplozoon paradoxum*, or twin worm, is very remarkable. The adult parasites produce eggs which have a size of

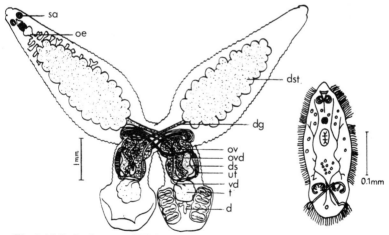

Fig. 3.15. Left: *Anatomy of* Diplozoon paradoxum *v. Nordmann.* sa, *sucking disc;* oe, *œsophagus;* dst, *yolk gland;* dg, *yolk tube;* ov, *ovary;* ovd, *oviduct;* ds, *yolk sac;* ut, *uterus;* vd, *vas deferens;* t, *testis;* d, *intestine (after von Nordmann).* Right: *Swimming larval stage (after Bychovsky). Both taken from Reichenbach-Klinke (1966)*

0.1–0.2 mm and which are provided with a long thread by means of which they are fastened to the gills of the fish. From these eggs the larvae hatch and maturate while swimming freely through the water until they find a fish. Then every two sexually ripened, but not yet adult, youngsters, which are called diporpa, combine with each other. About half-way along the body, each larva has a sucking

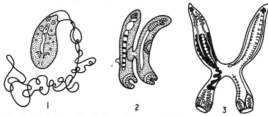

Fig. 3.16. Life cycle of the twin worm Diplozoon paradoxum *;*
1, *ovum (after Roth).* 2, *two larvae (diporpa) uniting to form a*
Diplozoon *(after Roth).* 3, Diplozoon paradoxum *after*
fusion of the two diporpa (after Nordmann)

disc and on the opposite side, a projection. Each larva puts its projection into the opening of the sucker of the other and in this way they grow into 'Siamese twins', which it is impossible to separate. Diporpa that can find no partner with which to combine die. At the time when combination to form a complete *Diplozoon* takes place, the diporpa have the size of 1.2 mm. The diporpa are hermaphroditic

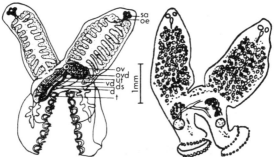

Fig. 3.17. Twin worms. Left: Diplozoon barbi *Reichen-*
bach-Klinke (after Reichenbach-Klinke). sa, *sucking disc;*
oe, *œsophagus;* ov, *ovary;* ovd, *oviduct;* ut, *uterus;* vd, *vas*
deferens; ds, *yolk sac;* d, *intestine;* t, *testis.* Right: Neodiplozoon barbi *(Tripathi) (after Tripathi)*

(male and female at the same time); after having united they mutually fertilise each other, having become one flesh in the most literal sense and not separable as long as they live.

Twin worms have been found on the gills of several species of fish, such as Eelpout (*Lota vulgaris*), Prussian Carp (*Carassius carassius*), Orfe (*Leuciscus idus*), Minnow (*Phoxinus phoxinus*), Bitterling (*Rhodeus amarus*), Bream, (*Abramis brama*), Rudd (*Scardinius erythrophthalmus*), Roach (*Rutilus rutilus*), Gudgeon (*Gobio gobio*), Miller's Thumb (*Cottus gobio*) and a few other species.

A new species, *Diplozoon barbi*, was discovered by Reichenbach-Klinke in 1951[25] on a golden variety of *Barbus semifasciolatus* that had been imported in Germany from the United States, but originally occurring in Eastern Asia. *D. barbi* causes the appearance of small grey pustules on the gills. Although it is much smaller than *D. paradoxum*, namely one millimetre only, it is more dangerous and may kill the fish. The diporpa of *D. barbi* combine with each other at the flat central side without 'crossing over' as in the other species. The adult specimens appear oval shaped at the anterior end, whereas the posterior part is much more elongated than in *D. paradoxum* and possesses eight suckers at the dorsal side.

A number of other species have been described, too. In the Genus *Neodiplozoon* a series of attachment hooks is present instead of four paired ones as in *Diplozoon* (Fig. 3.17).

Special treatments to remove twin worms are not known at the present time, but perhaps this is only because the parasite is not often met with in aquaria. Deducing from experiences with other worms, I should think that one or other of the following treatments would be successful: picric acid, methylene blue or the formaldehyde treatment recommended by Rankin (see pages 30–31, 34).

OX-HEAD WORM (BUCEPHALUS)

This is another sucking worm (Fig. 3.18) which may be found on the gills of fish. The name is given because of the typical shape of the larval form (metacercaria stage). The adult parasite is found in the intestine of Eel (*Anguilla anguilla*), Eelpout (*Lota vulgaris*), Perch (*Perca fluviatilis*), Pike-Perch (*Lucioperca sandra*), and Pike (*Esox*

Fig. 3.18. Right: *Drawing of* Bucephalus polymorphus, *showing the main anatomical features of the adult sucking worm (after Roth)*

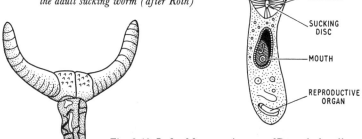

Fig. 3.19. Left: *Metacercaria stage of* Bucephalus dimorphus *(after Roth). The shape of this larval form gives the creature its appropriate common name*

lucius). The first larval stages (cercaria) develop in fresh-water mussels (*Unio* and *Anodonta*) and the typical ox-head shaped metacercariae (Fig. 3.19) parasitise on the gills, and occasionally on the skin, of the Cyprinid fish. These worms do not cause much harm and can easily be removed by giving the fish treatment with a $1-1\frac{1}{2}\%$ salt solution in which it should remain for 15–30 min. A bath of picric acid, 2–7 : 100 000 may alternatively be used.

PROTOZOAN PARASITES

Several other kinds of parasite may be found on the gills. Some of these, such as *Costia necatrix, Chilodonella cyprini* and others, have been dealt with previously, since these are mainly parasites of the skin and appear only occasionally on the gills.

Whereas *Cyclochæta domerguei* is a typical parasite of the skin and generally not found on the gills, a number of related organisms of the Family *Urceolariidæ* are obligatory parasites of the gills. They differ from other species by a shortened adoral spiral ($\frac{1}{2}-\frac{3}{4}$ of one turn), a different shape of elements of the adhesive disc and generally a smaller size. Lom[26] lists the following species:

Trichodinella epizootica, on gills of Perch, Pike-Perch, Ruff, Pike, Burbot, Trout (*Salmo fario*), Barbel (*Barbus barbus*) and a Bitterling

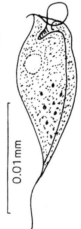

Fig. 3.20. Bodomonas rebæ   *Tripathi   (after Tripathi)*

0.01 mm

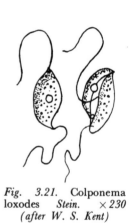

Fig. 3.21. Colponema loxodes   *Stein.*   × 230 (after W. S. Kent)

(*Rhodeus sericeus*); *Foliella subtilis*, on gills of Carp, Prussian Carp, Tench, Silver Bream and Bitterling; *Tripartiella copiosa*, on gills of Bleak, Silver Bream, Roach, Dace, Chub, Bitterling, *Leucaspius delineatus*, and the Spiny Loach (*Cobitis tænia*); *Tripartiella lata*, on the gills of Minnow; *Paratrichodina incissa*, on the gills of Stone Loach (*Cobitis barbatula*), Minnow, Roach, Rudd and Gudgeon.

On the gills of fishes in India, belonging to the Genera *Labeo* and *Cirrhina*, the parasite *Bodomonas rebæ* Tripathi (Fig. 3.20) has been observed, and on fishes in the U.S.A. its relative *B. concava* Davis. They belong to the Class *Mastigophora*, Sub-class *Zoomastigina* and thus are relatives of *Costia*. Size 15–18 µm. They attach themselves to the epithelium by means of the posterior flagellum. The related species *Colponema loxodes* Stein (Fig. 3.21) has been found on *Ictalurus punctatus*. These infections may be treated successfully with pyridyl-mercuric-acetate (P.M.A.), 2 mg/l, or acriflavin (4 mg/l).[27]

SUCTORIAN PARASITES

The Class of the *Protozoa* called *Suctoria* or 'sucking infusorians' consists of organisms that are mainly characterised for their attacking ciliated infusorians, which they suck out by means of hollow tentacles (Fig. 3.22). In recent years a number of species have been detected

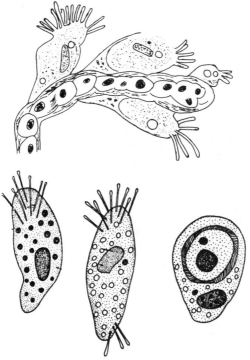

Fig. 3.22. Suctorian fish parasites. Upper: Trichophrya micropteri *Davis (after Davis).* Lower: Trichophrya intermedia *Prost (after Bychovsky). Both taken from Reichenbach-Klinke (1966)*

as parasites on the gills of fishes: *Trichophrya micropteri* Davis, on *Micropterus dolomieu* Lac.; *T. ictaluri* Davis, on *Ictalurus* species; *T. intermedia* Prost, on *Coregonus albula*; *C. wartmanni* and other *Salmonidæ* in Poland and Germany; *T. sinensis* Chen, on Amur Carp.

Infected fishes can be cured by formalin treatment during 1 h, according to Reichenbach-Klinke. It should be used in the same way as prescribed for treatment of *Costiasis* (page 75); duration of treatment to be prolonged to 1 h, if necessary, and provided that the fishes do not show effects of intoxication.

SPOROZOAN PARASITES

Sporozoans that infect the gills form small cysts which can be seen as little knots on the gill sheets, mostly in the respiratory folds. The size of such cysts may vary considerably, from microscopical dimensions to $2\frac{1}{2}$ mm. If there are only a few cysts the fish will not suffer much but, should their number increase, respiration will be hindered due to pressure on the blood vessels. Death may then occur with all the symptoms of suffocation. There are no known methods for healing fishes that are infected by sporozoans but, fortunately, these parasites do not often appear in tanks.

It would be worth while to try a treatment with mepacrine hydrochloride (atebrine), which is known to be very effective against

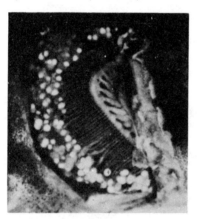

Fig. 3.23. Gills of a Tench, after removal of gill coverings (opercula), showing a number of Thélohanullus (Myxobolus) pyriformis *cysts (after Schäperclaus)*

sporozoan infections in human beings. This drug should be used in a concentration up to 300 mg per 100 l (0.2 gr/Imp. gal or 1.65 gr/U.S. gal), to be added in two or three parts at intervals of 48 h. Treatment should not be continued for more than 10 days. Compare also with page 333 and Chapter 4, pages 145–147.

The most important species of the *Sporozoa* parasites on the gills of fish are the following: *Myxosoma (Lentospora) dujardini* in Rudd and Roach: *Myxobolus pyriformis* in Tench (Fig. 3.23) and Weather-fish; *Myxobolus ellipsoideus* in Tench; *Myxobolus dispar* in Carp; *Myxobolus exiguus* in Bream; *Myxobolus mülleri* in Chub (*Squalius cephalus*) and other fresh-water fish; *Myxobolus anurus* in Pike; *Henneguya psorospermica* varieties in Pike and Perch, producing white cysts of up to 2 mm; *Henneguya lobosa*, producing oval cysts of 2.8 mm at the ends of the gill sheets of Pike; *H. minuta*, producing cysts of 0.15 mm in the gills of Perch; *H. creplini* Gurley [*H. acerinæ* Schröder], producing oblong white cysts of up to 1.1 mm in the gills of Ruff (*Acerina cernua*), *Dermocystidium branchialis* on the gills of Brook Trout (*Salmo fario*) and *D. vejdovskyi* on the gills of Pike (*Esox lucius*). For a further description, see Chapter 4.

UNICELLULAR ALGAE

A number of unicellular algae live as parasites. From this group the following parasites of fishes (Fig. 3.24) are known:
Mucophilus cyprini—Size 60–70 µm, mainly found on the gills, but also on the skin (see page 62).

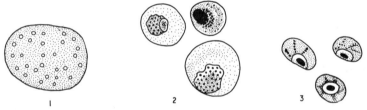

Fig. 3.24. Parasites of the Chytridiaceæ *Group which attack fish include:* 1, Mucophilus cyprini. 2, Oodinium ocellatum *(confined to salt-water fishes)*; *and* 3, Ichthyochytrium vulgare. *Nos. 1 and 3 attack both skin and gills. Drawn after appearance in stained smear preparations. Also see Fig. 2.36, page 60*

A case of sudden death of 30 Sword Tails (*Xiphophorus helleri*) and Kissing Gouramis (*Helostoma temmincki*), in which the gill sheets were completely cemented together by algal cells, was observed by Hofman, Bishop and Dunbar.[28] The algal cells closely resembled those of *Mucophilus cyprini*.
Ichthyochytrium vulgare—Size 5–20 µm. This parasite has a yellowish colour and contains many grains with a high refractive index. A few specimens on a fish will not do much harm. *Ichthyochytrium* attacks both the skin and gills (see Fig. 3.25).
Chlorochytrium piscicolens—Size 9–120 µm. Causes inflammation and cyst formation in the skin and the gills. Infected fishes show poor growth and emaciation (also see page 63).
Oodinium ocellatum Brown [*Branchiophilus maris* Schäperclaus]—Size 20–70 µm, nearly sphere-shaped and not transparent, when

living. The organism is surrounded by a membrane. The protoplasm seems to consist of a number of single drops when the organism is observed alive. In mounted slides it appears granulated giving a honeycomb effect. This parasite is only observed in sea-water aquaria,

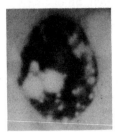

Fig. 3.25. Stained slide showing an Ichthyochytrium vulgare *parasite (× 2500)*

mainly on Coral Fishes. It has caused great epidemics among these species, with resultant large losses. The parasite forms oval cysts, about 0.3 mm in size. It is mainly a parasite of the skin.

A more detailed description of these parasitic unicellular algae and treatments against them have been given on pages 60–64.

HIGHER ALGAE

Schäperclaus has reported casualties in Trout that were due to penetration of blue-green algae (*Oscillatoriaceæ*) into the epithelium of the skin and the gills. Also see pages 301–302.

In a case of perforation of the operculum in Carp he found some threads of a common green alga of the Genus *Cladophora* and a larger amount of algae, probably of the species *Gommontia perforans* Acton.

FUNGUS INFECTIONS

Ordinary fungus (moulds of the Family *Saprolegniaceæ*) may attack the gills of fishes that have been weakened by lack of oxygen or that have been damaged by other parasites or by mechanical means or by corrosive chemicals. Treatment is the same as for fungus of the skin, but it is not advisable to treat the fungus by touching it with strong solutions of chemicals, as may be done in the case of an infection of the skin, since the gills are very delicate organs and could be affected by those chemicals. The remedy might be more harmful than the disease itself. Treatment consisting of bathing the fish in a solution of a suitable medicament is advisable.

For this purpose, the phenoxethol treatment, after Rankin as described on page 85, is recommended. As an alternative, potassium dichromate 1:25000–1:20000 may be used (see page 84), but this takes more time to clear the condition. It is important to keep the water clean and well aerated. Where other parasites are present, a phenoxethol treatment should be given first to eradicate the fungus and immediately afterwards a specific treatment for the primary infection must be employed.

GILL ROT

This is a dangerous disease caused by some of the lower *Fungi*, belonging to the Class *Phycomycetes*, Sub-class *Archimycetes*. The causative species are *Branchiomyces sanguinis* Plehn and *Branchiomyces demigrans* Wundsch. The former has been observed thus far in Carp (*Cyprinus carpio*), Tench (*Tinca tinca*), *Carassius carassius gibelio*, Stickle-backs and White Fish (*Coregonidæ*), while the latter has been found in Tench and Pike (*Esox lucius*). They may kill fish rather rapidly.

Both parasites produce branched hyphae 9–15 μm wide. They grow into the veins of the gill sheets where they cause stasis (complete stoppage of the circulation of the blood through the capillaries and smallest blood vessels in the part affected). Large areas of the gills

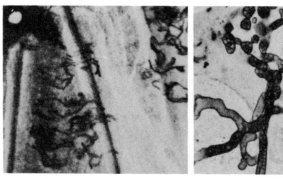

Fig. 3.26.
FUNGUS SPECIES CAUSING GILL ROT
The organisms which cause gill rot. Left: Branchiomyces sanguinis *in section of a gill sheet. A spore is shown in the top-left corner.* Right: Branchiomyces demigrans *in a part of a gill sheet (after photomicrographs by Schäperclaus)*

are cut off from the main bloodstream in this way. The gills become spotted; at some places they are devoid of blood, while elsewhere it is present in excess.

The places that are devoid of blood are liable to necrosis. They will decay and parts fall off. The affected fish dies from suffocation. The course of the disease is very rapid. When symptoms are first recognised it may already be too late to save the victims.

Diagnosis is easier with *Branchiomyces demigrans* infections than with *B. sanguinis*, since the former does not grow in the blood vessels only, but also produces hyphae extending to the outside at the surface of the gills, while the latter is confined to the blood vessels only. Both species produce a syncytium, i.e. a multinucleate complex without distinguishable cell walls; such structure may arise either from division without production of new cell walls or from concrescence of cells. In *Branchiomyces sanguinis* (Fig. 3.26) the tubes of the syncytium have a width of 8–30 μm, whereas in *B. demigrans* the ends of the syncytium reach a breadth of 22–28 μm, being much thicker than the ordinary hyphae (generally 13–14 μm). From the syncytia the spores are produced. These are globular in shape and have a size of 5–9 μm in *Branchiomyces sanguinis* and of 12–17 μm in *B. demigrans*.

In Rainbow Trout, gill rot may be caused by ordinary *Saprolegniaceæ*, according to investigations by Reichenbach-Klinke.

The occurrence of gill rot is furthered by high temperatures and the presence of much decaying organic matter in the water. Thus the infection is mainly confined to the summer months, especially following extremely hot days. The disease has not yet been observed in aquarium fish, which might be due to its rapid course only, symptoms passing by unnoticed before the victims die.

According to recent experience the disease may be eradicated by adding 1–2 g of copper sulphate per m^3 (1000 litres = 35.3 ft^3) of water, or for ponds even up to 8–10 g/m^3.[29] It must be emphasised, however, that copper treatments are very hazardous to fish, the lowest of these concentrations already being lethal to large trout in a few hours. See page 56.

INFLAMMATION OF THE GILLS

In this condition, the gills are enlarged and unusually red. The normal structure of the gills is destroyed to a large extent, the greater part of the gill sheets consisting of a great mass of inflammation cells. The disease may spread into other organs as well, such as those of the digestive tract. Thyroiditis may also occur as a complication.

The disease is contagious, so it is advisable to remove affected fish from the community tank. The condition is not very likely to occur in well-balanced tanks. It may show as a secondary complaint to other infections. The exact cause is not known, but from its contagious character it is most likely to be caused by bacterial or virus infections. Under favourable conditions, the disease may heal spontaneously.

In young *Salmonidæ* similar symptoms, with swelling of the gill sheets prevailing, have been thought to be due to an infection with slime bacteria of the Genus *Myxobacterium*, that could be combated with pyridyl mercuric acetate (2 mg/l; 1 h) or Lignasan X (1–2 mg/l) (these two are highly toxic to Rainbow Trout) or benzalkonium chloride (see p. 320).

The disease of young *Salmonidæ* is apparently not contagious; therefore some investigators doubt its bacterial origin and think it may be attributed to a lack of pantothenic acid (a vitamin).[30]

REFERENCES

1 HOFER, B., *Handbuch der Fischkrankheiten*, Munich (1904)
2 SCHÄPERCLAUS, W., *Lehrbuch der Teichwirtschaft*, Berlin (1933) and *Fischkrankheiten*, 3rd ed., Berlin (1954)
3 FINK, E., *Wochenschrift für Aquarien- und Terrarienkunde*, 55 (1934)
4 SMOLIAN, K., *Merkbuch der Binnenfischerei*, Berlin (1920)
5 FRY, F. E., 'The aquatic respiration of fish', in BROWN, M. E. (Ed.): *Physiology of Fishes*, Vol. I, Academic Press, New York (1957)
6 LEINER, M., *Die Physiologie der Fischatmung*, Leipzig (1938) (data compiled from other sources)
7 After SCHÄPERCLAUS, W., *Fischkrankheiten*, 3rd ed., Berlin (1954)
8 After SCHÄPERCLAUS, W. (1954), *loc. cit.*
9 LINDROTH, A., 'Zur Biologie der Befruchtung und Entwicklung beim Hecht', *Comm. Inst. Inland Fisheries at Drottningholm*, Stockholm, Sweden, No. 24 (1946)
10 SCHÄPERCLAUS, W., *Fischkrankheiten*, Braunschweig (1935)
11 MANNING, W. M., JUDAY, C. and WOLF, M., 'Photosynthesis of aquatic plants at different depths in Trout Lake Wisconsin', *Trans. Wis. Acad. Sci. Arts & Lett.* **31**, 377–410 (1938)
12 RABINOVITCH, E., *Photosynthesis and Related Processes*, New York, 961 (1951)
13 SYUZO EGUSA, 'The gas disease of fish due to excess of nitrogen' (Japanese with English summary), *J. Fac. Fish. and Animal Husbandry Hiroshima Univ.* **2**, 157–82 (1959)
14 ENGELHORN, O. R., 'Die Gasblasenkrankheit bei Fischen', *Zeitschrift für Fischerei* **41**, 297–317 (1943)
15 BUSCHKIEL, A. L., 'Doelmatic doorluchten', *Het Aquarium* **VI**, 116–20 (1935–36); DOWNING, A. L. and TRUESDALE, G. A., 'Aeration in Aquaria', *Zoologica (Scientific Contrib. N.Y. Zool. Soc.)* **41**, 129–43 (1956)
16 ATZ, J. W., *Aquarium Journal* (U.S.A.) **XXI**, 40–43 (Feb. 1950); KLEE, A. J., *The Aquarium* (U.S.A.) **XX**, 11–12 (Jan. 1951)
17 VAN DUIJN, Jnr., C., 'Effect of plants in aquaria', *Water Life* **VII**, 231–33 (Oct. 1952) and 289–90 (Dec. 1952)
18 STEINMANN, P., 'Toxicologie der Fische', in DEMOLL-MAIER (Ed.): *Handbuch der Binnenfischerei Mitteleuropas* **VI**, Stuttgart (1927)
19 After BANDT, H. J. (1936), SCHIEMENZ, F. (1937) and JONES, J. R. E. (1965); data taken from REICHENBACH-KLINKE, *Krankheiten und Schädigungen der Fische*, Stuttgart (1966)
20 DAWES, B., *The Trematoda*, Cambridge University Press (1946); also, BYCHOVSKY, B. E., 'Monogenitscheskye Sosalschtschiki ich Systema i filogenija', *Akad. Nauk. Moscow* (1957). English translation: 'Monogenetic trematodes, their systematics and phylogeny', by OUSTINOFF, P. C. and HARGIS, W. J., Washington (1961)
21 GLÄSER, H. J., 'Zur Kenntniss der Gattung *Dactylogyrus* Diesing 1850 (*Monogenoidea*)', *Z. Parasitenk.* **25**, 459–84 (1965)

22 PAPERNA, I., 'Studies on monogenetic trematodes in Israel: 2. Monogenetic trematodes of cichlids', *Bamidgeh* **12**, 1, 20–33 (1960)
23 PROST, M., 'Investigations on the development and pathogenicity of *Dactylogyrus anchoratus* (Duj. 1845) and *D. extensus* Mueller et. v. Cleave (1932) for breeding carps', *Acta Parasitol. Polon.* **11**, 17–47 (1963)
24 IZYUMOVA, N. A., 'Kislorodnyi rezhim vodoema kak odin iz faktorov, opredelyayushchikh biologiyu *Dactylogyrus solidus i Dactylogyrus vastator*', *Parazitol. Sb.* **18**, 295–303 (1958); *Referat Zhur. Biol.*, No. 6693 (1960)
25 REICHENBACH-KLINKE, H. H., 'Eine neue Art der Trematodengattung *Diplozoon* v. Nordmann', *Zeitschrift f. Parasitenkunde* **15**, 148–54 (1951)
26 LOM, J., 'The ciliates of the family *Urceolariidæ* inhabiting gills of fishes (the *Trichodinella* Group)', *Vest Českoslov. Spolecnosti Zool.* **27**, 7–19 (1963)
27 CLEMENS, H. P. and SNEED, K. E., 'The chemical control of some diseases of channel catfish', *Progr. Fish-Cult.* **20**, 8–15 (1958)
28 HOFMAN, G. L., BISHOP, H. and DUNBAR, C. E., 'Algal parasites in fish', *Progr. Fish-Cult.* **22**, 180 (1960)
29 REICHENBACH-KLINKE, H. H., *Bestimmungsschlüssel zur Diagnose von Fischkrankheiten*, p. 44, Gustav Fischer Verlag, Stuttgart (1969)
30 REICHENBACH-KLINKE, H., *Krankheiten und Schädigungen der Fische*, pp. 54–55, Stuttgart (1966)

4

DISEASES CAUSED BY
SPOROZOANS

Sporozoans are unicellular organisms, belonging to one Class of
the Sub-kingdom of the *Protozoa*.[1] Although some sporozoan infections are mentioned in other chapters, it is considered advisable to
treat the Class as a whole in a separate chapter, since otherwise it
would be difficult to get a clear impression of the natural history of
these organisms and their rôle as causative agents of fish diseases.
Generally, they do not confine themselves to one or two organs only.
    All members of the Class of the *Sporozoa* are parasitic. In the
principal phase of their life cycle they have no organs of locomotion
or they are amoeboid. They lack a meganucleus. After syngamy
they form large numbers of spores, each containing a sporozoite.
Apart from this propagative reproduction, a second process, the
so-called multiplicative reproduction, may occur, which consists of
simple division of the sporozoites. Both processes alternate.
    The Class is subdivided in two Sub-classes, the *Telosporidia* and
the *Neosporidia*. The *Telosporidia* only reproduce themselves at the
end of the vegetative period, whilst the *Neosporidia* may produce
sporozoites at any stage of their life cycle.
    The *Telosporidia* that are parasitic on fish all belong to the Order
Coccidiomorpha, Sub-order *Coccidia*. The *Coccidia* generally possess an
egg-shaped or globular body, surrounded by a thin membrane.
The vegetative stages live in the cells of the fish, preferably in the
epithelial cells. The young sporozoites are generally sickle-shaped.
These penetrate into the cells where they grow into their definite
globular or egg-shaped form. After some time they divide themselves,
producing a number of new sporozoites, but some part of the body
may remain as the so-called 'rest-body'. The sporozoites leave the
cell of the host and spread themselves in the tissue where they infect
further cells.

125

At one stage, two different types of sporozoites are produced. The smaller ones (microgametes) unite with the larger ones (macrogametes) and form oocysts. The oocysts produce a protective membrane. In the majority of cases the oocysts are removed from the fish with its excrements. The content of each oocyst divides into four parts, each of which forms a protective capsule. Inside the protective capsule further division takes place, producing sporozoites. In the Family *Tetrasporea*, to which all fish parasites of this group belong, each capsule or spore contains four sporozoites. Fishes become infected when they take up spores with their food. In the body of the fish the spore wall cracks and the sporozoites get their chance to penetrate the cells of the fish.

Species within the Family are (see Fig. 4.1):

Eimeria alburni Stankovitch: Cysts 19–21 μm, spores 13 μm $\times$ 6 μm. In the intestine and the surrounding adiposal tissue of Bleak, Rudd and Silver Bream.

Eimeria anguillæ Léger: Cysts 10 μm, spores 8 μm $\times$ 5 μm. In the intestinal epithelium of Eel (*Anguilla anguilla*).

KEY TO FIG. 4.1
1, Eimeria minuta *(after Thélohan)*. 2, Eimeria gasterostei *(after Thélohan)*. 3, *Three stages of sporulation of a Cnidosporid.* (Psb) *pansporoblasts;* (Sb) *sporoblasts;* (Sp) *spores (after Doflein)*. 4, *Next stage:* (a) *closed spore;* (b) *spore in the process of opening;* (c) *sporozoite (amoeboid form);* (p) *polar capsule (after Hofer)*. 5, *Third stage, Sporozoites penetrating into an intestinal cell;* (n) *nucleus (after Hofer)*. 6, Sphærospora masovica. (a), (b) *amoeboid stages;* (c), (d), (e) *spores (after Cohn)*. 7, Sphærospora elegans *spore (after Gurley)*. 8, Leptotheca perlata. (a) *fresh spore;* (b) *spore with pushed out nettle thread (after Hofer)*. 9, Myxidium lieberkühni. (a) *amoeboid stage;* (b) *specimen filled with spores;* (c) *spore;* (a) *after Bütschli;* (b) *after Hofer;* (c) *after Thélohan*. 10, Myxidium histophilum *spore (after Thélohan)*. 11, Myxosoma dujardini. (a) *normal;* (b) *abnormal spore (after Thélohan)*. 12, Chloromyxum fluviatile *spore (after Thélohan)*. 13, Chloromyxum mucronatum. (a) *top view of spore;* (b) *side view (after Hofer)*. 14, Thélohanellus pyriformis *spore (after Thélohan)*. 15, Myxobolus dispar *spore (after Thélohan)*. 16, Myxobolus exiguus *spore (after Thélohan)*. 17, Myxobolus ellipsoideus *spore (after Thélohan)*. 18, Myxobolus oviformis *spore (after Thélohan)*. 19, Myxobolus mülleri *spore (after Thélohan)*. 20, Myxobolus pfeifferi *spore*. 21, Myxobolus cyprini *spore (after Hofer)*. 22, Myxobolus cycloides *spores (after Gurley)*. 23, Myxobolus anurus *spore*. (a) *stiff thread;* (b) *polar thread (after Cohn)*. 24, Myxosoma cerebralis *spores (after Hofer)*. 25, Henneguya psorospermica *spore (after Thélohan)*. 26, Henneguya psorospermica minuta *spore (after Cohn)*. 27, Henneguya psorospermica lobosa *spore (after Cohn)*. 28, *Section through a kidney tubule of* Pygosteus pungitius *with spores of* Henneguya media. (ep) *epithelium cells;* (sp) *spores (after Thélohan)*. 29, Henneguya creplini *spore (after Gurley)*. 30, Henneguya schizura *spores*. 31, Hoferellus cyprini. (a) *spore;* (b) *three adult specimens, two of which contain a spore* (sp) *(after Doflein)*. 32, Glugea anomala. (a), (b) *fresh spores;* (c) *spore with pushed out nettle thread (after Thélohan)*. 33, Plistophora typicalis. (a) *fresh spore;* (b) *spore with polar thread (after Thélohan)*

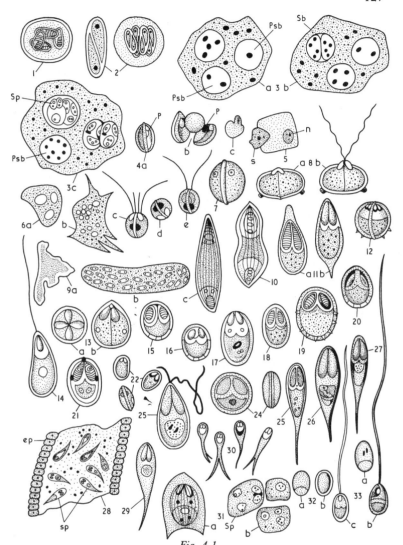

Fig. 4.1.
SPOROZOAN PARASITES OF FISH

Sporozoan parasites (Class, Sporozoa) *are divided into two Sub-classes,* Telo-sporidia *and* Neosporidia. *In both Sub-classes parasites of fish are found but in* Telosporidia *the fish parasites all belong to the Order* Coccidiomorpha, *Sub-order* Coccidia, *only and in the* Neosporidia *the sporozoans parasitic on fish are in the* Cnidosporidia *Order. Sub-orders* Myxosporidia *and* Microsporidia. *The* Cnido-sporidia *species are much the more widespread attackers of fish. Key to the illustration, which shows a number of sporozoan fish parasites, appears on the opposite page*

Eimeria cotti Gauthier: In the intestinal epithelium of Miller's Thumb (*Cottus gobio*). Cysts 10–11 μm, spores 7–8 μm × 5.1 μm.

Eimeria cylindrospora Stankovitch: Cysts 10–11 μm, spores 7–8 μm × 4 μm. In Bleak (*Alburnus lucidus*).

Eimeria cyprini Plehn: In the intestinal epithelium of young Carp (*Cyprinus carpio*) where it causes severe inflammation. If some pressure is exerted on the belly, a pus-like liquid will flow from the anal opening. The victims show severe emaciation and gaunt eyes. The intestinal mucosa contains oocysts of 8–14 μm in which four oospores are present; each oospore contains two sporozoites.

Eimeria cyprinorum Stankovitch: Cysts 12–13 μm, spores 7–8 μm × 5 μm. In the intestinal epithelium of fry of the following species: Barbel (*Barbus barbus*), Minnows (*Phoxinus phoxinus*), Roach (*Rutilus rutilus*) and Rudd (*Scardinius erythrophthalmus*).

Eimeria (*Coccidium*) *gasterostei* (Thélohan): This occurs in the liver of Sticklebacks (*Gasterosteus aculeatus* and *Pygosteus pungitius*). The cysts are 16–18 μm. The spores are spindle-shaped, measuring 10 μm in length and 4–6 μm in width.

Eimeria légeri Stankovitch: Cysts 10 μm, spores 7 μm × 5 μm. In the epithelium and subepithelial tissue of Bleak (*Alburnus lucidus*), Rudd and Silver Bream (*Abramis blicca* or *Blicca bjoerkna*).

Eimeria (*Goussia*) *minuta* Thélohan: This parajte has been found in the kidneys, the liver and the spleen of Tench (*Tinca tinca*). The cysts are spherical, 20–25 μm in size, and have a very thin membrane. The spores are oval, having a length of 15 μm and a breadth of 6–7 μm.

Eimeria (*Goussia*) *minuta* Thélohan: This parasite has been found in the kidneys, the liver and the spleen of Tench (*Tinca tinca*). The main symptom is a swelling of the liver. The cysts are thin and have a size of 9–10 μm. The four spores consist of two parts which open in the way of a pea-pod. The entire development occurs in the cells of the same host. The spores are spindle-shaped. There is no 'rest-body'.

Eimeria percæ R. D. de la Rivière: Spores 8 μm. In the epithelium and the submucosa of Perch (*Perca fluviatilis*).

Eimeria pigra Léger: Cysts 17–19 μm, spores 15 μm × 5 μm. In the intestinal epithelium of Rudd (*Scardinius erythrophthalmus*). Contrary to the condition in the other *Coccidia*, this species does not occur intracellular.

Eimeria piraudi Gauthier: Cysts 11–12 μm. Closely resembling *E. cotti*. In intestine of *Cottus gobio*.

Eimeria rouxi Elmassian: Cysts 10 μm, spores 6 μm. In the jejunum (middle part of the small intestine) of Tench.

Eimeria subepithelialis Moroff & Fiebiger: In the middle and end parts of the intestinal tract of Carp, where yellow knots of about 2 mm are produced. The main symptoms are the same as in *E. cyprini* infections.

Eimeria truttæ Léger & Hesse: Cysts 12 μm, spores 8 μm × 4.2 μm.

In the epithelium of the small intestine and the appendices pylorae of the stomach of Trout (*Salmo fario*).
Eimeria wierzejskii Hofer: Cysts 11–12 μm, spores 8.5 μm × 4.1 μm. In the intestine of Carp.

A number of *Coccidia* live as blood parasites that penetrate into the red blood corpuscles (erythrocytes). The infections may be transferred by leeches. Symptoms will be those of anaemia, with pale gill sheets and fading of colours, as well as emaciation and sluggish movements. Species are *Hæmogregarina acipenseris* Nawrotzky, found in Sturgeon, *H. esoci* Nawr. (in Pike), *H. bigemina* Lav. & Mesnil and *H. mugili* Carini in marine fishes. Further, *Dactylosoma salvelini* and *Leucocytozoon salvelini*.

FISH PARASITES IN THE *CNIDOSPORIDIA*

Most of the sporozoans parasitic in fish belong to the Sub-class *Neosporidia*, Order *Cnidosporidia*.

The *Cnidosporidia*, when in the adult stage, either possess an amoeboid form or they are surrounded by a cyst. The amoeboid stages can move by means of pseudopodia when they occur in free cavities of the body of the fish, such as the urinary bladder or the gall bladder. If, however, they are situated in the cells or between the tissue cells of the host, they generally become immovable or nearly so.

Sporulation occurs during the whole life cycle. In the cytoplasm pansporoblasts are produced, appearing as globular forms. Inside the pansporoblasts nuclear divisions take place till the number of nuclei has increased up to ten. Then each pansporoblast divides into two sporoblasts. The sporoblasts produce a fast membrane and a polar capsule, thus forming the spores.

Every spore consists of two valve-shaped parts, each of which contains a sporozoite, and two or more polar capsules. The polar capsules are pear-shaped bodies of high refractivity. They contain a rolled-up spiralised thread. If the spores reach the intestine of the fish they open in the way of a pea-pod. Then the polar capsules discharge the polar threads. These become attached to the villi intestinalis (the absorptive processes of the intestine). The sporozoites leave the spores and penetrate the intestinal cells, where they grow and multiply or swarm out to penetrate other organs of the host.

The Order *Cnidosporidia* is divided into two Sub-orders, namely, the *Myxosporidia* and the *Microsporidia*.

The *Myxosporidia* form two spores with one to four polar capsules in the pansporoblast. The polar capsules are always visible in live specimens, whereas in the *Microsporidia* they are not seen in the living state. In the pansporoblasts of the *Microsporidia*, four, eight or many spores with one polar capsule each are formed.

The Sub-order *Myxosporidia* is now divided into five Families, namely: (*a*) the *Myxidiidæ*, characterised by the possession of two polar capsules at opposite sides of the spores; the spore cytoplasm does not contain a vacuole; (*b*) the *Chloromyxidæ*, possessing four polar capsules in each spore. No vacuole in the spore cytoplasm; (*c*) the *Myxobolidæ* containing a vacuole in the spore cytoplasm. This vacuole stains with iodine. Generally, there are two polar capsules; (*d*) the *Unicapsulidæ*, with one polar capsule and lacking any glycogen-containing (with iodine staining) vacuole; (*e*) the *Ceratomyxidæ*, with two polar capsules; no glycogen-containing vacuole. Members of the *Unicapsulidæ* have been found in marine fish only.

There are so many species of the *Cnidosporidia* parasite in fish that it would be utterly impossible to deal with all of them in detail. I give a description of some of the more important examples of the group, while others will only be mentioned with name and occurrence. The review is, however, far from complete.

FAMILY MYXIDIIDÆ

Myxidium girardi Cépède: Spindle-shaped spores with longitudinal stripes and rounded ends; 9–10 μm × 5.0–5.5 μm. Produces white cysts in the kidneys of Eel (*Anguilla anguilla*).

Myxidium histophilum Thélohan: In the connective tissue of the kidneys and the ovaries of Minnows, where they occur in very large numbers. Spores 15 μm long.

Myxidium lieberkühni Bütschli: In the urinary bladder of Pike (*Esox lucius*) and Eelpout. Amoeboid stage shows much variability. Pseudopodia immovable, indented or thread-like. The endoplasm is yellowish-coloured and contains yellow or grey globules, while sometimes small crystals are also present. Spores 18–20 μm long, 5–6 μm wide.

Myxidium oviforme Parisi: Oval spores with longitudinal stripes; 10–13 μm × 8–9 μm. In the gall bladder of Salmon (*Salmo salar*) and Cod (*Gadus morrhua*).

A number of further species is found in the gall bladder of fishes: *Myxidium alosæ* in Twaite Shad (*Alosa finta*); *M. cristatum* in Tench (*Tinca tinca*); *M. rhodei* in Bitterling (*Rhodeus amarus*); *M. truttæ* in Trout (*Salmo fario*).

Zschokkella nova Klocacewa: In the gall bladder of Prussian Carp (*Carassius carassius*).

FAMILY CHLOROMYXIDÆ

Agarella gracilis Dunkerley: Induces cyst formation in the testicular tissues of South American fish.

Chloromyxum chitosense Fujita: Globular smooth spores of 8 μm × 9 μm. In Japanese Salmon.

Chloromyxum cristatum Léger: In the gall bladder of Tench.

Chloromyxum cyprini Fujita: Spores 10–12 μm × 10 μm; with 8–10 ribs on each scale. In the gall bladder of Carp (*Cyprinus carpio*). Fujita found this parasite in 20% of Carps in Japan.

Chloromyxum dubium Auerbach: In the gall bladder of Eelpout (*Lota vulgaris*).

Chloromyxum fluviatile Thélohan: Parasitic in the gall bladder of Chub (*Squalius cephalus*). Amoeboid adult parasites have a yellow colour, and are 25–30 μm in size. Spores globular, 7–8 μm.

Chloromyxum giganteum Fujita: Globular spores with ribs; 14–16 μm × 13–14 μm. In the gall bladder of Japanese Salmon.

Chloromyxum koi Fujita: In the gall bladder of Carp.

Chloromyxum légeri Touraine: Spores 7.5 μm. In the gall bladder of Carp.

Chloromyxum mucronatum Gurley: Parasitic in the urinary bladder and in the kidneys of Eelpout (*Lota vulgaris*), spores 8 μm, polar thread 7 μm.

Chloromyxum parasiluri Fujita: Spores 7.5 μm × 6 μm with 10–12 stripes. In Japanese fish.

Chloromyxum salvelini Fujita: Spores 10–13 μm with many ribs. In Japanese Salmonids.

Chloromyxum sphæricum Fujita: Globular spores of 8–9 μm with 9–10 stripes on each half of the scale. In the gall bladder of Japanese fish.

Chloromyxum truttæ Léger: In the gall bladder of Trout (*Salmo fario*). Produces jaundice (yellow coloration of the skin and body tissues) resulting from excess of bile pigment in the blood and the lymph, caused by obstruction of the bile ducts by the infection.

Trilospora californica Noble: In the gall bladder of American fish.

FAMILY MYXOBOLIDÆ

Henneguya brevis Thélohan: In the kidneys and ovaries of Sticklebacks. Spores have the shape of a pivot and possess a short tail, length 14–15 μm (including 4–5 μm of the caudal appendage), width 5–6 μm. Polar capsules 4–5 μm.

Henneguya carassii Fujita: With spores of 21 μm × 10 μm, and *H. spatulata* Fujita: With spores of 41–44 μm × 13–16 μm, have been found in Japanese fish.

Henneguya creplini Gurley [*H. acerinæ* Schröder]: Spores 70–82 μm × 8–9 μm with appendage of 30–40 μm; spindle-shaped. Produces oblong white cysts, 0.6–1.1 mm in size, in the gills of Ruff (*Acerina cernua*).

Henneguya lobosa Cohn: Spores 30–40 μm × 5–6.5 μm. Polar capsules 6–8 μm × 2–2.5 μm. Caudal appendage 22–28 μm. Produces oval cysts of up to 2.8 mm at the tips of the gill sheets of Pike (*Esox lucius*).

Henneguya media Thélohan: This is found in the kidney tubules and the ovaries of Sticklebacks (*Gasterosteus aculeatus* and *Pygosteus pungitius*). Spores spindle-shaped, 20–24 μm $\times$ 5–6 μm. Polar capsules 4–5 μm.

Henneguya minuta Cohn: Spores 28–45 μm $\times$ 10–11 μm. Polar capsules 11–14 μm $\times$ 2–3 μm. Caudal appendage 8–17 μm. Produces cysts of 0.10–0.15 mm in the gills of Perch (*Perca fluviatilis*).

Henneguya psorospermica Thélohan: This species is very variable and has been divided into several sub-species. They are mainly parasites of the gills of Pike (*Esox lucius*) and Perch (*Perca fluviatilis*), where they produce white cysts, a few millimetres in diameter. Spores 30–40 μm $\times$ 7–8 μm. The variety *H. ps. oviperda* L. Cohn attacks the eggs of Pike. Contrary to the other varieties, this one does not produce cysts.

Henneguya schizura Gurley: In the connective tissue of the eye muscles and the sclera (tough, fibrous outer coat of the eye) of Pike. Produces cysts of 440 μm up to 1 mm in length. The cysts are surrounded by a soft membrane. The spores are 12 μm long and 6 μm broad, with long forked tail ends.

Henneguya zikaweiensis Sikama: Produces globular cysts of up to 0.5 mm on the cornea of the eye of Goldfish (*Carassius auratus*).

Henneguya zschokkei Gurley: Oval spores, rounded at the anterior and pointed at the posterior end; 50–60 μm $\times$ 7 μm. Produces oval boils of 10–30 mm length and 7–20 mm width in *Coregonus fera*.

Hoferellus cyprini (Doflein): In the kidneys of Carp, where they can be found both in the epithelium and in the lumen of the tubules. In the latter, amoeboid stages can be encountered; these have a size of approximately 27 μm. If there are many of them in the tubules they may cause dropsy, followed by scale protrusion and exophthalmus. In autumn the amoeboid parasites leave the epithelium and the empty sites are filled with blood and secretions, which are gradually transformed to yellow bodies. The cause of the disease is slow. It may take up to one year before the infected fish dies. The spores of the parasite are 10–12 μm long and 8 μm wide; the tail ends are 2 μm long.

Myxobolus anurus Cohn [*Henneguya psorospermica anura* Labbé]: In the gills of Pike (*Esox lucius*). Produces cysts of 600 μm $\times$ 340 μm. Oval spores, 12–15 μm $\times$ 4–6.8 μm. Polar capsules 5.5–7 μm long, 2.1–2.5 μm wide. Polar thread 32–38 μm in length.

Myxobolus cycloides Gurley: In the pseudobranchia of Roach (*Rutilus rutilus*), and the gills of whitefish, Gudgeon (*Gobio gobio*) and Silver Bream (*Abramis blicca* or *Blicca bjoerkna*). Spores 11–15 μm $\times$ 8–10 μm.

Myxobolus cyprini Hofer and Doflein: In the kidneys, spleen, liver of Carp. On a few occasions it has also been found in Tench and Bream. Once it was believed that this organism was responsible for the pox disease of Carp, since Hofer found it in fish suffering from this affliction. Later investigations, however, showed that pox disease can occur independent of the presence of sporozoans. Spores 8–16 μm × 8–9 μm.

Myxobolus dispar Thélohan: In the skin, the gills and the intestinal epithelium of Carp (*Cyprinus carpio*), in the muscles and the spleen of Rudd (*Scardinius erythrophthalmus*), and in the muscles and the connective tissue of Bleak (*Alburnus lucidus*). Symptoms of the infection are large knots or boils appearing in different parts of the body. Length of spores 10–12 μm, breadth 8 μm. The two polar capsules are of unequal size, 7 μm and 5 μm, respectively.

Myxobolus ellipsoides Thélohan: In the gills, kidneys, spleen, liver, swim bladder and in the cornea of the eye of Tench (*Tinca tinca*). Spores 12–14 μm × 9–11 μm. Polar capsule 4 μm.

Myxobolus elongatus Fujita: Spores 15 μm × 6 μm. In Japanese fish.

Myxobolus exiguus Thélohan: Produces very small knots in the skin of Carp (*Cyprinus carpio*), whilst it also occurs as a parasite in the gills of Bream (*Abramis brama*) and in the stomach, the intestine and the kidneys of Grayling (*Thymallus thymallus*). In Carp, a very large number of small greyish- or greenish-white knots are produced. They may easily be confused with white spot (*Ichthyophthirius*). Spores 8–9 μm long and 6–7 μm wide. Polar capsules 3.6 μm; polar thread 15 μm.

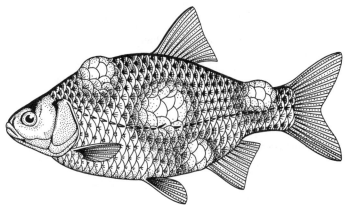

Fig. 4.2. Roach showing bumps, following infection by Myxobolus oviformis

Myxobolus luciopercæ Schäferna and Jirovec: Produces white cysts in the gill basket of Pike-Perch (*Lucioperca sandra*). Spores 8–11 μm × 7.4–9 μm. Closely related species are *M. sandræ* and *M. volgensis*.

Myxobolus mülleri Bütschli: The cause of knot or pimple disease in Chub (*Squalius cephalus*). The parasite also attacks the ovaries and kidneys of Minnows, and the gills of Chub. Spores 10–12 μm × 9–11 μm.

Myxobolus neurobius Schuberg and Schröder: Produces cysts in the nerves and the spinal marrow of Trout (*Salmo fario*) and Grayling (*Thymallus thymallus*). Oval spores, 10–12 μm × 8 μm.

Myxobolus notatus Mavor: Produces tumours in the cutis of Roach (*Rutilus rutilus*).

Myxobolus oviformis Thélohan: Knots are produced in the fins, the kidneys and the spleen of Gudgeon (*Gobio gobio*) and Eelpout (*Lota vulgaris*). It also occurs in the skin of Roach (*Rutilus rutilus*) (Fig. 4.2). White knots (cysts) are produced in the gills and other organs of Silver Bream (*Abramis blicca* or *Blicca bjoerkna*) and some other fish. Spores 10–12 μm long and 8–9 μm wide; polar capsules 6 μm.

Myxobolus pfeifferi Thélohan: Causes boil disease (*Myxoboliasis tubero-ulcerosa*) in Barbels (*Barbus barbus*) (Fig. 4.3). Large boils are

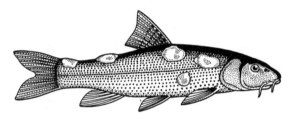

Fig. 4.3.
BOIL DISEASE VICTIM
Barbel (Barbus barbus) *affected by boil disease. Causative organism is* Myxobolus pfeifferi

produced on several parts of the body of the fish. These may vary from the size of a nut to that of a hen's egg. They may either be closed or they may open and ulcerate. Diseased fish move more slowly than normal and retreat to such parts of the river where the stream is more quiet. The body surface loses its lustre. Affected fishes gradually grow thin and emaciated. Later on the victims suffer from equilibrium difficulties; they come to the surface of the water and tumble 'head over heels', then they fall on to their side and finally die. The skin at the site of the boils is often stained, causing displacement and falling off of the scales. The flesh becomes straw-yellow in colour and has a bile-like, weak composition. The sporozoans can be found in large number in the boils (millions to some milliards of them in one single boil!), but they are also to be encountered in nearly all other parts of the body, such as the heart, the spleen, the kidneys, the ovaries and in the connective tissue of the intestine. The parasite has also been found in the neurolemma of Grayling (*Thymallus thymallus*) and in the ovaries of Prussian Carp (*Carassius carassius*). The spores are egg-shaped, 12 μm long and 10 μm wide. Secondary bacterial infections often occur. The disease manifests itself mainly in the hot season and is apparently latent in winter.

Myxobolus physophilus Reuss: In the swim bladder of Rudd (*Scardinius erythrophthalmus*), see page 236.

Myxobolus uniporus Fujita: Spores 12 μm × 3 μm. Polar capsules exceeding 7 μm, often unequal in length. In Japanese fish.

Thélohanellus fuhrmanni Auerbach: In the mucous membrane of the mouth of Roach (*Rutilus rutilus*).

Thélohanellus (Myxobolus) pyriformis (Thélohan): This forms thread-like cysts in the gills of Tench (*Tinca tinca*) and Weatherfish (*Misgurnus (Cobitis) fossilis*). The parasites also occur in the kidneys and the spleen. The spores possess only one polar capsule with a length of 16–18 μm and a breadth of 7–8 μm. The polar thread has a length of 30 μm.

Thélohanellus swellengrebeli Schuurmans-Stekhoven: In the muscles of Bitterling (*Rhodeus amarus*).

FAMILY CERATOMYXIDÆ

Ceratomyxa shasta Noble: Conical scale halves, that are bent at the back. Spores 14 μm × 6 μm. Destroys body tissues in young Rainbow Trout (*Salmo iridæus*) and has caused heavy losses in California.

Leptotheca perlata Gurley: This species has been found in the Gull (*Acerina cernua*).

Mitraspora cyprini Fujita: In the renal tubules of Carp and Prussian Carp in Japan.

Mitraspora elongata Kudo: In the renal tubules of *Lepomis cyanellus* in North America.

Myxosoma (Lentospora) cerebralis (Hofer) [*Myxobolus chondrophagus* Plehn; *Myxobolus cerebralis* Hofer]: This parasite is often found in the nervous system and the auditory organ of young Trout (*Salmo fario*, *S. lacustris*, *S. iridæus* and related species), further in Coho Salmon (*Oncorhynchus kisutch*), Chinook Salmon (*O. tshawytscha*) and Lake Trout (*Salvelinus namaycush*). Affected fish lose their sense of balance, they turn round in an awkward way and tumble 'head over heels' (**whirling or tumbling disease**). Further, a blackening of the tail, up to the anal pore, can be observed, while, later on, deformities of the skeleton are produced. Even if the victims recover from the infection, the deformities remain, thus affecting the fish for life. The deformities are caused by penetration of the sporozoans into the cartilage of the young fish, thus preventing normal ossification. Examples of deformities of this kind are a shortening of the gill covering or of the fins and deformities of the cheeks, which may grow together so that the fish cannot shut its mouth. This sporozoan does not produce cysts. The spores have a diameter of 7–9 μm and a thickness of 5 μm. The scale halves have a protruding rim. The polar capsules are 4 μm long.

The spores are not infective shortly after removal from the fish, but they become viable after four months of 'ageing' in spring water.[2] They are distorted and probably killed at 60° and 100°C, but not at 40°C, whereas they can stand freezing at −18°C. Spores are probably killed after 24 h exposure to 0.5 and 2% of calcium hydroxide, available chlorine (as sodium hypochlorite, NaOCl) at 1600 p.p.m. and benzalkonium chloride at 200 and 800 p.p.m.

Myxosoma (Lentospora) dermatobia (Ishil): Produces cysts of 0.1–0.3 mm in the skin of Japanese Eel.

Myxosoma (Lentospora) diaphana (Fantham, Porter & Richardson): Produces degeneration of the tissues of the ovaries and testicles in *Fundulus* species.

Myxosoma (Lentospora) dujardini Thélohan: In the gills of Rudd (*Scardinius erythrophthalmus*), Roach (*Rutilus rutilus*), Carp (*Cyprinus carpio*) and Perch (*Perca fluviatilis*), where they are present in white cysts of irregular form, sometimes branched, reaching a size of 1–1.5 mm. Symptoms of infection in fish are breathing difficulties and, finally, death from suffocation. The cysts are to be observed as tiny white or yellowish nodules. The same symptoms occur in infections of the gills with other *Myxosporidia*. The spores have a length of 12–13 μm and a breadth of 7–8 μm.

Similar diseases are caused by the related species *M. lobata* (Nemeczek) in Roach (*Rutilus rutilus*) and in *Aspius rapax*, and *M. funduli* (Kudo) in members of the Genus *Fundulus*.

Myxosoma (Lentospora) encephalica (Mulsow): Spores 5–5.5 μm. In the blood vessels of the brain in Carp.

Myxosoma (Lentospora) ovale (Davis): Produces cysts, 0.7 mm in size, in the gills of American fishes.

Fujita described and named the following species in Japanese fish: *M. elliptica*, *M. gigi*, *M. kawabatæ*, *M. leucogobiana*, *M. sacchalinensis*, *M. sphaerica* and *M. taiwanensis*.

Sinuolinea brachiophora Davis and *S. dimorpha* Davis have been found in the urinary bladder of American fishes.

Sinuolinea gilsoni Deraisieux: In the urinary bladder of Eel (*Anguilla anguilla*).

Sphærospora elegans Thélohan: This occurs in the tubules of the kidneys and in the connective tissue of the ovaries of Sticklebacks (*Gasterosteus aculeatus* and *Pygosteus pungitius*), further (but seldom) in the kidneys of Minnows (*Phoxinus phoxinus*) and Eelpout (*Lota vulgaris*). Amoeboid stage 20–25 μm. Cytoplasm with very fine granulations, fast homogeneous, containing several globules of high refractivity. Slowly moving pseudopodia. Spores 8–12 μm in length.

Sphærospora masovica Cohn: Amoeboid stages 10–38 μm; hyaline protoplasm. Pseudopodia lively moving. Spores, 8 μm, approximately sphere-shaped, but with a strong projecting equatorial brim. The spore cytoplasm contains two nuclei. It has been found in the gall bladder of Bream (*Abramis brama*).

Sphærospora reichnowi Jacob: Spores with delicate longitudinal striations; 9–10 μm. Produces tiny white knots in the mucous membrane of the intestine of Eel (*Anguilla anguilla*), whereas its

vegetative form induces morbid growth resembling pieces of cauliflower in the intestine itself.

Sphærospora tincæ Plehn: Spores 8–8.5 µm. Polar capsules globular;
thin scale with inconspicuous seam. This organism is responsible
for a disease of young Tench (*Tinca tinca*) in which the victims show
obesity in the region of the pectoral fins and where they persist in
an inclined position with the head pointing downwards. The main
site of the infection is the anterior kidney, lying between the swim
bladder and the gills. The young fishes are infected during the
first weeks of their life by spores of the parasite that are present in
the mud at the bottom. Starting from the intestine, the parasites
are transported by the lymphatic system to the lymphatic cavity
of the skull, from which place they invade the anterior kidney,
inducing proliferation and morbid growth. The affected kidney
becomes filled with spores and swells considerably; this condition is
the reason for the external symptom of local obesity. Later on, the
infection may spread to the serous membranes of the heart and the
belly, followed by the posterior kidney, the liver and the spleen.
In females, the ovary may also become affected. Generally, the
intestine is not affected. Spores may be excreted with the urine of
the infected fish.

The course of the disease is rather slow. The apathic inclined
position may last for weeks. Although recovery from the infection
by natural defensive powers is possible, many of the infected fishes
will die.

Wardia ovinocua Kudo: In the connective tissue of the ovaries and
in the eggs of North American fresh-water fishes.

SUB-ORDER MICROSPORIDIA. FAMILY NOSEMATIDÆ

The spores are generally very small. They contain a vacuole at one
end, opposite to the polar capsule. The latter is invisible when
living, but it can be demonstrated in stained slides.

Glugea acerinæ Jirovec: Spores 3.5–4.5 µm × 2.5–3 µm. Produces
cysts of up to 0.3 mm in the intestinal wall of the Gull (*Acerina
cernua*).

Glugea anomala Moniez [*Nosema anomalum* Moniez: *Glugea microspora*
Thélohan]: The cause of knot or pimple disease in Sticklebacks
(Fig. 4.4), and *Gobius minutus*. The knots (cysts) are 2–4 mm
in size. The parasite lives in the connective tissue of the cutis and in
the cornea of the eye, in the belly and in the walls of the stomach
and of the swim bladder, in the intestine and the testicles, whilst it
rarely occurs in the ovaries. The spores have a length of approximately 4–4.5 µm and a breadth of 3 µm; the polar thread is 30–
35 µm long.

Glugea hertwigi Weissenberg: Closely resembling *G. anomala*.
Produces knot disease in Smelt (*Osmerus eperlanus*). The spores are

4.6–5.4 μm × 2.3 μm. In Smelt under 10 cm (nearly 4 in) in size the
internal cysts can be observed when the fish is viewed against the
light.

Glugea pseudotumefaciens Pflugfelder: Produces *exophthalmus* (eye
protruding) and skin ulcers in exotic aquarium fishes. Knots are
produced in the ovaries, spleen, kidneys, liver, eyes and in the
nervous system. The parasite occurs mainly in the fibroblasts
(connective tissue cells) of these organs.

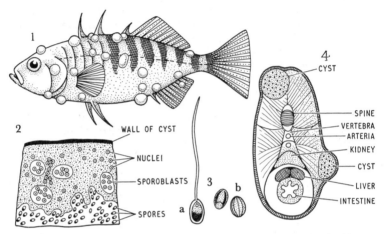

Fig. 4.4. 1, *Stickleback* (Gasterosteus aculeatus) *with knots, caused by* Glugea
anomala. 2, *Section of skin of Stickleback infected by* Glugea anomala. 3, *Spores
of* Glugea anomala; (a) *spore with polar thread;* (b) *fresh spores (after Thélohan).*
4, *Transverse section of Stickleback showing* Glugea *cysts*

Nosema girardini Lutz and Splendore: Spores 2–2.5 μm × 1–1.5 μm.
In the intestine of *Phalloceros caudimaculatus,* a Livebearing Tooth-
carp.

Plistophora acerinæ Vaney and Conte: Spores 3 μm × 2 μm. In
the mesenteron (mid-gut) of the Gull (*Acerina cernua*).

Plistophora ehrenbaumi Reichenow: Pansporoblasts 10–24 μm,
spores of variable size, dependent on the size of the pansporoblast,
larger ones 7.5 μm × 3.5 μm, smaller ones 3 μm × 1.5 μm. Produces
boil disease in European Catfish (*Siluris glanis*). The boils may vary
from hazelnut to fist-size. Has also been found in the dorsal muscles
of a Bullhead (*Cottus gobio*), whereas it occurs regularly as a parasite
of marine fishes.

Plistophora elegans Auerbach: Spores 10 μm × 4 μm. In Bream and
Roach.

Plistophora hyphessobryconis Schäperclaus: Pansporoblasts 30 μm;
spores 5–6 μm × 3.3 μm. Causes 'neon tetra disease' in exotic

aquarium fishes (Fig. 4.5), described in detail on pages 141–145. Has also been found in Minnows and Prussian Carp.

Plistophora longifilis Schuberg: Spores either 3 μm × 2 μm or 12 μm × 6 μm. In Barbel (*Barbus barbus*).

Plistophora macrospora Cépède: Spores 8.5 μm × 4.25 μm. In Stone Loach (*Cobitis barbatula*).

Plistophora mirandellæ Vaney and Conte: Spores 12 μm × 6 μm. In *Alburnus mirandella*.

Plistophora oolytica Weiser: Spores of variable size, either 8.4 μm × 4.2 μm, 5.5–6.5 μm × 3.5 μm or 3 μm × 1.5 μm. In Pike (*Esox lucius*), Roach (*Rutilus rutilus*) and Chub (*Squalius cephalus*) and in the soft-roes (*testes*) of River Char (*Hucho hucho*).

Plistophora ovariæ Summerfelt.[3] Fresh spores ovoid or ellipsoid, 8.42–10.7 μm × 4.24–0.15 μm. Not found in male fish, but only in ovaries, liver and kidneys of female Golden Shiners (*Notemigonus crysoleucas*).

Plistophora typicalis Gurley: On sporulation, the entire body divides into pansporoblasts. The sporoblasts are sphere-shaped, 25–35 μm in diameter. The spores are 5 μm long and 3 μm wide, whilst the polar thread reaches a length of 65–75 μm. The parasite has been found in the muscles of Ten-Spined Sticklebacks (*Pygosteus pungitius*), *Cottus scorpius*, *C. bubalis* and *Blennius pholis*. The volume of the muscles is increased, but the loosened muscle fibrils do not degenerate.

FISH PARASITES IN THE *HAPLOSPORIDIA*

The members of this Order, when in the adult stage, consist of a polynuclear plasmodium. The plasmodium encysts and produces spores by division into many parts. The spores lack any polar thread. In many species the spores possess a circular opening, which may or may not be closed by a lid. The membranes of the spores may bear appendages. All *Haplosporidia* parasitic in fish multiply by fission without preceding sexual processes (schizogony) and produce globular or oval spores of very simple structure.

These parasites generally produce rather big mesenchymal cysts, appearing as knots or pimples.

Fish parasites belonging to this Order are:

Dermocystidium branchialis Léger: Spores have a diameter of 7–8 μm. Produces globular knots at the gills of Brook Trout (*Salmo fario*).

Dermocystidium gasterostei Elkan: Spores 3–5 μm. Produces worm-like cysts in the skin of Stickleback (*Gasterosteus aculeatus* and *Pygosteus pungitius*). These cysts are 2–3 mm long and 0.2–0.3 mm wide. On the caudal fin the arrangement of the cysts follows the direction of the tail bones. No cysts appear on the gills, but in some attacked fish cysts also occur in the cornea of the eye, some of them being deeply embedded between the skull bones, close to the brain capsule. Morphologically, *D. gasterostei* closely resembles *D. percæ*, but it was found not infectious to Perch, and it penetrates much deeper, even to the skull, whereas the latter is restricted to the surface of the cutis. Also see page 66.

Dermocystidium percæ Reichenbach-Klinke: Produces globular or pear-shaped spores with a diameter of 3.5–13 μm. Next to the nucleus there are 2–4 small globular bodies in the sickle-shaped cytoplasmic area. Symptoms of the infection are the occurrence of oblong cysts, 1–2 mm long and 0.04–0.2 mm wide, in the cutis of Perch (*Perca fluviatilis*), especially at the fins, the head and the belly, at the border of the operculum and under the cornea of the eye.

The infection is not transferred from fish to fish. It is presumed that the life cycle of the organism includes some other host, such as a water flea or a cyclopid. The infection starts in the intestine of the fish, where the ripe spores release plasmodia, that are transported by the bloodstream and settle in the cutis. There each plasmodium becomes polynuclear and divides into a number of globular sporoblasts, 2–7.8 μm in size.

Dermocystidium vejdovskyi Jirovec: Spores 3.5–4.5 μm × 3–4 μm. Produces white globular knots at the gills of Pike (*Esox lucius*).

Lymphosporidium truttæ Calkins: This causes epidemics in Brook Trout (*Salmo fontinalis*). Symptoms are the occurrence of crater-like holes at the sides and the back of the affected fish. The holes may even extend as deep as the spine and the internal organs. The adult parasite resembles an amoeba, having a size of 25–30 μm. It does not contain a compact nucleus, the nuclear material being distributed over a number of small granules lying in the cytoplasm. For reproduction, the nuclear granules assemble and, in their neighbourhood, spores are produced.

The spores are very small, 2–3 μm only. They do not contain polar cells or polar threads. The contents of each spore fall apart into eight sporozoites. These leave their envelope and are expelled from the body of the fish with its excrements. When the spores are taken up by another fish the infection spreads. The spores can be found in all internal organs of the infected fish, but they are most numerous in the soft roes. The true systematic place of the parasite among the other Sporozoa does not seem to be entirely clear.

Sporozoon tincæ Volf and Dvorák: Oval spores 1.5–2 μm × 0.5 μm. The spores have a heavy membrane with great adsorptive power with regard to microscopical stains. There are two tiny globular nuclei that can be stained only with difficulty owing to the presence of the heavy membrane. Produces haemorrhages and ulcers in the skin of Tench (*Tinca tinca*), especially at the base of the fins. In the internal organs, white colonies, 1–3 mm in size, are produced.

NEON TETRA DISEASE (SPOROZOASIS MYOLYTICA)

This disease has got its popular name owing to its having been observed first in the Neon Tetra (*Paracheirodon* (*Hyphessobrycon*) *innesi*). It has been found in other species of fish, too, including Minnows and Prussian Carp. In Neon Tetra, the disease generally starts with the occurrence of some white blemish or spot in the blue-green line of the fish. This spot may occur anywhere along the length of the line. Gradually it will extend over a larger area and grow into a light-coloured band, which usually is perpendicular to the longitudinal axis of the body. The victims may die in the first stages of the disease but, if they are more resistant, the colour may be obscured further by a smoky white cloudiness, which may or may not be accompanied by emaciation and a sunken belly. Sometimes the red colour may be obscured, but this symptom is not often observed since the fish is not likely to survive long enough for this stage to be reached. However, other cases have been described where the whitish discoloration started at the tail and extended along the red areas towards the head.

In the muscles of the body and sometimes of the head, too, white or whitish translucent spots may appear. On cautious palpation or touching with a wooden spatula or a match these spots feel soft as compared to the unaffected parts of the body. Female Neon Tetras are more often affected than males.

In Glowlight Tetras (*Hemigrammus erythrozonus*) the smoky discoloration is seen inside the body, above the spine. The glow-line becomes pale and it gradually turns whitish. Breathing frequency increases. Death may occur in about one week.

The disease was first described by Schäperclaus in 1941.[4]

DEAD AND DYING CELLS DISCERNED

Upon microscopical examination of thin sections from the region of the pathological band in Neons it may be observed that its cells are necrotic, i.e. the tissue consists of dead and dying cells. In fish that have died in an advanced stage of the disease, the smoky area is found to be soft and of a spongy constitution. In this stage, pansporoblasts and sporocysts of a sporozoan may be found lying in the tissue, which on microscopical examination with a high-power objective can be seen as greyish-white globules. Free spores, that have been liberated, may also be observed.

The species of sporozoans responsible for the disease was not identical with species that were known already, so it has been described as a new one and named *Plistophora hyphessobryconis*.

The pansporoblasts of the organism are 26–33 μm in size. Generally they lie in groups of 3–30 specimens between the muscle

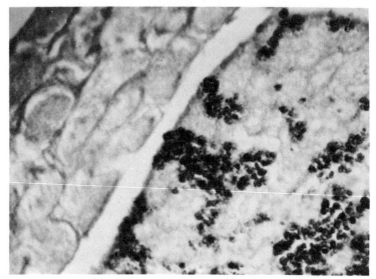

Fig. 4.5(a). Neon tetra disease. Numerous pansporoblasts of Plistophora hyphesso-bryconis *in necrotic muscle tissue of an infected* Barbus sumatranus. *Section stained with haematoxyline-erythrosin*

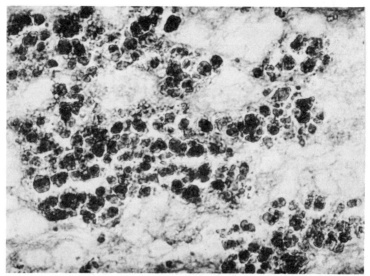

Fig. 4.5(b). Numerous pansporoblasts of Plistophora hyphessobryconis *in necrotic muscle.* × 400

fibres, that are liquefied. The pansporoblasts contain oval spores, 4–6 μm long and 3.5 μm wide. Each spore contains a polar capsule with a diameter of 3 μm.

The symptoms of the disease are in no instance sufficiently clear to allow certain diagnosis from external observation, and a postmortem and microscopical investigation is required to ascertain its cause. The easiest way is to make a smear preparation of the necrotic muscle tissue and to observe this first in the native state, keeping the smear moist and covering it with a cover glass. If available, phase-contrast optics are to be preferred for observation. Stained

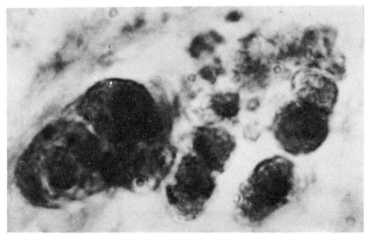

Fig. 4.5(c). Pansporoblasts of Plistophora hyphessobryconis. × *1500*

slides for further reference are best prepared by application of a histological staining technique intended for demonstrating connective tissue, such as Azan, Mallory or other modifications. Particulars can be found in any book on histological technique. The pansporoblasts may be surrounded by connective tissue, which is stained blue or blue-violet. Such enclosed pansporoblasts are often surrounded by black pigment. Since fixation and further preparation induces some shrinking in the specimens, the diameter of the pansporoblasts in the stained slide is reduced to approximately 23 μm.

ORGANISM FOUND IN SEVERAL SPECIES

This parasite has been found thus far in Neons, Glowlight Tetras, Rosy Tetras (*Hyphessobrycon rosaceus*), Flame Fish (*Hyphessobrycon flammeus*), *Hyphessobrycon gracilis*, *Hemigrammus ocellifer* and Pulchers (*Hemigrammus pulcher*), but also in entirely different types of fish,

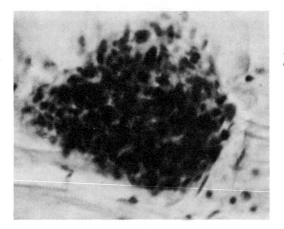

Fig. 4.5(d). Ripe cyst, releasing spores.
× 1000

namely, Swordtails (*Xiphophorus helleri*), Zebra Fish (*Brachydanio rerio*) and *Barbus sumatranus.*

Schäperclaus has observed *Plistophora hyphessobryconis* infections even in young Neon Tetras, only 3.5–4 mm in size. The victims often died within one week after hatching. Pansporoblasts could be detected at the edges of the fins and in the tail muscles. The youngsters showed heavily swollen bellies. Schäperclaus suggests that the infection may also be transferred from the mother to the ova,

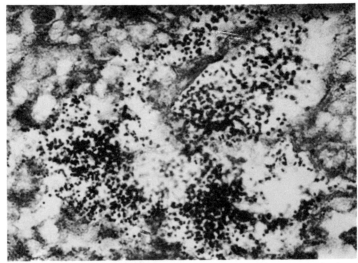

Fig. 4.5(e). Plistophora hyphessobryconis. *Scattered spores in necrotic tissue.*
× 400

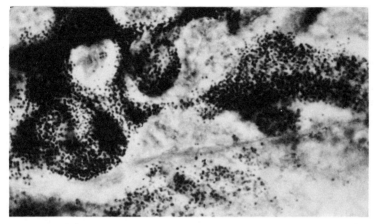

Fig. 4.5(f). Plistophora hyphessobryconis. *Huge aggregates of spores in necrotic muscle.* × 400

while the latter are in the ovary, either by spores entering the ova immediately, or by spores adhering to the ova and infecting the fry when hatching. In female Neons the ovaries are among the organs that suffer most from the infection.

CURES FOR SPOROZOAN INFECTIONS

It has been claimed in Holland that methylene blue in a concentration not less than 1 g/100 l should be effective against neon disease,[5] but others trying this treatment have not met with success. If one wishes to try this treatment, it should not be carried out in a fully planted tank. To avoid reinfection, the original tank should be disinfected and reinstalled completely.

Disinfection of a tank or pond in which an epidemic caused by sporozoan infection has occurred is performed most easily by means of potassium permanganate. A 1% stock solution is prepared in distilled water and so much of this solution is mixed with the water (after removal of all fish) as required to obtain a dark-coloured, but still transparent, solution. The bottom should be stirred up in order to kill any spores that could have sunk below its surface. After three days the permanganate solution is removed and replaced by fresh water. If brown precipitates of manganese (MnO_2 nH_2O) are observed, some phosphoric acid should be added and stirred through till they will have dissolved. Whether or not this phosphoric acid treatment is applied, the change of water should be repeated several times to remove the chemicals as complete as possible. Plants will not survive.

For disinfection of large ponds, as used for professional fish-breeding, permanganate is unsuitable. In such cases all fish of the infected water are to be destroyed, because even the survivors may remain carriers of living spores and spread the disease afterwards. The water of the ponds is drained off and disinfection performed by strewing 0.5–1 kg of calcium cyanamide per m^2 bottom area, to be added in two portions, the first at the end of November and the other at the end of March. Six weeks after the second treatment

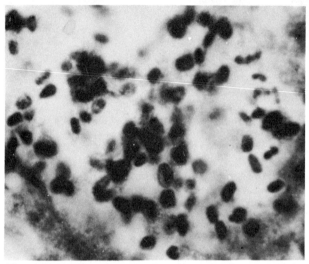

Fig. 4.5(g). Plistophora hyphessobryconis. *Spores at high magnification* × *3000. Haematoxyline stain (all photomicrographs by the author)*

the ponds may be filled and if the pH of the water proves correct, they may be put into use again; otherwise the water must be changed one or more times before setting fish. This treatment was originated by E. Tack.[6]

For disinfection of ponds in which infection with *Myxosoma cerebralis* (see p. 135) has occurred, addition of 10 g of malachite green per m^3 (1 mg/l) has been recommended.[7] Probably this dye could be of use for eradicating the spread of other sporozoan infections as well.

Infected fishes may be treated by administering acetarsone mixed with the food at a rate of 10 mg/kg fish during 3–4 successive days.

Boils, knots or pimples in fishes that are large enough for handling, may be opened by means of a flame-sterilised scalpel and scraped out; then the wounds are swabbed with a 0.1% solution of nitrofura-zone. The fishes are then put in a permanent bath of 1 g/50 l, to be added in three portions at intervals of 8–12 h, for 1–2 weeks, and they are also given this drug in the food at a rate of 0.01% during 2 weeks.

Any infected material should be thoroughly destroyed, either by burning it or using strong disinfectants such as 1% potassium permanganate, calcium cyanamide or sodium hypochlorite. Do not forget disinfection of your hands and of any instruments used!

Since mepacrine hydrochloride (atebrine) is known to be a very efficient anti-sporozoan agent in human medicine, it would seem worth while to give it a trial for treatment of sporozoan infections in aquarium fish. It should be used in a concentration up to 300 mg per 100 l, in the same way as described for treatment of stubborn cases of *Ichthyophthiriasis* (white spot) (see page 47). Success will depend on whether the drug will be adsorbed in the body of the fish and reach the encysted parasites which as yet cannot be predicted. The best chances may be expected in infections of the gills, since the gills are most capable of taking up dissolved substances from the water and then a good concentration of the drug in the circulating blood could be built up. It may also be tried as a food additive; a daily dosage of 1 mg per 100 g fish is suggested.

Another drug that might have some effect is furazolidone, to be administered mixed with the food. See page 327.

REFERENCES

1 VAN DUIJN, Jnr., C., 'Protozoan parasites of fish, sporozoan infections', *The Microscope* **9**, No. 9, 227–37 (Sept.–Oct. 1953), but completely revised and extended
2 HOFFMAN, G. L., and PUTZ, R. E., 'Host susceptibility and the effect of ageing, freezing, heat and chemicals on spores of *Myxosoma cerebralis*', *Progr. Fish-Cult.* **31**, 35 37 (1969)
3 SUMMERFELT, R. C., 'A new microsporidian parasite from the Golden Shiner [*Notemigonus crysoleucas (Cyprinidæ)*]', *Trans. Amer. Fish. Soc.* **93**, 6–10 (1964)
4 SCHÄPERCLAUS, W., 'Eine neue Microsporidienkrankheit beim Neonfisch und seinen Verwandten', *Wochenschrift für Aquarien- und Terrarienkunde* **38**, 381–84 (1941)
5 STOLK, A., *Het Aquarium* **21**, 187 (1950)
6 TACK, E., 'Bekämpfung der Drehkrankheit mit Kalkstickstoff', *Der Fischwirt* **1**, 123–30 (1951)
7 REICHENBACH-KLINKE, H., *Bestimmungschlüssel zur Diagnose von Fischkrankheiten*, Gustav Fischer Verlag, Stuttgart (1969)

5

DISEASES CAUSED BY
BACTERIA AND VIRUSES

Bacteria are micro-organisms of very small dimensions; usually between 0.5 and 10 μm. Thus a microscope with high power is required for their study. In the living state, bacteria show little contrast, due to the fact that their refractive index differs but little from that of water. It is, therefore, usual to stain preparations of bacteria.

The easiest way to obtain a good preparation is to make a smear of the material, containing the bacteria, on a microscope slide. It should be allowed to dry, and after this the preparation is fixed by drawing it through a flame (with the film-side upwards). Then the smear is covered with some drops of carbol fuchsine for three to five minutes. Following this it is washed under the tap until the water does not remove any more dye. The slide is dried again and is now ready for examination. If it must be preserved over a long period, it is advisable to place a very small drop of Canada balsam dissolved in xylene, or one of the modern synthetic resin mountants, on the smear and cover it with a cover glass, pressing the glass down so that only a very thin film of mountant remains. Should this film be too thick, observation with high-power microscope objectives is impossible.

An important method of staining is that of Gram. The bacteria are first stained with a 1% solution of crystal violet (5 min) and then immediately (without washing) treated for 1–2 min with an iodine solution (1 g of iodine mixed with 2–3 g of potassium iodide (KI) in a mortar and dissolved in a small volume of water. After the solids have been completely dissolved water is added to make the volume 300 cm^3). The preparation is then thoroughly washed with alcohol (96%) and the alcohol washed away with water. After this, a second staining is done with watery fuchsine (1% solution), the smear being subjected to it for about half a minute. The surplus dye is washed away with water, and after drying the preparation is ready for examination. With this method of staining, some bacteria will lose the violet dye when treated with alcohol while others will retain it. The former will then take the second dye and consequently some bacteria will appear with a violet colour, and the others, red. Bacteria that appear violet with the staining of Gram are called Gram-positive, and the others Gram-negative. This is an important feature in identifying bacteria. The majority of bacteria pathogenic to fish are Gram-negative.

Although a great number of species of bacteria are known, there are but slight differences in the shape and size of these organisms, so that, as a rule, it is impossible to identify them by microscopical examination.

To identify a bacterium it is necessary to cultivate it in different media and to observe which chemical changes it produces in these. Several precautions must be taken to make sure that a pure culture is obtained and that this remains pure, that is, only contains one single species and not a mixture of different kinds of bacteria. Therefore, bacteriological investigations can only be done by those who have had a special training in bacteriology and have access to a fully equipped laboratory.

Microscopical examinations of material from sick fishes can be done by laymen, if they possess a microscope with a $\frac{1}{12}$ in oil immersion objective, but in this way they can only determine the presence of bacteria and to which morphological group they belong. It is *impossible* by this means to say which species is present, whether it is pathogenic or harmless.

This must be kept in mind when investigating bacteria. Bacteria are found practically everywhere, in water and air, on plants and in the bodies of men and animals, etc. Most of them, however, are saprophytes (i.e. they feed on dead organic material and not living tissue) whose activity is of great importance in nature. Thus, if bacteria are found in the slime of the skin of a fish, or in its intestines, these may be saprophytes and it would be a great mistake to regard them as the cause of a disease without further evidence. The internal organs (except the intestine) of healthy fishes contain no bacteria; thus if bacteria are found in the heart, liver or ovary these may be the cause of the disease. This may only be concluded, however, if the material is taken from a fish which has been killed for examination and dissected immediately, or that has been dissected immediately after a natural death. This precaution is necessary as bacteria from the intestine (where they are normally present in large numbers) spread, soon after death, to other organs and their discovery would then be no indication that they were the cause of disease.

Fortunately, most bacterial diseases show characteristic symptoms which enable us to recognise them with sufficient accuracy for practical purposes, without making a complete bacteriological examination. Bacterial infections may occur in the internal organs, in the muscles and in the skin, including the fins. In nearly all cases where the skin or the muscles, or both, are affected, red spots show, which are called ecchymoses.

Fishes that are not weakened by bad conditions, or by infections with other parasites, generally have a great resistance to bacterial infections. This is due to the presence of a large amount of bactericidal substances in the blood which helps them to overcome an infection. But if they are wounded, or their resistance is decreased by other causes, bacterial infections may not be conquered easily. Consequently the best precaution against the occurrence of illness among fish is the keeping of them under the best conditions, i.e. in clean tanks

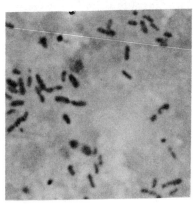

Fig. 5.1. Bacteria in a smear preparation from the liver of a diseased   Acara   (× 2500 approx.)

which are well planted and receive enough light (natural or artificial) to enable the plants to produce plenty of oxygen and the provision of suitable food. Cleanliness of the tank is important, especially in the case of bacterial and fungus infections, since these organisms thrive in water that contains much dead organic material. Decaying of such substances is due to the activity of bacteria and fungi.

Most of the bacteria (Figs 5.1 and 5.2) that cause diseases of fish can only attack if the fish have been injured or weakened, but some

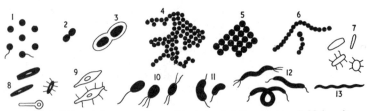

Fig. 5.2. The more important forms of bacteria: 1, Micrococcus. 2, Neisseria. 3, Diplococcus. 4, Staphylococcus. 5, Sarcina. 6, Streptococcus. 7, Bacterium. 8, Bacillus. 9, Clostridium. 10, Pseudomonas. 11, Vibrio. 12, Spirillum. 13, Spirochæte. Note the shape and arrangement of each

species have greater pathogenic capacities and may even attack completely healthy undamaged fishes. It is often difficult to say whether or not bacteria are the primary cause of a disease. Our knowledge of bacterial diseases of fish is still incomplete. With regard to the identification and nomenclature of bacteria pathogenic to fish, considerable confusion exists. This is partially due to deficiencies in the description of bacteria isolated from diseased fishes, and on the other hand, to the difficulties in obtaining reliable experimental material from animals that are surrounded by a medium in which all kinds of bacteria closely related to pathogenic species are present. Furthermore, experimental fishes, as required for artificial infection tests for proving the pathogenicity of isolated strains of bacteria, cannot be kept under aseptic conditions. Consequently, knowledge is still scanty and often controversial.

VIRUS INFECTIONS

Viruses are infectious agents of very small dimensions, which pass through filters that retain bacteria. Although some of the larger ones form particles that can just be seen in the optical microscope with the highest magnification, the exact shapes and dimensions can only be determined by means of the electron microscope, while further information is obtained from electron diffraction microscopy. The group is heterogeneous, some of them showing some differentiation so that they could be regarded as living organisms, while others consist of autocatalytic crystals only.

Viruses multiply locally in the cells of the body and form inclusion bodies in the cells. Very little is known about virus disease in fish, which is not surprising since for investigating viruses even more elaborate and expensive laboratory equipment is required than in dealing with bacterial infections.

TREATMENT OF BACTERIAL INFECTIONS

Until the introduction of modern drugs, such as the sulpha compounds and the antibiotics, very few bacterial diseases of fish could be treated with reasonable chance of success. Today the position is different and we are able to combat a number of these infections successfully, at least in theory, since often the actual use of the curative agent may be prevented by prohibitive cost or by Government regulations not permitting its being sold to laymen. In Great Britain, especially, restrictions are severe. In consequence of this, most experimental work with antibiotics for the treatment of fish diseases has been done in the U.S.A. where it seems to be rather easy to obtain any antibiotic at the chemist's even without a doctor's prescription. This has resulted in the use of antibiotics for treatment of all kinds of fish diseases, which is a rather dangerous situation.

Antibiotics should never be used for treatment of diseases which can also be cured by ordinary chemicals. It is now a well-established fact that indiscriminate application of antibiotics may result, and often does result, in producing resistant strains of bacteria so that infections may spread that can no longer be eradicated by the antibiotic. This is most likely to occur if too low dosages are given. With these drugs it is generally more harmful to use them in a too low dosage than in a too strong one.

Indiscriminate use of antibiotics may also result in a serious disturbance of biological and biochemical equilibrium in a tank, since non-pathogenic bacteria, which are necessary to break down waste products of animal and plant metabolism, are also killed. Treatments should not, therefore, be extended over longer periods than are required to obtain a cure.

Since treatment of bacterial diseases of fish follows principally the same lines, a general survey of such methods will be given before dealing with specific infections.

'SULPHA DRUGS'

From the group of the sulphonamides, or sulpha drugs, there are several which can be used for treatment of fish. Among these are sulphanilamide, sulphadiazine, sulphamerazine, sulphamethazine, sulphaguanidine and sulphisoxazole. The first mentioned is less expensive than the others. There is no difference in efficaciousness to be expected between these compounds.

Sulphanilamide may be used in amounts of 10–25 g to 100 l (0.45–1.1 g/Imp. gal or 0.37–0.95 g/U.S. gal). Fishes can stand this concentration very well for several days, but the cure should not be extended over a longer period, otherwise toxic reactions may occur, consisting in renal damage, anaemia and leukopenia. Generally, three days' treatment should be sufficient. If no recovery is observed after five days, the drug must be considered to be ineffective, and no further treatment of this kind given. After treatment, a complete change of water should be made.

In America, sulphamerazine has been used extensively, mixed with the food, for treatment of bacterial infections in Trout. Dosage 8 g of sulphamerazine per 100 lb of Trout per day (about 175 mg per kilogram Trout). Extensive medication with this drug, giving it regularly as a prophylactic to control endemic furunculosis, for a period of eight months, caused massive kidney damage, similar to that observed in humans with sulpha drug intoxication.[1] In female Brook Trout, treated in this way for two years, sterility was produced. Feeding sulpha drugs for periods up to 13 weeks did not produce renal damage.

Growth of fingerling Brook Trout (*Salmo* or *Salvelinus fontinalis*) was somewhat retarded by sulphamerazine, but no such effect was observed in the Rainbow Trout (*Salmo gairdneri*).[2] Sulphisoxazole did not retard growth of these species and of Brown Trout (*Salmo trutta*); on the contrary, growth stimulation was observed on prolonged treatment of juvenile Chinook Salmon.[3] With present knowledge, this appears to be the best suited sulpha drug for treatment of fishes. The growth of Brown Trout was retarded by sulphamerazine, but as soon as the medicated food was replaced by normal, growth was resumed. Snieszko warns that caution is recommended, since chemotherapeutic agents are species-specific with regard to their side-effects on the hosts and the control of pathogenic bacteria; therefore results obtained in treatment of one disease in one species of fish should not be generalised without experimental support.

All sulpha drugs appear to make the fishes liable to a secondary superficial fungal growth on the gills with prolonged treatment (up to 30 days); this may cause casualties.[3] This risk, too, is least with sulphisoxazole.

Whereas in large fish ponds and hatcheries adding the drugs to the food appears to be the only suitable method of treatment, in small garden ponds and in aquaria addition of sulphonamides to the water is to be preferred. With this way of application, the risk of renal damage in the fish is decreased, whereas the pathogenic bacteria that are spread into the water are attacked also.

Sulphisoxazole can also be used in marine aquaria. Daily addition of 0.96 mg/l for one month did not impair general health of Killifish (*Fundulus heteroclitus*), although adrenal inactivity was indicated in some as well as a slight effect on the liver.[4]

'ANTIBIOTICS'

Among the antibiotics, penicillin is not a promising substance for treatment of bacterial infections in fish. Penicillin is highly active against a number of Gram-positive bacteria but has less or no activity against most Gram-negative species, and, as previously stated, the latter are the most common infectious agents in bacterial diseases of fish. Further, penicillin is destroyed comparatively rapidly in aquarium water. In fact, the only report known of a case where penicillin has cured a bacterial infection in fish refers to local treatment of tuberculous wounds with penicillin ointment, although it has been claimed to be effective against fungus and also against white spot (a protozoan infection) in a concentration of at least 100 000 units to 100 litres, or approximately 5000 units to the gallon. A more promising compound seems to be ampicilline (a synthetic penicillin-derivative, a.o. sold under the trade name Penbritin[R]) which may be administered as a food additive. A capsule of 250 mg is equivalent to one million I.U. of penicillin, but it attacks many more bacterial species than penicillin; among these are *Proteus* infections.

Chloromycetin^R (chloramphenicol) and Aureomycin^R (chlortetracycline) are active against many Gram-positive and Gram-negative bacteria and some viruses, while chlortetracycline is also known to be efficient for killing certain protozoans. Chloramphenicol should be used in a dosage of not less than 25 mg, preferably 30–50 mg per Imp. gal. As previously stated, with antibiotics strong dosages are always to be preferred lest resistant strains of bacteria should develop. Too low dosages would do much more harm than good.

Another method of application of chloramphenicol is by adding it to granulated food, at a rate of 1 g/1 kg of food. This treatment was found effective in preventing epizootics of infectious dropsy in Carp in Russia, whereas adding the drug to the water with a concentration of 1 g/l had no effect. Healing of Carps with manifest dropsy was accomplished by three injections given in the intestines.[5]

According to H. R. Axelrod, chlortetracycline should be used in a concentration of 600 mg/Imp. gal (500 mg/U.S. gal). While lower dosages may be lethal to many pathogenic bacteria, there are likely to be some survivors which become resistant to the drug; thus, although the first infection may be successfully combated, in a later outbreak of disease the same antibiotic would be of no use.[6]

Axelrod stated that toxicity tests have shown that chlortetracycline is harmless to fish in concentrations up to 2.4 g/Imp. gal (2 g/U.S. gal). Nevertheless, after recovery the fish should be placed in fresh water, since the same would not hold in the long run.

Chlortetracycline acts as a growth factor for pigs, chickens and turkeys. If young fish are given foods containing chlortetracycline growth rate is accelerated and they show more intense colour at an earlier time, but it has been shown that this will result in a *loss of fertility*, unless a supply of several vitamins is added to the food at the same time. Chlortetracycline causes a *deficiency* in vitamins of the B-complex, especially of vitamin B_{12}, together with vitamins E and K. Vitamin E is required for fertility, so it is not astonishing that sterility should result from continuous feeding or other contact of fish with chlortetracycline. Although this phenomenon can be prevented by supplying the deficient vitamins (as is done in certain proprietary foods) the writer thinks that caution is needed in experimenting with these drugs. See also the article by *Water Life Analyst*.[7]

Dr. Aaron Wold observed serious secondary effects of chlortetracycline treatment in a concentration of 300 mg/Imp. gal (250 mg/U.S. gal). After four days of continuous contact with this concentration, the fish became hollow-bellied, refused to eat, swam at the surface and finally died.[8] It is not reasonable to let fish remain in contact with chlortetracycline for such a long period; using a heavy dosage, 48 h should be sufficient to obtain a cure. Contrary to

Axelrod, Wold recommended low dosages of 60 mg/Imp. gal (50 mg/ U.S. gal). Since chlortetracycline has no advantage over chlor- amphenicol with respect to action against bacteria pathogenic to fish, whereas chloramphenicol apparently lacks the unwanted side- effects described for chlortetracycline, this latter drug cannot be recommended but should always be replaced by chloramphenicol for antibiotic treatment of bacterial infections in fish.

Axelrod has also suggested the use of oxytetracycline (generally known under the trade name 'Terramycin', registered by the manufacturers Messrs. Pfizer). I found it reasonably effective against fish tuberculosis when applied dissolved in aquarium water, but it is not very stable under aquarium conditions and develops toxic properties on prolonged treatment.[9] The method of applica- tion by mixing it with the food, although more laborious, seems to be more appropriate and was found successful in treatment of *Aeromonas* (formerly *Pseudomonas* or *Chromobacterium*) *punctata* infec- tions in Golden Shiners by F. P. Meyer.[10] A ration containing 0.83 g Terramycin activity per pound of feed (approximately equivalent with 1.8 g per kilogram of feed) at the rate of 3% of body weight each day for eight days effected a cure. The virulence of the bacteria was proved in infection experiments at the laboratory. More recently Terramycin (oxytetracycline) has also been applied for injection therapy, at a rate of 3 mg/150–400 g fish.

Addition of Terramycin to the food caused an enhancement in growth rate of some fresh-water fishes.[11]

Robert G. Piper tried erythromycin thiocyanate for treatment of kidney disease in the American Rainbow Trout (*Salmo gairdneri*), caused by unidentified *Corynebacterium* species (Gram-positive), but found it toxic. The drug was administered orally by mixing it with the food at the rate of 45 mg of drug per pound of fish per day for 21 days.[12]

D. A. Conroy has experimented with kanamycin and found it highly effective against infections with bacteria belonging to the *Pseudomonadaceæ* and for treatment of tail- and fin-rot.[13] It was applied by intraperitoneal injection of 20 µg of kanamycin per gram fish (1 microgram = µg = 0.001 milligram). Oral administra- tion (mixed with the food) did not give favourable results in his experiments, although Hering in South Africa in a personal communication mentioned by Conroy has been successful in curing tail-rot and 'red mouth' disease in this way. Experiments with kanamycin dissolved in the water of the tank in which the fishes are swimming were not promising, except in later investigations where *Aeromonas punctata* was the principal invader (see p. 178). Treatment of fishes by injection requires special skill and is probably illegal in Britain if performed by unqualified persons, since it may be regarded as constituting some kind of surgery.

Streptomycin, the first antibiotic detected after penicillin, has been suggested by Schäperclaus for treatment of bacterial infections in fish, either by injection or by adding 10 mg/l of water. For injection 10–20 μg/g fish could be tried. Actual results, however, were inferior to those obtained with kanamycin.

Streptomycin has proved to be highly toxic to *Tubifex* worms, the medium tolerance limit being 0.5 mg/cm^3 which is much lower than the tolerance of blue-green algae and Gram-negative bacteria.[14]

The addition of antibiotics to the food did not influence the reproductive ability of Guppies (*Lebistes reticulatus*) if *Tubifex* was fed, but if peas were given as the main food, the number of offspring increased by 28% after application of chlortetracycline with vitamin B_{12} ('Aureovit'), 31% after procain-penicillin and 20% after oxytetracycline (less convincing).[15] A positive result occurred especially with a plant-feeding ration, where the antibiotics apparently had the effect of allowing a better utilisation of less-valuable proteins.

Ghittino[16] found antibiotic therapy of virus-infected Sockeye Salmon helpful against secondary infections.

PHENOXETHOL

While antibiotics may be the most effective substances against the majority of bacterial diseases of fish, there are other chemicals available which have proved effective against some of these infections. They are inexpensive compared with drugs such as Chloromycetin^R (chloramphenicol) and Aureomycin^R (chlortetracycline).

Phenoxethol and some of its derivatives have proved to be good cures for tail- and fin-rot and other bacterial complaints.[17]

Stock solutions of the substances are made up as follows: phenoxethol: 1 cm^3 phenoxethol + 99 cm^3 of water (1% v/v). Propylene phenoxethol: as for phenoxethol (1% v/v). *Para*-chloro-phenoxethol: 0.1 g of *para*-chlorophenoxethol dissolved in hot water with vigorous shaking, and diluted to 100 cm^3 (0.1% w/v). Allow to cool.

Phenoxethol, it is pointed out, may be used in the concentration 10 cm^3 of stock solution per litre of aquarium water, and the same applies for propylene phenoxethol. *Para*-chlorophenoxethol has been used at 50 cm^3 of stock solution per litre or, for greater convenience, the required weight is calculated (0.05 g/l), dissolved in hot water, and slowly added to the tank water. *However, this latter compound has been found to be highly toxic to some species of fish, so it cannot be recommended for general use*; see page 340.

The dose may be added direct to the tank (it should not damage plants) if epidemic conditions exist, or single cases may be treated in glass or enamel containers. It is important that the fish receive an adequate supply of oxygen, especially if propylene phenoxethol is used. None of the phenoxethols decomposes rapidly, so it is unnecessary to make further additions unless the disease proves resistant. The temperature should be maintained at or above 16°C (approx. 60°F). Generally fin-rot cases improve after three days of treatment but, if no progress is apparent after this period, the affected portion of the fin should be cut away.

Cases of white fungus normally improve within 24 h in phenoxethol and 4 to 5 h in *para*-chlorophenoxethol. This will depend on the kind of fungus causing the infection. The therapeutic action of the phenoxethols may be accelerated by the addition of a small quantity of calcium chloride or sodium chloride (salt). It should be remembered that both fin-rot and fungus may occur as secondary conditions to other diseases, and treatment will not cure them unless the primary disease is dealt with also.

It is difficult to assess the reaction of all fish to treatment with the phenoxethols, and most of the research has been connected with varieties of Goldfish. Where tropical fish are concerned it is advisable to add the total dose in two parts, with a 24-hour interval between each. This is especially important with *para*-chlorophenoxethol, where a slow drip addition is probably the best method. Young Veiltails remained in phenoxethol for a month without showing signs of discomfort and Red Swordtails were 'dropped' in *para*-chlorophenoxethol and were growing well. Phenoxethol has been used in conjunction with quinine dihydrochloride for the treatment of white spot and its complications in adult Veiltails. All three phenoxethols may be used in conjunction with acriflavine and penicillin (doses not yet known) but not with formaldehyde. As has been stated previously, however (p. 153), penicillin is quite useless for treatment of bacterial diseases in fish.

Other diseases for which Rankin suggested the phenoxethols may be effective are: *Ichthyophonus*, bacterial dropsy, cotton wool disease ('mouth fungus'), 'bloom' disease, scale protrusion and bacterial and fungal diseases generally. The phenoxethols can generally be regarded as ineffective against diseases of animal origin and *para*-chlorophenoxethol is the only one that shows some activity in this field, but this proved highly toxic to some species of fish, such as Guppies and Kissing Gouramies. It should be remembered that these drugs were designed for use against the fungi and bacteria, which are included in the Plant Kingdom.

Propylene phenoxethol in higher concentrations acts as an anaesthetic. Bagenal used it on Plaice (*Pleuronectes platessa*) in seawater and found a 0.01–0.025% solution a useful anaesthetic for periods up to 1 h in aquarium fish of a wide range in size.[18] In a 0.01% solution Plaice were limp after 20 min and could recover after having been in it for 2 h, but not after 3 h. In a 0.025% solution complete anaesthesia occurred after 5 min and fishes were able to recover after 30 min, but not after 1 h of contact with the drug. In the anaesthetised condition, surgery on fish may be performed by qualified persons.

Phenoxethols may also be mixed with dried food and given orally, as described for treatment of *Ichthyophonus* infections (see page 258).

OTHER CHEMOTHERAPEUTICS

Another powerful modern drug is furazolidone. It has been found effective against furunculosis in trout when applied in the feed.[19] Force feeding of up to 500 mg per kilogram body weight per day for 14 days did not produce pathological effects, but even at lower dosages indications of toxicity have been noted. A dosage of 25 mg per kilogram body weight of fish per day for 14 days was sufficient to control mortality and prevent recurrence of the disease after withdrawal of medication, whereas at 10 mg per kilogram body weight per day, while checking mortality, furunculosis recurred when treatment was stopped.

Furazolidone is successfully employed in veterinary practice for treatment of diseases of poultry, caused by bacteria of the *Salmonella* group, by sporozoans and flagellates (*Hexamita*). Therefore it may be expected to prove of more general value in treatment of diseases of fishes than can be indicated now.

A chemically related compound, nitrofurazone, is effective against many Gram-positive and Gram-negative bacteria and sporozoans. It may be used as a 0.1% solution for local treatment of skin lesions (swabbing wounds and inflamed parts), avoiding contact with the healthy parts of the skin, with the gills and the eyes. Internally, it may be given in the food at a rate of 0.01%, for one week to maximally two weeks. As a permanent bath the recommended strength is 1 g in 50 l of water (or 1.37 gr/Imp. gal, or 1.14 gr/U.S. gal), to be added in 3 portions at intervals of 8–12 h; total period of treatment from 3 days up to 3 weeks. This treatment seems promising but is still in the experimental stage. Stolk has reported that at 1 g in 40 l it should be effective against white spot as well.

Pyridyl mercuric acetate (PMA), technical quality, has been used successfully for treatment of bacterial infections of the gills in Salmon and Trout, and of external protozoan infections in all fishes. It is used at a concentration of no more than two parts in a million (2 mg/l) for 1 h.[20] Sockeye, Chinook and Coho Salmon, and Brook Trout can stand this treatment perfectly well, but the chemical proved to be toxic to older Rainbow Trout.[21] One should therefore be cautious when treating other fishes, especially small aquarium fish. Treated fishes will accumulate mercury in their internal organs.

Acriflavine has been successfully applied against tail- and fin-rot, and seems to be promising for the effective treatment of other infections as well.

For local treatment of inflamed parts of the body, some further chemicals can be useful, such as merthiolate and iodine. These should never be used for bathing the fish since they are very toxic and would kill it when applied in this way.

Fish eggs may sometimes be carriers of fish pathogenic bacteria, especially if the spawning adults bear an infection. This holds for *Aeromonas salmonicida* (causing fish furunculosis) and *A. liquefaciens*. Viable bacteria do not enter the eggs, but they are carried on the outer surface of the eggshell only, enabling surface disinfection, which has been successfully performed with the organic iodine compound povidone-iodine, whereas washing with sulphomerthiolate, merthiolate or acriflavine proved unreliable.[22]

COTTON WOOL DISEASE ('MOUTH FUNGUS'), COLUMNARIS DISEASE

This disease is characterised by the occurrence of a fungus-like growth resembling white cotton or cotton-wool at the mouth and cheeks of the fish. Whitish-grey spots may appear at the head, the fins, the gills and the body. The lips may become swollen and gradually take on an almost macerated appearance. The fins may get ragged, too. The infected fishes lose their appetite. Their movements may become sluggish. If no adequate treatment is given, serious damage is done. The whole frontal part of the head is sometimes eaten away and finally the fish dies. The popular name 'mouth fungus' is inaccurate and should be discarded, since this complaint has nothing whatsoever to do with true fungus infection.

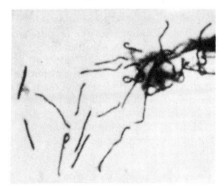

Fig. 5.3. Myxobacteria *found in columnaris disease (after a photomicrograph by H. S. Davis in Reichenbach-Klinke, 1966)*

Cotton wool disease is caused by slime bacteria (*Myxobacteria*), either *Chondrococcus columnaris* or another species, *Cytophaga columnaris*—see Fig. 5.3. Both species consist of Gram-negative slender rods. The disease is contagious. *Chondrococcus columnaris* has also been described as infecting the skin, fins and gills of *Fundulus heteroclitus* in brackish and sea-water, as well as in other marine fishes.[23]

For treatment, good results have been obtained by phenoxethol, and also by sulphonamides and by pyridyl mercuric acetate. Of these, I would recommend phenoxethol, for aquarium fishes in early stages of the infection, as being the safest with respect to the fish. Pyridyl mercuric acetate should be used with caution, because it may produce toxic reactions in some species of fish (dosage 2 mg/l for 1 h).

Chloromycetin (chloramphenicol; 5–10 mg/l) and Aureomycin (chlortetracycline; 10–20 mg/l) have both proved to be effective. Using a full dosage in an early stage of the disease, successful recovery can be expected at the end of 48 h.

Other treatments having been advocated are a 'dipping' treatment with copper sulphate 1 : 2000 for 1–2 min only (to be used with utmost caution, see page 56), or malachite green 1 : 15 000 for 10–30 sec (not recommended for small aquarium fishes).

For treatment of ponds, addition of 1 mg copper sulphate per litre has been recommended for disinfection. Heavily affected pond fishes may be successfully treated by feeding them drugged food, prepared by admixing sulphamerazine or preferably sulphisoxazole (see p. 352) at a rate of 200–240 mg/kg fish. Sulphamerazine is rather toxic to Brown Trout.

Swabbing the mouth with Lilly's tincture of merthiolate seems to arrest the disease instantly, according to Clarence H. Butler.[24] Disinfection of the tank is accomplished by adding 1 cm³ to 2.5–4 Imp. gal (or 3–5 U.S. gal) after the fishes have been removed. Following such disinfection, the water must be changed completely.

Arthur S. Campbell recommended a treatment with Brilliant Green.[25] Four grains of the dye are dissolved in just sufficient ethanol (alcohol) and this amount is added to one U.S. gallon of water. The fish is caught in a small net and, while it is in the net, it is dipped into the dye solution for 45 sec. It has been claimed that one treatment would cure the most stubborn cases. However, from the very short duration of the treatment, it might be taken to be a rather drastic procedure. It is suggested that it would be better to swab the mouth with a small pencil or brush dipped into the dye solution, rather than dip the whole fish.

Hydrogen peroxide treatment has also been stated to be effective. For details, see page 328.

TAIL- AND FIN-ROT (*BACTERIOSES PINNARUM*)

This disease is completely characterised by its name, symptoms being putrefaction of the tail or other fins, or both, and in most cases ecchymoses are visible. The tail becomes torn and is gradually consumed by the activity of the bacteria (Fig. 5.4). Frequently a secondary fungus infection occurs. Fishes that have much pigment are more susceptible to this pest than others, e.g. Black Mollies.

The condition is generally associated with fish who are in low health. Protracted low temperature, dirty living conditions, gas embolism, damage and weakness caused by other disease, may be predisposing causes. In Veiltail stock, even if a cure is effected, it may cause permanent malformation of the all-important caudal fin. Although not normally an infectious condition the disease may attain epidemic proportions in the tropical tank, sometimes attacking the

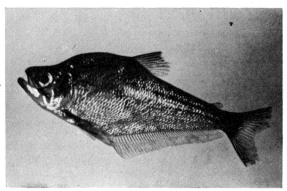

Fig. 5.4.
CHARAX
WITH TAIL-
AND FIN-ROT
Photograph by C.
J. M. Timmerman
showing a species of
Charax *infected by*
fin- and tail-rot.
With these diseases,
primarily bacterial
in origin, fungus
may appear as a
serious secondary
infection

members of one particular species. Black Mollies appear very susceptible to contamination of this kind, and have been known to die within 24 h of their inclusion in a tank where Platies were suffering from fin-rot.

Excessive illumination or ultraviolet irradiation has also been reported to induce the condition, the damage done to the fin tissues probably opening the way to bacterial infections. It has also been shown that susceptibility to fin-rot is increased by lack of inositol in the food.

It has not yet been possible to clear the aetiology of the disease or to ascribe its cause to any single species of bacteria. Snieszko[26] could isolate *Hæmophilus piscium* and *Aeromonas salmonicida* along with other undetermined species from Trout showing symptoms of fin-rot, whereas Conroy[27] could produce tail- and fin-rot experimentally by injecting fishes with pure cultures of *Aeromonas punctata*. From spontaneous cases of the disease Conroy isolated *Pseudomonas putida*, *Aeromonas punctata* and *Aeromonas liquefaciens*. Reichenbach-Klinke also mentions *Pseudomonas fluorescens, Ps. granulata, Aeromonas hydrophila* (a close relative of *A. punctata*) and *Myxobacterium* species. Other, but unidentified, strains of bacteria have been isolated by other investigators. It would appear that the infection may be caused by a number of different kinds of bacteria that just happen to be present when the resistance of the fins or tail of fishes has been weakened by mechanical damage (such as wounds obtained in fights) or other undue conditions.

Tail-rot is a serious complaint. If the infection spreads on to the body of the fish it will be too late to effect a cure, so early treatment is very important.

Until recently, there was but one reliable method to cure a diseased fish and that was surgical. Although surgical treatment still may be required in advanced cases, we are now in a position to be able to save many fishes from death by less drastic methods, especially by treatment with phenoxethol, with acriflavine and with the antibiotics kanamycin and chloramphenicol (Chloromycetin[R]). It has been stated that ozone for 1 h, repeated three to four times a day, will effect a cure in 10 days[28] (see also page 338).

PHENOXETHOL AND ITS DERIVATIVES

C. E. Bowers reported successful treatment of fin-rot by means of phenoxethol (there is an error in this statement regarding the dosage; '10 milligrams' of stock solution should read '10 cm^3'.[29] At an earlier date I had suggested that phenoxethol might be valuable in the treatment of bacterial infections, in a personal communication to Rankin. He has reported that he also has succeeded in curing fin-rot with it.[30]

Phenoxethol and related compounds are active against penicillin-resistant, Gram-negative organisms of a similar kind to those associated with many fish diseases. The compounds referred to are phenoxethol B.P.C., propylene phenoxethol and *para*-chlorophenoxethol. (The official name of these drugs is spelt with 'th', but in some papers it is spelt 'phenoxetol', which is a registered trade name according to *The Merck Index of Chemicals and Drugs*, 7th Edn., Rahway, N.J., U.S.A., 1960.)

Cultures from fin-rot sections revealed motile Gram-negative organisms which were easily destroyed by the phenoxethols. An extract from Rankin's casebook illustrates this: Fin-rot, Case 2: Goldfish, caudal fin almost completely lost. Successfully treated in tank with phenoxethol. Initial culture on blood agar. Result of test on culture two, carried out by Dr. Erich Boehm. The organisms were killed by 1.25% phenoxethol within 5 min, 0.75% propylene phenoxethol within 5 min, 0.30% *para*-chlorophenoxethol within 5 min, 0.75% phenol after 2 h.

The test shows that *para*-chlorophenoxethol was the most effective agent against these organisms *in theory*, as was also shown in actual practice. It is a peculiar property of phenolic bactericides that halving a given dose more than halves the antibacterial activity, thus *para*-chlorophenoxethol was a great deal more effective than the other chemicals.

It is of interest to note that the organisms must be very hardy to resist the strong phenol solution for 2 h. Dr. Boehm also pointed out that they survived a temperature of 100°C (moist heat) maintained for 20 min and that they caused an infection of the eye in guinea-pigs. Rankin's *in vitro* results show that more than ten times the therapeutic dose of phenoxethol is necessary to inhibit the growth of these organisms, and yet the fish are obviously cured by the normal amount. The reason for so large a disparity is not yet understood.

ACRIFLAVINE TREATMENT

In America, acriflavine has been found to be effective against tail- and fin-rot. This treatment should be applied as follows: A stock solution is prepared by dissolving one tablet in 330 cm^3 of water. At first the sore spots are swabbed with a small pencil or brush dipped into this stock solution, and then the fish is placed in a container with 10 cm^3 of the stock solution per Imp. gal for three days (8 cm^3/ U.S. gal).

The water is then changed and the diseased places are swabbed again with the stock solution, after which the fish is placed in clean, fresh water for one or two days. If necessary, next day the fish is again placed into the acriflavine solution for a further three days' (maximum up to four days') treatment. If, after this period, complete recovery should not have been attained, only surgical treatment remains.

SURGICAL TREATMENT

Take the fish in the hand and cut the affected fins with a pair of scissors. The fins must be cut through where they are not yet rotten so that it may be quite certain that the remaining part is free from the infection. It is better to cut a part that is too large than one that is too small for, if the infected part is not completely removed, putrefaction will continue and then it will be much more difficult to cure the fish by another operation. After surgical treatment the wounds must be disinfected to avoid fresh infection. This may be done by touching them with a small pencil or brush dipped into a 1% solution of silver nitrate ($AgNO_3$) in distilled water, followed by touching the wound in the same way with a 1% solution of potassium dichromate.

After this has been done the fish is placed in clean, fresh water, to which potassium dichromate (1 : 25 000) is added (2½ gr/Imp. gal or approximately 2 gr/U.S. gal), where it must remain for a week to ten days. After this time the wounds will have healed. If the wounds are seen to have healed earlier, do not prolong treatment, but change the water at once.

Take care to give the fish the best possible conditions during the period of recovery; give it plenty of oxygen, using artificial aeration when necessary, and supply good, nourishing food. The cut fins will regenerate, but this will take time.

In advanced cases of tail- or fin-rot it is advisable to resort to surgical treatment at once and apply acriflavine during 3–5 days as an after-treatment. I must add, however, that surgery on animals, even for the purpose of curing them from a dangerous disease, is illegal in Britain if it is undertaken by persons who are unqualified.

CHLORAMPHENICOL (Chloromycetin). Small aquarium fishes may be treated with the usual dosage of 13 mg/l (60 mg/Imp. gal; 50 mg/U.S. gal), combined with feeding them with a suitable food to which 1 mg per gram of food has been added.

For fishes of at least 10 g weight, dosage may be increased to 50 mg/l for up to 24 h only, or (according to Reichenbach-Klinke) to 80 mg/l for not more than 8 h.

KANAMYCIN

Recent experiments by Conroy have shown that good results can often be achieved with kanamycin added to the water at a rate of 3.1 mg/l (14 mg/Imp. gal or 11.7 mg/U.S. gal).

Fishes that are sufficiently big to handle may be treated by intra-peritoneal injection of 20 μg (0.02 mg) of kanamycin per gram fish. The treatment can be combined with chloramphenicol, to be added to the food at a rate of 1 mg per gram of food. Combined treatments with different types of antibiotics is generally employed in human and veterinary medicine in cases where bacterial infections exist that easily develop resistance against antibiotics and chemo-therapeutics; this unwanted phenomenon is less likely to occur when drugs are applied in combination with each other.

OTHER TREATMENTS

Other drugs that have been reported to be effective are sulphadiazine (see page 351) and a German commercial product called Aquarol (see page 319).[31]

APPEARANCE OF TAIL-ROT IN NEWTS

Tail-rot may also appear in newts. Bathing them in a solution of any drug cannot be expected to be effective with these animals, however, since chemicals administered from the outside will not reach the tissues in which the infection has spread. Therefore, with newts, surgery is the only reasonable treatment. Since the tail of a newt is much stronger in build than the tail fin of a fish, it is better to cut it with a razor instead of using scissors. For disinfection a 1% solution of silver nitrate $(AgNO_3)$ (1 g dissolved in 100 cm^3 of distilled water) may be recommended, followed by touching the wound with a 1% solution of potassium dichromate. After this, the animal is placed in a 1 : 25 000 solution of potassium dichromate, as mentioned previously.

Newts are excellently suited for treatment with antibiotics by injection and *per os* (in the food). Kanamycin is to be used in a dosage of 1 mg per gram of newt (weighing them on a letter scale is not too difficult) and this is injected at the root of the tail, the hypodermic needle to be inserted pointing in the direction of the tail-end.

This treatment is to be combined by adding 1 mg of chloramphenicol per gram of food, which is accomplished most easily by injecting the required amount into small earth-worms or enchytrae, to be swallowed by the newt immediately afterwards.

The methods of treatment listed will bring success in all cases where the infection has not been allowed to penetrate to the body of the victim.

TAIL- AND FIN-ROT IN MARINE FISHES

In fish kept in salt-water aquaria tail- and fin-rot is very common and often occurs epidemically. Generally, the first symptom is the occurrence of a haemorrhagic area under the scales near the peduncle and this is followed by progressive erosion and fraying of fins and tail and later on by roughening, raising and a general sloughing-off of the tail region. Bacteria isolated from diseased fishes include *Vibrio* (*Pseudomonas*) *ichthyodermis* (ZoBell and Upham) and not further identified *Pseudomonas* species.

According to Oppenheimer,[32] effective treatment may be obtained by injecting a mixture of penicillin and streptomycin at the concentration recommended per unit weight. Addition of oxytetracycline (Terramycin[R]) to the food has also been reported to be effective.[33]

Riseley advocates a combined treatment with iodine and chlortetracycline (Aureomycin[R]).[34] The infected parts are gently touched with an iodine solution (commercial 10% solution in ethanol diluted ten times with sea-water). Then the treated fish are allowed to recover for a short time in well-aerated sea-water until the shock of this treatment has diminished. Next they are placed in a clean tank with chlortetracycline (one capsule containing 250 mg in 18 l—or 4 Imp. gal or 5 U.S. gal—of sea-water). Treatment should not be continued for more than 3–4 days; the causative bacteria should be effectively defeated during that period and the fins should have started to grow. In bad cases the strength of the antibiotic solution is increased by 50%.

For big fishes Riseley recommends swabbing the diseased parts with a strong solution of Aureomycin in sea-water and then putting them directly in the stronger bath.

Although Riseley does not discuss the pH of the sea-water in the tropical marine aquaria where he applied these treatments successfully, it should be pointed out that chlortetracycline rapidly loses its antibiotic effect in sea-water at pH 8.2.[32] Therefore I advise checking the pH value of the water prior to deciding on the best policy of treatment in a specific case.

Riseley further reported to have used Achromycin (= tetracycline) in the same way and with the same dosage and to have found it effective.

PEDUNCLE DISEASE

This is essentially a variety of tail-rot in which the caudal fin is eroded away, the caudal part of the body being attacked next (Fig. 5.5). Among tropicals, fishes with high amounts of black pigment, such as Black Mollies, appear most susceptible. This condition is the

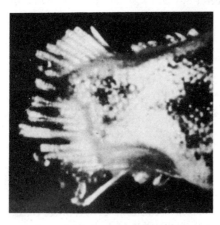

Fig. 5.5. Tail end of an American Sea Trout, suffering from peduncle disease caused by Myxobacteria *(after a photograph by Snieszko, taken from Reichenbach-Klinke, 1966)*

most severe form of tail-rot, requiring drastic treatment at once, either by intramuscular injection of kanamycin into the affected area or, where this is impossible, by giving minced meat drugged with chloramphenicol and sulphadiazine as the food, and applying a silver nitrate and potassium dichromate treatment locally as described for treatment of eye fungus (pages 213–214).

DROPSY (*HYDROPS* OR *ASCITES*)

This trouble consists of an accumulation of liquid in one or other of the internal organs or the tissues. In human beings dropsy often occurs in heart or kidney disease. In fish, the disease usually affects the belly, which may swell to a considerable extent so that the victim looks like a balloon and one rather expects it to burst. However, the fish dies long before the pressure becomes great enough for this to happen.

A thorough investigation into dropsy disease in fish has been made by Wilhelm Schäperclaus.[35] He discovered that in all cases of dropsy the intestines were highly inflamed and, in the majority of cases, the liver was also badly affected. In animals which were very severely affected the kidneys were also diseased. However, most victims die before this stage is reached. The content of the belly is an almost watery liquid, colourless or sometimes light green or pinkish. A little reddish colour only occurs if the blood-vessels in the belly are also inflamed.

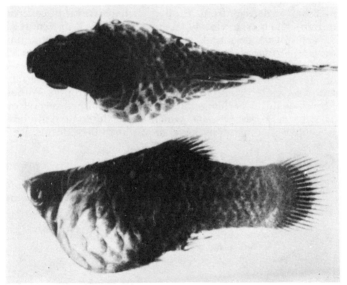

Fig. 5.6. Top and side view of a Livebearing Tooth-carp affected by dropsy (after Amlacher). It is possible that a virus may be the primary cause with bacteria secondary invaders

Although it is generally believed that the disease is not infectious, this is not quite true. It is more or less contagious. On the European continent (especially in Germany) Carp breeders regularly experience large losses due to dropsy (Fig. 5.6). Perhaps tropicals have a higher resistance to this disease. Among the exotic fishes, the Dwarf Gourami (*Colisa lalia*) is the most common victim.

Serious epidemics of dropsy have occurred in Poland and Germany, causing heavy losses. The epidemics have started in Poland and spread westward. They occur in spring or early summer, when the weather is growing warmer. Symptoms of the disease may vary somewhat. W. Wunder[36] distinguishes the so-called German form of dropsy, which conforms to the description as given above, and the Polish form, which is characterised by the occurrence of ulcers and lesions in the skin with only small amounts of exudate, or even without exudate formation. If the fish are dissected, they give off a disagreeable, sweet smell. Apart from the inflammation of the intestines, discoloration of the liver can be observed, while several internal organs may grow together. Fish that have recovered may show deformities of the skeleton and the finnage. If ulcers in the skin have been present, they will leave scars.

In aquarium fish, secondary symptoms may often occur, such as scale protrusion, due to the internal pressure, or to inflammation of the scale pockets. Ecchymoses do not always show.

In fishes suffering from dropsy, Schäperclaus discovered a bacterium which is a variety of an already well-known species, which can always be found in water and milk. This bacterium is *Aeromonas (Pseudomonas) punctata (Chromobacterium punctatum)*. The typical form of this bacterium is completely harmless. The variety which has been found in fishes suffering from dropsy has been named *forma ascitæ* (from Greek-Latin: *ascites* = dropsy). Although Schäperclaus in his earlier publications distinguished several other varieties of *Aeromonas punctata*, which cause different symptoms of disease, later investigations have shown that these forms are not

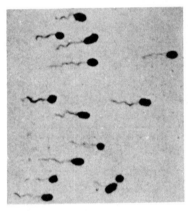

Fig. 5.7. Aeromonas punctata. × *1000.*
After a photomicrograph by Schäperclaus

constant and thus they cannot be regarded as separate varieties but merely as modifications whose features are dependent on the conditions in which they are living.[37] Although such modifications may be of great scientific interest they have little practical value for the average fish-keeper.

Aeromonas punctata (Fig. 5.7) is a small, rod-shaped micro-organism with one flagellum at the end of its body. Its length is 1–1.5 μm.

The ends of the rod are rounded, and the flagellum is about three times longer than the body.

From the investigations of Schäperclaus it is obvious that the bacterium is normally dormant and can only harm fish if they are not in a perfectly healthy and well-fed condition. Further, the parasitic forms of *Aeromonas punctata* do not seem to be particularly common and a diseased fish is not contagious to others unless the liquid, which contains bacteria, escapes into the water. This only happens when the body of the fish is decaying after its death so that in an aquarium there is but a very small risk of infection. Nevertheless, it is advisable to remove a diseased fish from the community tank.

Although generally, but not always, *Aeromonas punctata* can easily be isolated from the liquid in the belly and from the organs of the diseased fish, later investigations have given rise to some doubt whether this bacterium is the true primary cause of the disease. Scientists in Russia and Yugoslavia (Pjessov, Goncarov, Tomasec, Ljajman and Spoljanskaja) have gathered evidence in favour of the opinion that a virus is the primary cause of the disease (Fig. 5.8), the bacteria coming into play as secondary invaders.

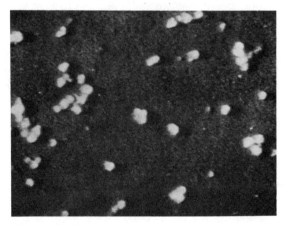

Fig. 5.8. Electron photomicrograph of virus particles found in Carp suffering from dropsy (× 9000). After Roegner-Aust and Schleich (photograph by Deubner). Aeromonas punctata, *acting as secondary invaders, are shown in Fig. 5.7*

This opinion has been confirmed by investigations made with the aid of the electron microscope and other experiments that have been carried out by Sophia Roegner-Aust and F. Schleich.[38] They found virus globules, having a size of up to 0.1 μm, in the liquid taken from the belly and also in that pressed from the internal organs of diseased Carp. These liquids were filtered through ultra-filters, retaining all ordinary cell constituents and bacteria as well. If the filtrate was injected into healthy Carp, these developed the exudate form of dropsy.

The incubation time of the disease depends on the temperature of the water and on the age of the fish. At 20°C (68°F) the course of the disease is rather rapid, the fish dying a few days after having been injected with the virus suspension. At 10–12°C (50–55°F) infected fish may survive for months. Further, the course of the infection is more rapid in young fish than in adults. This agrees with observations made in the study of other virus infections, namely, that viruses multiply most rapidly in tissues that are themselves still in full growth.

Further evidence was brought forward by Goncarov in 1959.[39] The viral aetiology was confirmed by finding eosinophilic (heavily staining with the dye eosin) inclusion bodies in the glia of the brain and in the epithelium, by the data of electron microscopy, and by the production of active artificial immunity by vaccination of Carp in the absence of *Aeromonas punctata*.

It has also been found possible to produce cytopathological changes in kidney tissue *in vitro* (tissue culture) by addition of ultra-filtrate of dropsy liquid, and when this affected tissue was inoculated into normal healthy Carp the symptoms of dropsy could be induced again.[40]

Heuschmann-Brunner failed to find bacteria in some cases of dropsy, although specific bacteria were sometimes found in fish that did not show any symptoms of dropsy, whereas those symptoms did occur in Carp that had been in contact with diseased specimens for 16 h, or that had been treated with ultrafiltrates of organs from diseased fishes.[41]

From these investigations it has to be concluded that dropsy is due to a primary virus infection, which is generally further complicated by a secondary infection with *Aeromonas punctata*.

Tets, another Russian investigator, subjected Carp to infection with dropsy by injecting them with pathological material from fish suffering from an ulcerous form of the disease, and also by contact with fish having the ulcerous form. From the end of June to autumn, the experimental fish did not develop the disease. It was concluded that the ulcerous form of dropsy is not contagious in summer.[42]

TREATMENTS FOR DROPSY

Most treatments which have been suggested in the past are unreliable. Although it seems to have been possible to rescue one or two fish from death, generally the most to be hoped for was some lengthening of the victim's lifetime.

In recent years, however, good results have been obtained in aquarium fish by application of the antibiotic chloramphenicol

(Chloromycetin), using a dosage of 60 mg to 1 Imp. gal (50 mg/ U.S. gal; 13 mg/l) during a longer period, or even up to 230 mg/ Imp. gal (190 mg/U.S. gal; 50 mg/l) for 24 h only, for fishes of at least 10 g of weight. Chloramphenicol is known to be effective against some virus infections as well as against bacteria.

In Russia, good results were obtained in Carp by giving them three injections with levomycetin (the Russian brand of chloramphenicol).[43] Ninety Carp of two years old, suffering from dropsy, were treated in this way. Sixty-eight of them recovered (76%), whereas only 10% of the control group of untreated fish survived. Adding 0.5 g/l to the water did not prevent the spread of the disease, but adding granulated food containing 1 g of the antibiotic per kilogram of food prevented further outbreaks of dropsy and the yield of two-year-old fish was 86%.

Since the rate of multiplication of the virus is increased at higher temperatures of the water, it is advisable to keep cold-water fish at as low a temperature as possible. For tropicals, it will be difficult to make temperature adjustments. Certain species of fish that can stand relatively low temperatures, such as most Livebearing Toothcarps, *Barbus conchonius* and Paradise Fish, can be kept at 16°C (60°F) until recovery. No food should be given. Chloramphenicol may cure the infection in a period of 3–7 days.

Injection of 3 mg oxytetracycline (Terramycin[R]) per 150–400 g fish weight has been reported to be efficacious in cases of dropsy in Carp in their second year of age.

Schäperclaus reported that mortality decreased about 20.4% through the injection of antibiotics such as chloramphenicol, streptomycin and patulin.[44]

In very bad cases of dropsy, where a great volume of exudate has accumulated in the belly, surgical treatment could be applied to remove the liquid before starting the chloramphenicol treatment. This should only be done by qualified persons and if the fish is large enough to allow manipulation of a hypodermic needle without damaging internal organs. A syringe with a very thin hypodermic needle is used. The fish is taken in the left hand, and, with great care, the needle is pricked into the belly. Then the liquid is drawn away. The needle must be introduced a few millimetres before the anal opening and into the belly in the direction of the head. After this operation, the fish is given treatment by bathing it for 15–30 min in a $2\frac{1}{2}$% salt solution. It is then placed in clean, fresh water to which the required amount of chloramphenicol is added. And some chloramphenicol is added to granulated dry food at a rate of 1 mg/g food. To reduce the expense of this treatment, the container in which the fish is to be treated can be quite small.

Ian M. Rankin found *para*-chlorophenoxethol effective in treatment of dropsy; 50 cm^3 of a 0.1% v/v stock solution per litre of aquarium water were added gradually in a period of 24 h. Prior to putting the fish in this solution, the belly was punctured with a hypodermic needle and syringe to remove the accumulated liquid. The fish recovered after seven days. For four months after recovery no signs of recurrence of the disease were observed, which is a long enough period to make sure that a complete cure had been obtained and not a mere temporary improvement. However, several species of fish cannot stand this treatment, see p. 340.

SCALE PROTRUSION (*LEPIDORTHOSIS CONTAGIOSA*)

In aquaria, cases of a disease frequently occur in which the scales of a fish project and fall off. From numerous investigations it is evident that this symptom is not always due to the same cause, although in all instances bacteria are found to be present. In most cases all the scales of the body stick out, while in the others only some of them are in this condition. Besides the protrusion of the scales, there are generally some red spots on various parts of the body or fins (ecchymoses). In some cases the fins are torn as well. The scales may be so loose that they fall off if the body of the diseased fish is rubbed. If the scales are pressed a little, a watery exudate appears. This has been formed in the pockets of the scales. The pressure of this fluid causes the scales to rise. Generally the exudate is colourless or slightly yellowish. This scale infection may occur as an accompanying symptom of another disease, generally dropsy, or it may appear as an independent complaint. Here I shall deal only with the latter case, since this is the more important.

In fresh-water fishes there are two species of bacteria that cause this raising and falling off of the scales. One of these is *Vibrio piscium*, a comma-shaped bacterium, discovered by David. This micro-organism is the cause of a dangerous infectious disease. All the scales of the victim stick out, and large areas of the skin become blood-coloured as a result of swelling of the blood-vessels. Post-mortem examination reveals that the belly and the pericardium contain a colourless or blood-flecked exudate, while the muscles show numerous small haemorrhages. In aquaria, however, this disease is not common; in fact, I have not seen a single case.

It should be noticed that in male *Pachypanchax playfairi* scale protrusion at the back is a normal phenomenon, not due to any pathological condition.

I now come to my own investigations on this subject.[45] In all cases of independent scale disease in tropical aquarium fishes I have found a small rod-shaped bacterium, conforming closely to the description of *Bacterium astaciperda*, which was first discovered as the cause of scale infection by Dr. Marianne Plehn at the beginning of this century, and has been described by Prof. Bruno Hofer and later by Prof. Lehmann and Prof. Neumann. Unfortunately these descriptions are very indefinite, while it has been proved that this bacterium is not the cause of the disease in fresh-water Crayfish

(*Astacus fluviatilis*) which is known as 'lobster-pest' and from which disease the name has been derived (*astaciperda* = a cause of lobster-loss). I have therefore given a new description of this bacterium and proposed to give it the name *Bacterium lepidorthosæ*.

Bacterium lepidorthosæ is a small, very motile rod, which can live at any temperature from 4–37°C. Since the organism is motile, it must have flagella but unfortunately I could neither determine how many there are present, nor how they are situated. However, on account of its physiological features, it is permissible to put the organism in the Genus *Bacterium*. It is Gram-negative and facultatively anaerobic, i.e. it can live either in the presence or absence of free oxygen.

Gelatine media are liquefied and then have a strong smell of amines (later ammonia is produced). In peptone media indole and hydrogen sulphide are produced. Milk becomes acid and coagulates at temperatures from 22°C to 37°C in four days. The following sugars are fermented with the production of both gas (a mixture of carbon dioxide (CO_2) and hydrogen (H_2)) and acid: glucose, fructose, galactose, sucrose, lactose, maltose; and the sugar alcohols: mannitol, dulcitol, adonitol, while from inositol only acid is produced. In McConkey medium growth takes place, with production of gas and acid. Methyl red test: positive. The organism grows both in uric acid and citrate media. On potato, yellow colonies of sappy appearance are formed, while ammonia production takes place. Nitrates are reduced to nitrites and ammonia. Starch is liquefied, while the formation of amylodextrin and maltose can be demonstrated. The test of Voges-Proskauer is negative.

The symptoms of the disease caused by *Bacterium lepidorthosæ* differ somewhat according to the intensity of the infection. In most cases it progresses very slowly. Sometimes it is three to four weeks before the scales protrude all over the body. At first the victims do not seem to suffer much discomfort but later their movements become slower, while the frequency of breathing increases. The tail next becomes paralysed and immovable. Hanging near the surface of the water, the animals die in a few days. If a fish has been infected very badly, the course of the disease is quite different. The characteristic symptom of scale-raising does not occur at all but the red patches on the skin of the belly and on the fins are very obvious. Such badly infected fish generally die a few days after the outbreak of the infection. The bacteria can be found in all internal organs of the victims.

The disease caused by *Bacterium lepidorthosæ* (Fig. 5.9) is more or less contagious, although epidemics never occur. It has been experimentally shown that infection takes place from the skin. Completely healthy and undamaged fishes could not be infected simply by putting them in an infected tank, but infection soon occurred if their skin had been injured. Most of the diseased fishes which I investigated belonged to the Labyrinths (especially Fighting Fish

174

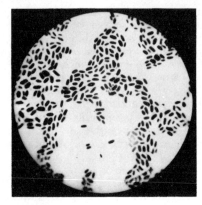

Fig. 5.9. Bacterium lepidorthosæ *from a pure culture. Magnification* × 580

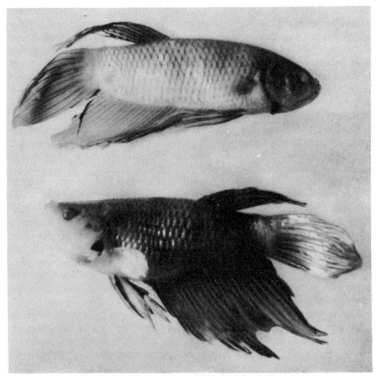

Fig. 5.10. Siamese Fighting Fish (Betta splendens) *with scale protrusion. The author has found that* Bacterium lepidorthosæ *is present in all such cases*

(*Betta splendens*) (Fig. 5.10) and Paradise Fish (*Macropodus opercularis*))
and Livebearing Tooth-carps.

A sure cure is not yet known. However, it might be expected
that chloramphenicol in a dosage of 10 mg/l (60 mg/Imp. gal or
50 mg/U.S. gal) or sulphanilamide (1 g/Imp. gal) would be effective.
To avoid infection of other fishes in the tanks, those with the disease
should be removed and treated separately. Treatment of a large
community tank would be prohibited by the extensive cost of the
drugs. For disinfection of large tanks nitrofurazone is suggested in a
strength of 1 g in 50 l of water (1.37 gr/Imp. gal or 1.14 gr/U.S. gal),
to be added in three portions at intervals of 8–12 h; total duration
three days if only disinfection is needed, or up to three weeks if
required for curing diseased fish.

It would also be worth while to experiment with the phenoxethols,
as described on pages 156–158. Kanamycin also looks promising
(p. 329).

Bacterium lepidorthosæ is also pathogenic to other living beings.
Mice that had been injected with 1–5 mm^3 of a pure culture of
the bacteria showed signs of paralysis after 18 h. They were sitting
with scarcely any movement and with completely stiffened limbs,
while breathing frequency was increased. 24 h after the infection
the animals died. Fishes have a much higher resistibility. A female
Swordtail, after having been injected with 8 mm^3 of a pure culture
of the bacteria, lived for four days.

To avoid the occurrence of scale protrusion in aquarium fishes
it is important that the fishes are not kept at too high a temperature, since this weakens them, while it increases the reproductive
rate of the bacteria. Further, avoid lack of oxygen, keep the tank
clean and take care that fishes are not damaged by handling. Do
not place in the tank stones that have sharp edges on which the
fishes could injure themselves.

SPOTTINESS OF THE SKIN IN LABYRINTHS

I once investigated a very contagious disease in a tropical aquarium
which only affected the different species of the Labyrinth group of
fishes—other species remaining immune.[46] The symptoms were that
the skin showed 'corroded' spots, sometimes blood-coloured, while
red spots on fins and skin could be very clearly seen. Further, there
were spots which were badly infected by a fungus of slimy consistency. These outward signs varied somewhat; in some cases the
'corroded' spots predominated whilst in others the ecchymoses or
the fungus infection were more prominent.

A thorough investigation of this disease proved that it was caused
by *Pseudomonas fluorescens* (Fig. 5.11). This is a rod-shaped bacterium 1.6–3 μm long and about 0.5 μm wide. It is Gram-negative.
When grown on culture media containing peptone a characteristic

yellow-green fluorescence is produced. Growth takes place up to a temperature of 37°C. The organism has 2–6 cilia situated at the ends, with which it can move through the water. Bacteria could only be isolated from the skin of the diseased fish; none could be found in the internal organs, since an abundance of oxygen (readily found on the skin) is essential to their growth.

There have already been published earlier accounts concerning the pathogenic nature of *Pseudomonas fluorescens*, e.g. by Schäper-

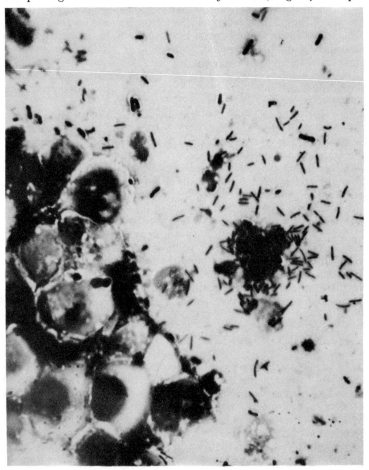

Fig. 5.11.
BACTERIAL INFECTION
Bacteria between the epithelial cells in the skin of an infected Gourami. Most are
Pseudomonas fluorescens *but some encapsulated saprophytic bacilli are also
present. Magnification × 1500*

claus, who found this bacterium in cases of diseases in Eels that had been injured and subsequently developed tumours and ulcers. In the cases of *Pseudomonas fluorescens* infection in Labyrinth Fishes which I investigated, no ulcers or tumours were found. The fungus is evidently only a secondary parasite, which can only attack the skin of a fish when its resistance has been weakened by the activity of the bacteria.

The organism is, just as *Aeromonas punctata* (Fig. 5.7), one of the commonest aquatic bacteria, and were it always virulent it is possible that there would be no fishes at all in the waters. However, it is only facultatively parasitic, and the non-pathogenic strains are by far the commonest. It appears also that the organism can exist on the fish in a latent state.

The species of fish which I saw affected in the tropical aquarium were Three-spot Gouramies (*Trichogaster trichopterus*—see Fig. 5.12) (including the Blue variety), Paradise Fish (*Macropodus opercularis*),

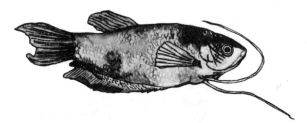

Fig. 5.12. Blue variety of Trichogaster trichopterus *with spottiness of skin due to* P. fluorescens *and secondary fungus infection (photograph from original water-colour by the author)*

and all species of the Genus *Colisa*. Other Labyrinth Fishes were not present in the tank. Species which were not affected in the same aquarium were various kinds of Livebearing Tooth-carps, several Barbs and Characins and two young specimens of *Æquidens pulcher* (*Æ. latifrons*), representing the *Cichlidæ*. All these fishes remained completely healthy, although there is no reason to conclude that they have a natural immunity to the disease, for it has appeared that the members of the Carp Family (*Cyprinidæ*) can also be attacked, although the symptoms are not the same as in the *Labyrinthici*. I have tried several treatments but all affected fishes died in a relatively short period. However, prospects of curing fishes from this infection are much better now that the modern antibacterial drugs are available.

Conroy[47] found kanamycin treatment by injection (see page 329) very effective against *Pseudomonas fluorescens* infections in *Cyprinidæ*.

SPOTTINESS OF THE SKIN IN PIKE[48]

Generally, the symptoms of this condition are inflammated reddish spots and ulcers, either all over the body or restricted to the mouth region. Soon after the beginning of the disease the victims become languid. Death rate is high. The outer parts of the liver show an accumulation of blood. Sometimes the characteristic external symptoms may be lacking.

The true cause of this disease has not yet been convincingly established. In several cases bacteria have been found, including *Aeromonas salmonicida, Ae. punctata, Ae. hydrophila, Pseudomonas fluorescens* and members of the Genus *Vibrio*, but in other cases bacteria were absent. Therefore it has been suggested that the primary cause of the disease might be a virus, bacteria only acting as secondary invaders, as in dropsy. This requires further investigations.

SPOTTINESS OF THE SKIN IN OTHER FISHES

In other species of fishes, a bacterial disease may occur which shows symptoms resembling those described for the Labyrinth Fishes. 'Corroded' spots, ecchymoses and, later, secondary fungus infection, are the chief symptoms and they may be caused by different kinds of bacteria, such as *Pseudomonas fluorescens, Aeromonas punctata* or *Proteus vulgaris (Bacterium vulgare)*.

Conroy infected common Goldfish (*Carassius auratus*) experimentally by intraperitoneal injection with 0.1 ml of a suspension of *Pseudomonas fluorescens* per gram of body weight. In order to eliminate the possibility of being misled by any aspecific effect of the inoculation *per se*, a group of control fishes were inoculated with a similar quantity of sterile Ringer's frog physiological salts solution. The symptoms produced in the infected fishes closely resembled those described by me in Labyrinth Fishes, except for the ecchymoses, which were restricted to the opercula.

Snieszko[49] has reported epidemics of pond fish due to *Pseudomonas fluorescens* infections.

Fishes are most susceptible to such diseases at pairing time during the spring. Infections take place from the skin, through which the bacteria penetrate into the subcutaneous connective tissue and the muscles. In the skin a collateral oedema is formed, producing a local protrusion of the scales. The 'corroded' spots soon become infected by fungus, too, and, when this stage is reached, there is not much chance of recovery.

In cases of *Aeromonas punctata* infection it is possible that a treatment with salt could have some good effect, since growth of this bacterium is hampered by the presence of salt. In solutions containing up to about 0.8% of salt, growth of the bacteria is abundant, but in stronger solutions development decreases proportionally with increase of salt concentration. Above 2.5%, growth is very poor, while above 4.2% it is completely inhibited. Such strong solutions may not be used for treatment of fishes, since they cannot stand them; 3.5% of salt is the greatest strength that may be used in practice and then for only 15 min. In fishes that had been infected experimentally by injections with suspensions of *Aeromonas punctata*, *Ae. hydrophila*, *Ae. liquefaciens*, *Pseudomonas fluorescens* or *Ps. putida*, effective cures were obtained by injections with kanamycin.[47]

Other investigators have found chloramphenicol (Chloromycetin) added to the water (50 mg/l) and sulphamerazine (see page 351) effective.[50] It is recommended that experiments also be carried out with other modern drugs, as described on pages 152–158.

In the case of infection with *Proteus vulgaris*, spots of a yellowish colour are formed. The scales in these areas become very loose so that they may fall off or be exfoliated when lightly touched. Red spots (ecchymoses) may be showing too and will sometimes occur alone, without the typical yellow spots of this disease. Diseased fishes swim to and fro in a dull manner. In one or two days they fall on their sides and breathing frequency decreases more and more until death follows from complete exhaustion.

As in most cases of bacterial disease in fishes, the typical form of *Proteus vulgaris* is harmless, while only some strains, that show slightly different features in bacteriological investigation, are pathogenic. *Proteus* infections can be treated by administering ampicilline (Penbritin[R]) in the food (2 mg/g) for at least eight days. To prevent occurrence of intestinal catarrh arising from an induced avitaminosis, vitamin B-complex should be incorporated in the food at the same time (a good yeast preparation may do). This treatment must not be combined with chloramphenicol.

Strains of *Proteus vulgaris* can also be pathogenic to human beings, where they may cause inflammatory processes in the urinary tract.

The related species *Proteus morganii* (Winslow *et al.*) has been isolated from the heart blood of the Chub variety *Squalius cephalus cabeda*.

RED PEST OF CARP AND TENCH

This disease (*Purpura cyprinorum*) has not often been observed in aquaria up to the present but it may sometimes occur in ponds that are crowded. The skin of the belly in infected fishes shows a dark red colour. The ventral and anal fins, and the lower part of the tail, may also be red-coloured, while the gills show haemorrhages and necrotic places. The reddening of the skin is due partly to abnormal widening of the blood vessels and partly to haemorrhages in the skin.

Often the intestine is badly inflamed and this is recognisable if a section of the organ is examined. The intestine will also show blood coloration, while sometimes a bloody and slimy exudate is formed and large sections are covered with small ulcers. The heart also becomes affected; the pericardium thickens and becomes fused with the heart muscle. Diseased fishes are dull and they frequently come near the surface where they lie without movement (often on their sides) till they die. The disease may be very contagious, but in good conditions recovery is possible. This can be furthered by ample aeration and streaming the tank through with fresh water.

The disease may be caused by varieties of *Pseudomonas putida*, namely, *Pseudomonas putida forma cyprinicida* and *Pseudomonas putida forma Davidi*. The former has 1–6 cilia, while the latter is normally not motile. Both are about 1 μm long and 0.8 μm broad.

Conroy[51] infected Goldfish experimentally by injection with a suspension of *Pseudomonas putida* and observed them to develop similar symptoms as described here as characteristic for red pest. The generalised desquamation was accompanied by the production of ecchymoses on the opercula and body. The intestine was covered with haemorrhagic spots. However, in these experimentally infected fishes, Conroy found that the disease was not contagious, since both the control fishes (having been injected with a salt solution instead of with the bacterial suspension) and one of the inoculated fish failed to develop symptoms, even when in close contact with diseased specimens. This might be another indication of the generally high resistance of healthy fishes against bacterial infections, or it could be that the strain of *Ps. putida* employed could have had a low virulence against fish.

In other cases of red pest, *Aeromonas* (formerly *Pseudomonas*) *plehniæ* has been found which is closely related to *Aeromonas punctata*. Its size is 1.6–3.6 μm in length, and 0.6–0.9 μm in width. The organism usually has one polar flagellum, but in some cases two polar cilia may be found.

For treatment, chloramphenicol or kanamycin are recommended; they may also be combined. Sulpha drugs have been found ineffective in experiments of my own.

RED PEST OF EELS
AND RED SORE OF PERCH AND PIKE

This is *Pestis rubra anguillarum*, a very serious epidemical disease, which is caused by a comma-shaped bacterium, named *Vibrio anguillarum*. In fresh-water aquaria this disease is not likely to occur, since *V. anguillarum* is adapted to waters that contain much salt, its optimum being a salt concentration of 1.5–3.5%. Below 0.25% of salt, growth is completely inhibited. Thus, this bacterium cannot live in pure, fresh water, but occurs in brackish water and in the sea. It has been detected as the cause of epidemics in sea-water aquaria.

Symptoms of the disease are the formation of extensive blood-coloured areas on the skin, especially on or near the fins ('red fin disease'), as well as a swelling and reddening of the muscles near the heart. Occasionally, red boil-like ulcers appear, too ('red boil disease'). According to investigations by Schäperclaus only Eels that are going from fresh water into brackish waters and into the sea to their spawning places are attacked. *Vibrio anguillarum* has also been found in other fish, such as Perch and Pike in the Baltic, where scale protrusion may be one of the symptoms caused; this disease is also known as 'red sore'. A special variety has been found in Finnock (immature *Salmo trutta*), Plaice and Saithe.[52] In Pike, inflammation of the cheeks may also be caused. In these fishes no special conditions, except the salt concentration of the water, are required for the outbreak of the disease.

In *Vibrio* infections of marine fishes in Japan, effective cures have been obtained by adding sulphisoxazole or nitrofurazone to the food and by injecting chloramphenicol, tetracycline or streptomycin.[53]

RED PEST AND BOTCHES DISEASE OF EELS

In fresh water, a disease closely resembling the former may appear. The same symptoms may occur, while also botches showing a red colour appear. These botches are produced by ulceration of the cutis (Fig. 5.13) and the subcutaneous connective tissue. The ulcers may open and discharge their content of pus into the water. Consequently, the disease is very contagious. In good conditions, however,

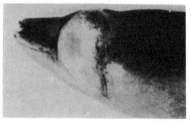

Fig. 5.13. Head of an Eel with large ulcer due to botches disease (illustration after Schäperclaus)

healing is possible. This can be furthered by good aeration and frequent changes of water. Constant running water is better.

The disease is supposed to be due to infection with a strain of *Aeromonas punctata*, which has also been found in tumours in other species of fish, but then the botches generally do not show a red colour. Sometimes eye protrusion is produced. The strains of *Aeromonas punctata* found in these infections have been distinguished as *forma sacrowiensis* by Schäperclaus, but later on it has been shown that the type was not sufficiently constant to permit regarding them as separate varieties.

Recently, some doubt has arisen as to bacteria being the primary cause of this disease. It has been suggested that the primary cause might be a virus, *Aeromonas punctata* being a secondary invader only, analogous to what happens in dropsy. A decision cannot yet be made.

RED SPOT DISEASE

Conroy[54] has described an interesting case of red spot disease in *Barbus partipentazona*, caused by *Pseudomonas putida*. The infection was confined to this one species of fish, all others in the same tank (the public aquarium of Buenos Aires) remaining unaffected.

Symptoms were the appearance of rather big red spots of well-defined area and boundaries at the flanks and the belly.

The infection was resistant to penicillin and to Terramycin[R] (oxytetracycline), but it could be cured by treatment with kanamycin at a concentration of 20 μg per gram fish, administered by intra-peritoneal injection of an aqueous solution.

RED MOUTH DISEASE OF TROUT

This is an infectious disease occurring in young Trout. The symptoms are reddening of the mouth, the opercula, the fin bases and the rectum.

Aerobacter liquefaciens and *Pseudomonas fluorescens* have been found in such cases, as well as unidentified other bacteria in the internal organs.

The infection responds well to treatment with sulphamethazine, according to Reichenbach-Klinke[55] (dosage as for sulphamerazine, see p. 351).

SEPTICAEMIA OF CALLICHTHYIDAE AND POECILIIDAE[56]

Septicaemia is the invasion of the bloodstream by bacteria and their multiplication therein. In tropicals of the Families mentioned, severe infections with *Paracolobactrum aerogenoides*, another member of the *Pseudomonadaceae*, causing this condition, have been observed. The bacteria were found everywhere in the body cavity. Diseased fishes died within one week. In *Catostomus catostomus commersonii* Lac. wounds and haemorrhages in the skin have been observed.

The causative organism was found pathogenic to Goldfish, Trout, Mice and Caviae in infection experiments. All artificially infected animals died within 19 h.

ULCER DISEASE

Although a number of infectious conditions in fish are characterised by external ulceration, in fresh-water fishes the term 'ulcer disease' is restricted to those cases that are due to *Hæmophilus piscium*. The disease starts with a minor local lesion. After some days a papule forms, which gradually develops into an open ulcer. Both symptoms and cause of the infection are remarkably similar to a human disease, namely, the ulceroglandular type of *tularæmia*, caused by *Pasteurella tularense*. *Hæmophilus piscium* is a small oval rod-shaped Gram-negative organism. It is non-motile. On first isolation a rich culturing medium containing blood is required; it is this condition which has led to the generic name of this and related species, *Hæmophilus* meaning 'blood-lover'. The disease is mainly restricted to Trout. In North America it causes large losses.

Treatments with dips in copper sulphate solutions, with sulpha drugs and with aureomycin have been reported to be unsuccessful, but chloramphenicol and oxytetracycline added to the food at a rate of 50 mg per kilogram of fish per day were equally effective in treatment of fingerling and adult Brook Trout, but Chloromycetin (chloramphenicol) gave fewer recurrences.[57] It may be expected that the newer tetracycline derivative, doxycycline (Vibramycin[R], see p. 338) will be even more effective.

ULCER DISEASE OF MARINE PUFFER FISH

In marine Puffer Fish (*Tetraodon* species) an ulcer disease may be produced by a *Vibrio* infection or a mixed infection by *Vibrios* and secondary invading other bacteria. These infections may be treated by adding nitrofurazone or sulphisoxazole in the food or by injecting chloramphenicol, tetracycline or streptomycin (see last chapter).

PASTEURELLOSIS

Pasteurella pfaffi (Hadley *et al.*) Hauduroy *et al.* has been found as the causative organism of a highly contagious infection in White Perch (*Roccus americanus*) in the Potomac river (U.S.A.), where large numbers of fish suddenly died.[58] *P. pfaffi* is an immotile Gram-negative organism, 1–2 μm in length and 0.5–1 μm in width. They produce haemorrhagic septicaemia and necrotic enteritis. The isolated bacteria could be cultivated at 20°C and at 30°C, but not at 37°C; in this respect they differ from strains of bacteria that have been described as the same species, but isolated as a pathogen from birds (doves, sparrows and canaries), which have a body temperature of approx. 40°C, and also pathogenic to mice (body temperature 40°C, too) and guinea-pigs (caviae).

TUBERCULOSIS DISEASE[59]

A number of instances of disease in fishes in which the main symptoms are lack of appetite, progressive thinness, and sluggish movements may be caused by fish tuberculosis. It has been found that a number of other symptoms may also be due to this infection, namely, skin defects including blood spots and wounds that may ulcerate and

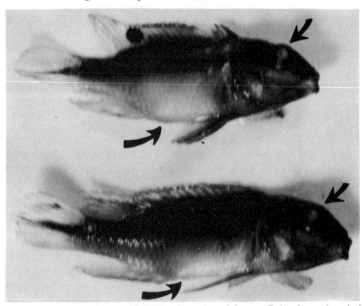

Fig. 5.14. Male and female of Pelmatochromis pulcher, *suffering from tuberculosis, as shown in post-mortem histological examination after killing them for investigation. External symptoms are:* Exophthalmus *(eye protrusion, also see page 214) and abnormal shape of the belly. Internally, tuberculous lesions were found in the liver and other organs and behind the eyes*

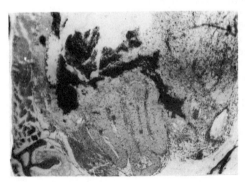

Fig. 5.15. Darkly stained tuberculous lesions near the intestine of one of the fishes of Fig. 5.14. Iron-haematoxyline stain. Photomicrograph by the author. × 50

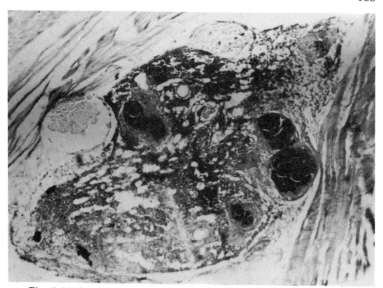

Fig. 5.16. Large, almost tumour-like, tuberculous masses in the liver of a Pelmatochromis pulcher, *showing external symptoms of* Exophthalmus *also. Gram-staining of a longitudinal section.* × 100

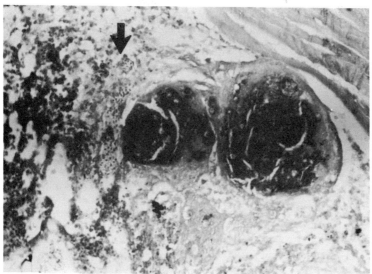

Fig. 5.17. Similar lesions to Fig. 5.16 at higher magnification. Bacteria are already recognisable, especially in the region below the arrow. Gram-staining. × 250 *(photomicrograph by the author)*

produce cavities and some type of fin-rot, characterised by the outer fin rays falling out. Further, scales may loosen and fall out.

These symptoms do not occur in the opening stages of the infection, however, but only when the disease has reached a more progressive stage. With delicate fishes such symptoms will seldom or never be observed, because death of the victims will generally occur before such a stage is reached.

Diseased fish generally show faded colours and may keep their fins folded. However, since all these symptoms can also occur in other diseases, a certain diagnosis can only be accomplished after a post-mortem examination has demonstrated the presence of tuberculous cysts and acid-alcohol fast bacteria. The latter term indicates that the bacteria, after having been stained with a phenolic solution of fuchsine, retain this stain on treatment with a dilute mineral acid and ethanol, as will be specified later on.

In the internal organs tuberculous cysts are formed, appearing as small, dirty-grey knots (tubercles), often containing necrotic tissue of blackish colour. These tubercles may have rather different sizes and, in small fish, they will often only be found on examination with a microscope. Normal tissue is pushed aside by the growing tubercles and if the latter grow near or even into blood-vessels, the bloodstream can be hindered and sometimes bleeding may occur.

The infection may also spread into the skeletal system and then deformities are caused, such as a crooked spine (either *skoliosis* or *lordosis*), deformed cheek and seriously damaged fin rays (Fig. 5.18). Finally death is caused as a result of the ever-increasing weakening of the victim's resistance and consequent emaciation.

Tubercles may occur in all internal organs (e.g. the intestine, kidneys, liver, spleen and in the heart) where they are much more dangerous than when their appearance is confined to the skin and the muscles.

The disease may occur epidemically and cause great losses. I personally investigated a case of tuberculous epidemic in half-grown Black Widows (*Gymnocorymbus ternetzi*), where about 800 fishes had died within a few weeks.

Wood and Ordale[60] have described cases of fish tuberculosis in Pacific Salmon and Trout, namely, in Chinook Salmon (*Oncorhynchus tshawytscha*), Silver Salmon (*O. kisutchi*), Blueback Salmon (*O. nerka*), and the Rainbow Trout *Salmo gairdneri*. Lesions were found most frequently in the liver. They varied from small miliary tubercles to huge necrotic areas, that were filled with acid-fast bacteria. Fish tubercle bacteria could be observed in stained smears from the heart, kidneys, brain, muscles, the intestines, the pyloric caeca, and roe.

Fish tuberculosis is mainly caused by bacteria that only cause tuberculosis in cold-blooded animals. Also human tubercle bacteria are not pathogenic for fishes, although these bacteria can survive for some period if fishes are infected with them experimentally.

Fishes that show symptoms of tuberculosis must be removed

187

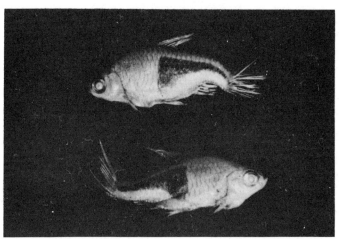

Fig. 5.18. Harlequin Fish (Rasbora heteromorpha) *with crooked spines and other symptoms of fish tuberculosis (by courtesy Prof. Dr. H. Reichenbach-Klinke)*

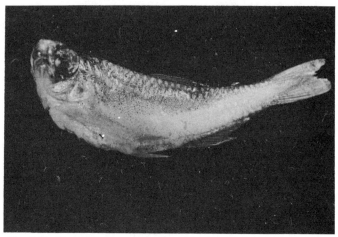

Fig. 5.19. Neon Fish (Paracheirodon (Hyphessobrycon) innesi) *with lordosis due to fish tuberculosis (by courtesy Prof. Dr. H. Reichenbach-Klinke)*

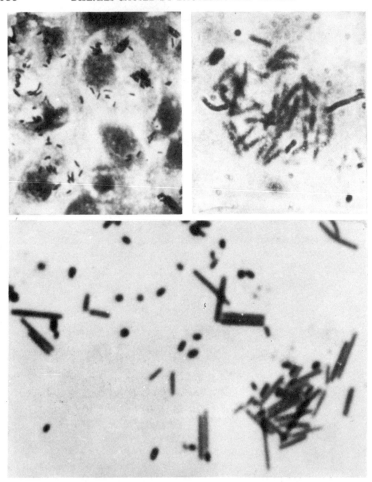

Fig. 5.20. Fish tubercle bacteria. Left: *In a smear preparation from the liver of a* Danio malabaricus *with tuberculous knots (after Jahnel).* Right: *In the spleen of a diseased* Nannacara anomala *(after Amlacher).* Lower: *In a smear preparation from the eye of a* Pelmatochromis pulcher, *suffering from double-sided* Exophthalmus. *Both types of bacteria shown showed positive staining after Ziehl-Neelsen.* × 4000 *(photomicrograph by the author)*

from the tank to avoid infection of other specimens. Thorough study of such cases, accompanied by a complete bacteriological investigation, if possible, should be of great importance for adding to our knowledge of bacterial diseases of fish. A microscopical investigation of smears from the internal organs, stained according to the method of Ziehl-Neelsen, is sufficient to make diagnosis certain (Fig. 5.20).

All members of the Genus *Mycobacterium*, to which all tubercle bacteria belong, are acid-fast, i.e. if they are stained with hot carbol fuchsine for about 5 min (the slide is heated with the dye until it vaporises, then taken away and reheated after vaporisation decreases; this is repeated until the slide has been in contact with the hot dye for 5 min) they hold the stain against an alcoholic solution of a strong acid, while other bacteria will lose it. After staining, the slide is washed with water and then it is treated with a 1% solution of hydrochloric acid (HCl) in alcohol until no more dye is extracted (which usually takes 15–30 sec). Then it is immediately washed with water.

Since focusing of the preparation would be difficult if only the few acid-fast bacteria were visible, the smear is stained afterwards with a 1% aqueous solution of methylene blue for half a minute. Then the preparation is washed under the tap, dried in the air and examined with an oil-immersion objective. A large area must be searched before the investigation may be considered as negative. Material must be taken from all internal organs, but especially from the intestines, liver and kidneys. In taking the matter from which to make a smear, notice parts of the organs that show a different appearance (use a magnifying glass in doing this). Microscopists who have the means to work on histology may do valuable work in cutting sections of the organs and studying pathological changes. If positive results are obtained, these should be recorded in full (illustrated by photographs or drawings, if possible) and made known.

At present several species of fish tubercle bacteria are known, mentioned below, and there are indications that even more species must exist.

Mycobacterium piscium (Bataillon, Dubard and Terre): This species has so far been found in most cases of tuberculosis in fish. It is also pathogenic to frogs and reptiles. Its size depends on the size of the cells of the host and it has been found to vary from 3–12 µm length and 0.3–0.5 µm width.

In Swordtails (*Xiphophorus helleri*) its length is less than 3–5 µm; in *Cichlasoma meeki* it is 3–5 µm; in Black Widows (*Gymnocorymbus ternetzi*) 3–3.5 µm; in Neon Tetras (*Paracheirodon* (*Hyphessobrycon*) *innesi*) (Fig. 5.19), *Tanichthys albonubes* and *Apistogramma ramirezi* 5–7 µm; in *Danio malabaricus* 3–7 µm; in *Haplochromis multicolor* 4–9 µm; and in Angel Fish (*Pterophyllum*) and Guppies (*Lebistes reticulatus*) 6–10 µm. In the Mosaic Gourami (*Trichogaster leeri*) a length of 6–12 µm was found but, on isolation in a pure culture, the size range was only 3–5 µm. These figures have been taken from investigations by J. Jahnel and H. Reichenbach-Klinke in Germany.[61]

In *Danio*, *Gymnocorymbus* and *Hyphessobrycon* species *M. piscium* may sometimes produce tubercles in the eye cavity leading to eye protrusion (*Exophthalmus*) and blindness. In such cases the colours of the fish will get dark instead of fading. Platies (*Xiphophorus maculatus*) seem to be resistant. *M. piscium* has also been found in *Barbus tetrazona*.

In cold-water fish this bacterium has been found in intestines of Golden Carp (Hi-Goi) (*Cyprinus carpio* var. *auratus*), Goldfish (*Carassius auratus*), Pike-Perch (*Lucioperca sandra*) and European Catfish (*Siluris glanis*); also in the intestines of the Axolotl, and in frogs.

Mycobacterium platypoecilis (Baker and Hagan) was isolated for the first time from *Xiphophorus* (*Platypoecilus*) *maculatus* (Platies) by J. A. Baker and W. A. Hagan in 1942.[62] It is a short, rod-shaped organism that does not show size variation in different hosts. It is highly pathogenic for Platies, but Goldfish are resistant, while for *M. piscium* it is just the other way round. *M. platypoecilis* has its temperature optimum at 30°C and flourishes at 25°C, but it is killed at 37°C (human body temperature). In cultures it produces an orange pigment when illuminated, or a cream-coloured one in darkness.

Mycobacterium anabanti Besse: This species was isolated for the first time from Paradise Fish (*Macropodus opercularis*) in France.[63] *M. anabanti* multiplies at temperatures between 12°C and 33°C, but not at 37°C. Its temperature optimum is 25°C. In cultures an orange-yellow or cream-coloured pigment is produced. The organism has also been found pathogenic to *Lepomis* (*Eupomitis*) *gibbosus* and Bettas.

Mycobacterium fortuitum Cruz: This organism appears as short rods or coccoid forms. It multiplies at temperatures from 18° up to 42°C and is pathogenic to a range of cold-blooded animals as well as to cattle and humans. In 1953 Nigrelli isolated a strain of fish tubercle bacteria from diseased Neon Fish *Paracheirodon* (*Hyphessobrycon*) *innesi*; this strain was identified as *M. fortuitum* by Ross and Brancato in 1959.[64] The organism has also been found in Plaice (*Pleuronectes platessa*), Cod (*Gadus morrhua*) and other fishes, and in tortoises as well. Grey or whitish tubercles, that may become necrotic, appear in the kidneys and in the liver, but generally the spleen is not affected. In advanced cases the skeleton is attacked and deformed.

Mycobacterium salmoniphilum Ross:[65] Straight or curved rods, producing colonies at artificial culturing media in only 3–4 days at the optimal temperature of 25°C. At 10°C and at 37°C no growth takes place. Pigments ranging from yellowish to violet are produced. The organism is pathogenic to *Salmonidæ* and has been found in *Oncorhynchus gorbuscha* and *Salmo gairdneri*.

Mycobacterium marinum Aronson:[66] Infects marine fishes only. It was discovered in 1926 in the liver, spleen, kidneys, ovary, pericardium and eyes of tropical Coral Fishes, namely, *Abudefduf mauritii*, *Micro-*

pogon undulatus and *Centropristes striatus*. It has also been found in other marine fishes, in frogs and in caymans. It consists of small fragmented rods. Optimal temperature 18–20°C. No growth at 37°C. In cultures a citron-yellow pigment is produced, changing to orange on ageing. As in *M. piscium*, the size of the organism varies with the size of the cells of the host.

M. marinum is also pathogenic to humans, where it causes ulcerous and tuberculous skin lesions; such infections have been reported from the Baltic region, the Hawaiian coasts and Florida. The isolated bacteria grown in culture media were 1.5–2.5 μm in length. They grow optimally at 30–33°C in 7–10 days and slower at 37°C (14 days), in which respect they differ from those isolated from infected fishes. This variety of tubercle bacteria is resistant against streptomycin, *para*-aminosalicylic acid (PAS), *iso*-nicotinic acid hydrazide (INH) and thiacetazone, but it was found to be susceptible to thyrothricin, cycloserine (D-4-amino-3-isoxazolidinone) and iridocin. The latter two prevented any growth of this bacterium at 5 μg/cm^3.[67]

Occasionally other acid-alcohol fast bacteria have been found in diseased fish, but generally investigations were not carried on far enough to enable the organisms either to be identified with species already known or to be recognised as new species. In 1962 Conroy and Valdez[68] described strains of fish tubercle bacteria isolated from *Paracheirodon* (*Hyphessobrycon*) *innesi* and also pathogenic to *Macropodus opercularis* and *Trichogaster trichopterus*, but not to Goldfish (*Carassius auratus*). Growth takes place from 18°C to 37°C. Development of colonies on first isolation takes 21 days, which may be shortened to 6–7 days when using a liquid medium incubated under continuous shaking. In suitable culture media an orange-yellow up to orange pigment is produced. Conroy and Valdez provisionally named it *Mycobacterium species indeterminata*, but later it was identified by R. E. Gordon as *Nocardia asteroides* Blanchard, belonging to the Family *Actinomycetaceæ*. *Nocardia* infections have been observed in Trout and other species, too.

TREATMENT OF TUBERCULOSIS IN FISH

Reichenbach-Klinke has experimented with penicillin ointment (as sold in tubes for medical or veterinary use) for treatment of Mosaic Gouramies (*Trichogaster leeri*) suffering from deep tuberculous wounds in the skin. The ointment was rubbed into the wounds, which contained large numbers of fish tubercle bacteria. As a result of this treatment the acid-fast bacteria disappeared 'as by magic'. However, in cases where no wounds or ulcers are present, such treatment cannot be given, while application in the form of a solution in the aquarium water is not promising, owing to penicillin being destroyed comparatively rapidly in aquarium water.

Conroy's kanamycin treatment, consisting of intraperitoneal injection of 20 μg (0.02 mg) per gram fish, may be expected to be effective in several cases where fishes are big enough to handle for injection, since kanamycin is a specific anti-tuberculous drug in human medicine, too.

Streptomycin has been expected to be effective when applied by injecting 10–20 μg/g fish or by adding 10 mg/l of water, as advocated by Schäperclaus. Streptomycin is the first antibiotic with very high activity against human tubercle bacteria that has been detected and it is still the most widely used in combination with other drugs, such as para-aminosalicylic acid (PAS), iso-nicotinic acid hydrazide (INH), viomycin, a.o., but its results in treatments of fish tuberculosis have been disappointing. It is certainly inferior to kanamycin and also to chloramphenicol for treatment of bacterial infections in fish.

The cheapest and most simple treatment in cases that are unsuited to Reichenbach-Klinke's penicillin ointment cure, appeared to be one with iso-nicotinic acid hydrazide (INH, Isoniazid, Nidaton or a great many other commercial names). This drug does not need to be injected, but can be given orally (in the food) at a rate of 3–5 μg/g fish per day. Since this drug is sufficiently stable in aqueous solution, it may also be added to the aquarium water at a concentration of at least 3–5 mg/l of water. The fishes will stand up to ten times this concentration for three days. However, INH has already been proved ineffective against Mycobacterium marinum and against unidentified Mycobacteria found in an epidemic of Exophthalmus.

A CASE OF FISH TUBERCULOSIS TREATED WITH TERRAMYCIN[R] (OXYTETRACYCLINE)[69]

I personally investigated a case of a tuberculous epidemic in half-grown Black Widows (Gymnocorymbus ternetzi) where about 800 fishes had died within a few weeks. The bacteria found differed in size and in form from Mycobacterium piscium, being more oval in shape and much smaller; they might have been identical with Mycobacterium fortuitum or with Nocardia asteroides as investigated by Conroy and Valdez, but since no special bacteriological investigations could be made at that time, no true identification is possible.

Typical small tubercles, which were also acid-fast, were found in longitudinal sections of the diseased fishes (see Figs 5.21–5.23).

With the few specimens of fish that were still alive when I was called in I experimented in an attempt to effect a cure. Owing to the small number of fish it was impossible to try several drugs, so I confined myself to one I had in hand to test its value for treatment of fish diseases, namely, Terramycin[R] (oxytetracycline), kindly placed at my disposal by Mr. H. R. Axelrod. The stuff used was 'Terramycin, Animal Formula, Soluble Powder', manufactured by Chas.

193

Fig. 5.21. Fish tuberculosis. Two tubercles in section of Gymnocorymbus ternetzi. × 1000 (Ziehl-Neelsen staining)

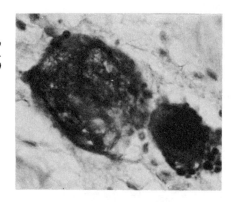

Fig. 5.22. Two small tubercles in the internal organs of Gymnocorymbus ternetzi; the one to the right is pressing upon a blood vessel in which blood corpuscles can be seen. × 1000 (Ziehl-Neelsen staining)

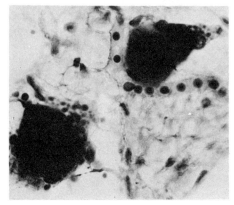

Fig. 5.23. Bacteria of fish tuberculosis found in Gymnocorymbus ternetzi. Smear preparation stained after Ziehl-Neelsen. × 2000 (all photomicrographs by the author)

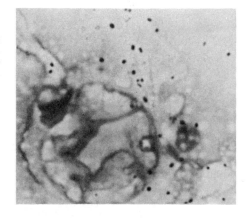

Pfizer & Co., Inc., New York; this was a crude product of low cost as compared to the purified crystalline drug, which by that time sold at $4 per capsule in the veterinary grade and at $8 in the medical grade (these prices have gone down considerably in later years). Each pound of the crude powder represented 25 g of active oxytetracycline hydrochloride.

The amount for treatment of fish diseases, recommended by Axelrod, was 13 mg/l of pure oxytetracycline, which is equivalent to 227 mg/l of the crude powder. The water turns rather dark and may get cloudy after the drug has been added.

After a treatment of three days a real improvement in the condition could be observed; the fishes looked normal in coloration again, having an appetite and swimming normally. Treatment was discontinued and the water changed. Then it appeared that a cure had not yet been effected and a further casualty occurred.

A second treatment for another three days was given, which had to be discontinued owing to deterioration of the solution, which seemed to have attained toxic properties. Having been put in fresh water again, after some days a number of fishes again began to show symptoms of fading, and folding of fins, therefore a third three-day treatment with a fresh oxytetracycline solution was given. This seemed to be effective, for symptoms disappeared and there were no further casualties or recurrences.

Although from this preliminary experiment it would seem that oxytetracycline could be useful for curing fishes suffering from tuberculous infections that have not yet advanced too far, this treatment cannot be recommended any more, it obviously being more risky and inferior to the treatments described before. It should also be stated that a used oxytetracycline bath is very toxic to fishes that are brought into it afterwards, although fishes that have been in it from when it was still fresh can stand it for some period. Application as a food additive seems more promising, but now a newer related antibiotic, namely doxycycline (trade name Vibramycin[R]) that has a much better penetrating power into cells and tissue and is more stable, should be preferred for further experimentation.

FURUNCULOSIS

This disease does not occur in aquaria but it may be very serious in free waters. First symptoms occur in the internal organs. The intestine is heavily inflamed and shows a blood-red colour. In very bad cases, fishes will die in this stage of the disease, without showing characteristic external signs. Sometimes the peritoneum becomes inflamed as well. If the fish has sufficient resistance to survive this stage, diffuse haemorrhagical processes in the muscles occur. They can be recognised easily by their colour when a dead fish is dissected. These processes penetrate to the surface and produce swellings or boils, which contain a bloody, pus-like substance consisting of destroyed muscle tissue, leucocytes and numerous bacteria. These boils or furuncles are the most characteristic feature of this disease, from which it has its name. They are usually seen as rounded swellings on the sides of the victim's body. Sometimes the furuncles will burst and discharge their content of pus and blood into the water. About 8–14 days after the appearance of swellings fishes become sluggish in their movements, separate themselves from the others and may be caught in the hand.

Furunculosis is caused by *Aeromonas salmonicida*, a rod-shaped micro-organism of 2–3 μm in length. It is immotile and Gram-negative. Optimum growth takes place from 10°C to 15°C (50–60°F). Infection may occur within a few hours when a healthy fish is placed into infected water and, in very bad cases, death may follow even within 3–4 days. The infection takes place from the gills, the alimentary tract and from wounds. *Aeromonas salmonicida* may be present in a latent stage in healthy fish for a long time. If

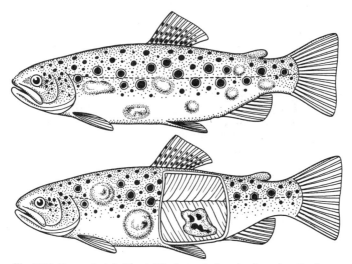

Fig. 5.24. Furunculosis in Trout. The lower specimen has been opened to show how the muscles are attacked

such fishes are weakened by bad conditions, the disease will break out, while they will already have been a constant source of infection to other fishes.

Especially, a preceding or successive infection with *Rabiesvirus salmonis* aggravates the seriousness of the disease (see pages 202–206).

Furunculosis occurs in Salmon (*Salmo salar*) and several species of Trout (*Salmo fario*, *Salmo salvelinus*, etc.—see Fig. 5.24). Even *Salmo iridæus*, considered immune for a long time, can develop this disease when in unfavourable conditions, as was shown by Schäperclaus. From Lough Neagh Pollan (*Coregonus pollan*) a strain of *Aeromonas salmonicida* has been isolated which differs from the regular form by lack of indole production in broth cultures.[70]

In Japan, bacteria have been isolated from the Salmonid fishes *Oncorhynchus masou* and *O. gorbuscha*, believed to be a variety of the ordinary furunculosis organism, namely *Aeromonas salmonicida masoucida*.[71] This variety easily acquired resistance against nitrofuran derivatives that are otherwise highly effective against furunculosis.

Other species of fish, especially those of the Carp Family, are relatively immune. There are but very few cases known at present in which fishes other than *Salmonidæ* were affected. This is obviously the reason why the disease does not occur in aquaria and ponds, for Trout and Salmon are not often kept under such conditions.

Furunculosis of fish has nothing to do with the human disease that bears the same name, so that infection of humans has not to be feared. Furunculosis may break out at any time, but it is always worse in hot weather in summer and during the breeding season (autumn).

If cases of this disease occur, it is especially important to take precautions to prevent the infection from spreading. Diseased fishes must be removed as soon as possible and the carcasses must be destroyed either by burning them or by burying in lime as far away from the water course as possible; every dead fish is a source of infection. Nets used in catching diseased fishes must be disinfected. Potassium permanganate in a strong solution may be used for this, but since this has a very bad effect on the material of which the nets are made, it will be better to disinfect nets and other things that have been in contact with infected water by putting them in a 5% solution of formaldehyde (1 part by volume of commercial Formalin with 5 parts by volume of water) for some hours, and after that they should be washed with fresh water.

TREATMENT OF FURUNCULOSIS

Nowadays furunculosis can be successfully treated by either sulpha drugs, chloramphenicol or oxytetracycline, or with furazolidone.[72]

A multiple sulphonamide therapy was advocated by Flakas.[73] During the first three days, a mixture of 12 g of sulphamerazine with 6 g of sulphaguanidine per 100 lb (45.4 kg) of fish per day was given in the food, followed by giving 6 g of sulphamerazine and 4 g of sulphaguanidine per 100 lb of fish in the food daily for seven days. *This treatment must not be used on Brown Trout any more.* For general use this treatment may be considered now to be superseded by sulphisoxazole, as described on p. 352.

Oxytetracycline or Chloromycetin (chloramphenicol) may be applied by giving 1 gram of each per kilogram food and feeding the whole stock of fish with it for a sufficiently long period (up to 10 days).

These antibiotics are recommended if ulcer disease is also present, or when the disease should prove resistant to sulphonamide treatment. Antibiotics are much more expensive than sulpha drugs.

Furazolidone is applied by feeding of 25–75 mg/kg body weight of the fish per day for a fortnight. This dosage must not be reduced, otherwise the disease will recur after treatment will have been stopped owing to resistant strains having been developed. It is recommended to start treatment with the highest dosage at least during the first one or two days.

PSEUDO-FURUNCULOSIS

In young Sockeye Salmon (*Oncorhynchus nerka*) a contagious disease has been observed where the external symptoms closely resembled those of furunculosis. However, instead of *Aeromonas salmonicida*, a bacterium belonging to a rather different group, the *Streptomycetaceæ* (a Family of the *Actinomycetales*) was found. This has been

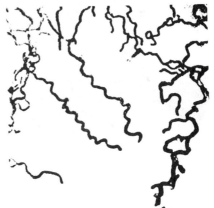

Fig. 5.25. Hyphae of Streptomyces salmonicida *from the liver of a young Sockeye Salmon.* × 1000 (after Rucker)

named *Streptomyces salmonicida* (Fig. 5.25).[74] Apart from heavy skin lesions, the main infectious herds were observed in the liver, whereas knots occurred in the body cavity. In the kidneys secondary infections with *Pseudomonadaceæ* were demonstrated.

VIRUS DISEASES

In the earlier part of this chapter a virus has been described as the primary cause of dropsy, with bacteria as secondary agents. Some diseases are due to virus infections only. Research of fish diseases has not yet advanced to any appreciable extent in respect of viruses. Probably in the future a number of other diseases of doubtful origin will be proved to be caused by them.

LYMPHOCYSTIS DISEASE

This disease is characterised by the formation of proliferous growths of connective tissue in the skin and the fins of fish, somewhat resembling small pieces of cauliflower. These growths incorporate a typical net-shaped body in their interior. Most of them will be found on the fins. They grow slowly and it may take several months for them to reach a size of 0.5 cm (approx. 0.2 in). Infected fish will gradually grow thin. Secondary fungus infections may occur in advanced cases. The course of the disease is slow; it takes at least two months after the infection before the first external symptoms begin to show.

The causative virus could not yet be isolated and purified, but it has been demonstrated by electron-microscopy, ultrafiltration and infection experiments. It has a hexagonal shape, size 200 ± 20 nm and should crystallise in rows.[75]

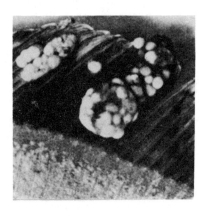

Fig. 5.26. Lymphocystis growth on the dorsal fin of a Plaice (Pleuronectes platessa) (after Schäperclaus). This disease may also show itself on the fish's skin. It is caused by a crystallisable virus with hexagonal profile, about 0.2 μm long

In aquaria, the disease has been observed in Paradise Fish (*Macropodus*). In free waters it has been found in Smelt (*Osmerus eperlanus*), Flounder (*Pleuronectes flesus*), Plaice (*Pleuronectes platessa*— see Fig. 5.26) and Sole (*Solea vulgaris*). Further, it has been observed in *Sargus* in sea-water aquaria.

POX DISEASE (*EPITHELIOMA PAPULOSUM*)

This is mainly a disease of Carp (*Cyprinus carpio*—see Fig. 5.27) and Prussian Carp (*Carassius carassius*), but it is sometimes also observed in other species, namely, Tench (*Tinca tinca*), Rudd (*Scardinius erythrophthalmus*), Bream (*Abramis brama*), Pike-Perch (*Lucioperca sandra*), Smelt (*Osmerus eperlanus*), and in aquarium fish. The disease has been known since the Dark Ages, according to the

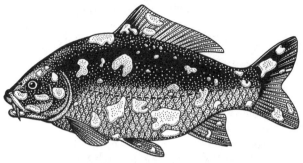

Fig. 5.27. Carp with pox disease (redrawn after colour-plate by Hofer). This complaint has been known to exist for hundreds of years and was recorded in the sixteenth century

'Fischbuch' ('Fish Book') published by Konrad Gessner in 1563 at Zürich (Switzerland). Carp breeders in Germany regularly experience large losses due to pox disease.

SYMPTOMS OF POX DISEASE

The main symptoms of the condition are the occurrence of small milky-white spots, somewhat resembling opal glass or tallow, which gradually increase in size. They may merge till finally large areas of the fish's skin are covered with them. In very bad cases the fish may have the appearance of having been immersed in stearin. The

Fig. 5.28. Section of a pox in a Carp specimen, stained with haemalum and eosin (after Roegner-Aust and Schleich with photomicrograph by Chorman). Magnification × 36, approx. The pox consists of proliferating epithelium with enlarged cutis papillae

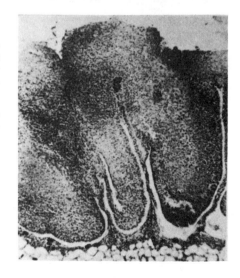

milky-white spots are raised 1–2 mm above the surface of the skin. The surface of the spots themselves is smooth, although on rare occasions some may show tiny furrows. Sometimes the whitish appearance may be clouded by the presence of tiny strings of black pigment. Thick growths may get a reddish-grey lustre. The spots are solid and harder than the normal surrounding parts. They cannot be removed by rubbing.

In the ordinary course of the disease, the pox may fall off after having reached a certain thickness, but they will reappear after some time. In aquaria, it has been observed that new spots appeared 6–8 weeks after the old ones had fallen off. The pox disease of fish does not bear any direct relation whatsoever to the smallpox disease of men. The pox of fish consists of a proliferous growth of cells of the epidermis (epithelium cells) with enlargement of the papillae of the cutis (Fig. 5.28). In the epithelium cells inclusions can be found, resembling the bodies of Guarnieri and cell inclusions occurring in pox diseases of poultry and sheep, which are virus diseases.

In 1896, Hofer found sporozoans in Carp suffering from pox disease and he considered them to be the causative agents of the

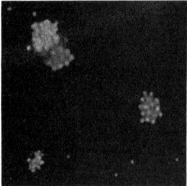 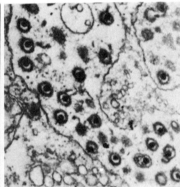

Fig. 5.29. Electron micrograph (after Roegner-Aust and Deubner) of the isolated pox disease virus in Carp. Magnification × 10 000

Fig. 5.30. Carp pox virus in ultra-thin section of tissue. × 300 000. Detail of an electron micrograph by Schubert

disease, although these organisms did not occur in the skin, but in the internal organs only. The symptoms of pox were then considered to be due to disturbances of metabolism, especially of excretion, caused by renal damage. Later on, it was proved that this sporozoan infection had been incidental and could not be the real cause of the pox disease. For some time the disease has been regarded as a result of disturbance of metabolism caused by a faulty diet, lack of vitamins or certain minerals, skin damage and others, while some influence of hereditary factors has been suggested in addition to such adverse conditions.

Sophia Roegner-Aust and F. Schleich[76] and Sophia Roegner-Aust and B. Deubner[77] have made new investigations of the disease with the methods of virus research. They have been able to find a virus in Carp pox. This virus has a globular shape with a diameter from 0.07 μm up to 0.22 μm. Generally, the particles lie in groups together (Figs 5.29 and 5.30). These results have been confirmed by later investigations on pox disease in Barbel (*Barbus barbus*) by Schubert and Meyer.[78]

If healthy Carp were injected in the lymphatic system with a suspension of virus-containing material, a number of them would develop pox disease, but others remained unaffected. Therefore, it seems that some other factors, as yet unknown, would be required to allow the virus to affect the fish. These factors might be hereditary or environmental, or both. Further investigations will be required to answer these questions.

SPONTANEOUS HEALING WITH GOOD CONDITIONS

Pox disease may heal spontaneously if the fish are kept under good conditions, such as not too high a water temperature and clean water with a high content of oxygen. In running water the chances of recovery are better than in standing water.

Generally, the disease is not lethal and, if the infection does not attack large areas of the body, the victims do not suffer much. However, in bad cases, normal growth of the fish is inhibited, the affected fish will grow thin and may suffer from skeleton weakness owing to incomplete ossification of the bones, especially of the vertebrae. After the latter condition has healed, the spine may remain crooked.

TREATMENT OF POX DISEASE

Intraperitoneal injection of affected Carp with 1 ml of a 1% solution of the arsenic compound Arycil, followed by three injections with a 5% solution at successive days, has proved efficacious, but is scarcely economically applicable.

KRYO-ICHTHYOZOOSIS

This disease has been discovered for the first time in South America by G. Pacheco and J. R. Guimaraes.[79]

Swellings at the base of the fins occur, especially at the base of the pectoral fins. Infected fishes swim awkwardly; wallowing in the water they try to reach the surface, where they remain as long as their body powers allow. Sometimes they sink to the bottom, falling to their sides or lying on their back. The disease is fatal and takes a very fast course; the victims die after a few hours.

Post-mortem examination reveals discoloration of the gill sheets and of the internal organs. The gall bladder shows a red colour instead of the normal green, and contains a slimy amber-coloured liquid. In the mouth and the stomach abnormal amounts of slime are found. The disease can only occur at temperatures below 16°C (60°F), since at higher temperatures the virus is inactivated.

CAULIFLOWER DISEASE

Symptoms of this condition are morphologically somewhat resembling those of Lymphocystis diseases, but the cauliflower-like growths (Fig. 5.31) occur mainly at the head (and particularly the mouth), whereas generally they show a brownish-red colour. Sometimes, however, the growths may appear white with red spots and stripes. They have the character of tumours of the collagenous connective tissue, called *papilloma*. The disease has been observed in Eel (*Anguilla anguilla*), Smelt (*Osmerus eperlanus*), Bleak (*Alburnus alburnus*) and Cod (*Gadus morrhua*). Schäperclaus suggests that the condition may be due to virus infection, which seems likely from its similitude with *Lymphocystis* disease, for which the viral origin has been proved. However, thus far a cauliflower disease virus has not yet been demonstrated.

INFECTIOUS VIRUS-SEPTICAEMIA IN TROUT (INFECTIOUS KIDNEY AND LIVER DISEASE; INul; Egtved-disease)

This is a disease of Salmonid fishes, especially of different species of Trout. The belly of affected fishes is distended as a result of swelling of the kidneys, combined with the accumulation of fluid in the abdominal cavity. This fluid may either be of light amber colour and half-transparent, or it may be opaque and show a red colour. It may exert considerable pressure on the abdominal wall, but not to such an extent as in ordinary dropsy (see page 166). Some amount of eye protrusion (*Exophthalmus*, see page 214) is often present, too. Blisters filled with clear amber or turbid liquid occur in the skin, most frequently on the sides. Sometimes the anal region appears swollen and the intestine may contain a yellow purulent liquid.

In the course of the disease symptoms proceed in a regular order, starting with discoloration (either darkening or fading of colours!), withdrawal from the main swimming space, apathy, eye protrusion, spottiness of the skin followed by secondary fungus development,

203

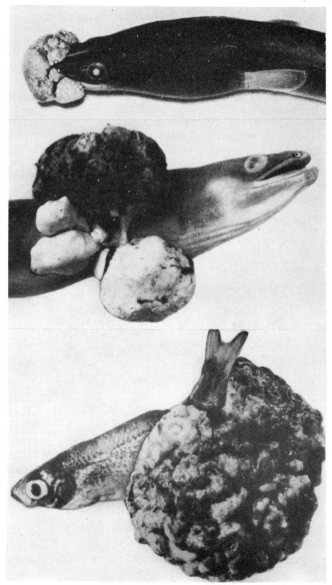

Fig. 5.31. Cauliflower disease. Upper: *At the mouth of an Eel (most common site); photograph* Bayerische Biologische Versuchsanstalt, *taken from Reichenbach-Klinke, 1966.* Middle: *In the pectoral fin region of an Eel, with dark pigmentation and hyperaemia at the dorsal side and whitish-yellow and pink coloration in its lateral and ventral parts (after Amlacher).* Lower: *In the ventrocaudal region of a Bleak (after Amlacher)*

fin-rot and fungus, bloody inflammation of the mouth and the internal organs, swimming round in circles, anaemia and production of exudates in the belly or heavier inflammation of the internal organs, yellow or marblish discoloration of the liver, appearance of bloody exudate in the swim bladder, swelling of the kidneys accompanied by haemorrhages. The muscles are affected last of all.

In the anaemic condition, the number of red blood corpuscles may be only $300/mm^3$ instead of the normal value of 1–2 million.

The swelling of the kidneys is due to dilation of the interstitial tissue, which squeezes the renal canaliculi (small channels in the kidney) and the black pigment cells, that are characteristic for Trout kidneys, nearly to disappearance. The canaliculi become necrotic, giving rise to small and large necrotic areas. In advanced stages the whole kidney appears enlarged and necrotic. Generally the dorsal kidney is affected first. Its thickness may be 1.5–2 times its normal value. The head kidney is taken in only when the disease progresses into advanced stages. The anterior parts of the kidneys often appear speckled brown and whitish, whereas the midline of the organ is bloody red. The surface of the affected kidney appears waved instead of being completely smooth as in the normal condition.

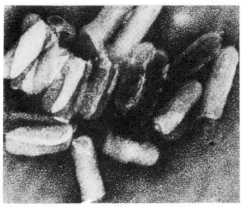

Fig. 5.32. Rabiesvirus salmonis. × *100 000. Electron micrograph of a negatively stained preparation, by Zwillenberg and Jensen*

The muscles above the kidneys often show a soft consistency owing to the presence of abscesses. The swim bladder may show wavy scarifications, too; it may or may not be filled with the same liquid as is found in the abdominal cavity.

Sometimes the heart and the spleen are covered with opaque false membranes, making them appear whitish. Very often the liver shows an abnormal pale or yellowish, sometimes speckled, appearance. In about half of the cases the gall bladder is of reduced size and is found to contain a yellowish fluid and yellowish congelations. At times additional lesions may appear as small papillae projecting from the outer walls of the gullet or the stomach, whereas in advanced cases the intestines and appendices pylorae may be surrounded by proliferating white glistening tissue, resembling soft roe. Such tissue consists of typical tubercles. Small miliary tubercles may be found in the liver, spleen, kidney, eyes, gills, muscles and the anterior part of the intestinal tract. However, the disease has nothing at all to do with fish tuberculosis (see page 184).

According to the main course of the disease some varieties of the affliction are distinguished.[80] In the so-called neurovegetative variety abnormal swimming movement prevails. This form and the muscle-attacking variety are not very contagious and may heal spontaneously, but they can develop into the lethal haemorrhagic and exudative forms.

The disease is caused by a virus that has been isolated in 1965 and described as *Rabiesvirus salmonis* (Fig. 5.32). It contains ribonucleic acid (RNA), characteristic for *Myxoviruses*, whereas its dimensions of 0.180 μm length and 0.06–0.07 μm (depending on the preparation method) width, and structural details show it to be related to the viruses of measles and mumps in humans, of the Sub-Group *Paramyxoviruses*.[81]

Mixed infections by this virus and *Aeromonas salmonicida* (the fish furunculosis organism, see pages 194–196) often occur.

The disease has been observed in Brook Trout (*Salvelinus fontinalis*), Brown Trout (*Salmo trutta*), Rainbow Trout (*Salmo gairdneri, Salmo iridæus*), Salmon (*Salmo salar*), Sockeye (Blue-back) Salmon (*Oncorhynchus nerka*) and Coho (Silver) Salmon (*Oncorhynchus kiustch*). Outbreaks of the disease have a seasonal character.

TREATMENT. Extensive investigations have been performed by Snieszko, Griffin, and collaborators.[82] They experimented with the sulpha drugs: sulphamerazine, sulphadiazine, a mixture of sulphamerazine and sulphathiazole, and with sulphisoxazole (gantrisin) (3,4-dimethyl-5-sulphanil-amido-isoxazole), mixed with the food, and also with the antibiotics Aureomycin, chloramphenicol (Chloromycetin) and oxytetracycline (Terramycin).

All sulpha drugs arrested the disease, whereas of the antibiotics only chloramphenicol delayed its progress. However, whereas the sulpha drugs stopped the progress of the infection, they did not provide a cure, since after prolonged treatment the disease reappeared within 40–50 days after the last administration.

To keep the disease under control in hatcheries, Snieszko *et al.* advocated administration of gantrisin or sulphamerazine at a rate of 8–10 g per 100 lb of fish per day, well mixed with the food. Therapy should be continued until mortalities drop to a very low level. Then it should be repeated for weekly periods every month, till the cold season for the disease is over. The other sulpha drugs, although effective, should not be used because they retard the growth of the fish. For Brown Trout, only gantrisin should be used since in this species sulphamerazine shows a growth-retarding effect, too, which does not occur in the other *Salmonidæ*.

It has also been found, however, that efficaciousness of these sulpha treatments may only be achieved in cases where a mixed infection with *Aeromonas salmonicida* exists, success depending on the effect of the drugs on this bacterial infection only. A sure cure of the viral infection itself has not yet been achieved. Prophylaxis consists of increasing health condition of the fishes by adding vitamins of the B-group, axerophtol (vitamin A) and vitamin T to the food.[80]

Increasing the pH value of the water into the alkaline region decreased the number of casualties, too, whereas anaemic cases improved by injections with methylene blue.[83]

PANCREATIC NECROSIS IN TROUT[84]

Fishes affected by this disease show intermittent whirling or cork-screwing movements. Rotation occurs along the longitudinal axis of the body, as also occurs in *Hexamita (Octomitus)* infections, whereas in tumbling disease caused by *Myxosoma cerebralis* the turning is 'head over heels'. Swimming speed is often highly increased. In the entire intestinal tract no food is found, whereas a nearly colourless mucus is present in the more or less distended gut. Bile flow is nearly completely stopped. The spleen and the liver appear pale. The disease is contagious and may cause large losses, especially in young Trout. Histological investigations show hyaline degeneration and necrosis of the voluntary muscles and pancreatic lesions. The disease has an incubation period of 6–14 days. Brook Trout (*Salvelinus fontinalis*) is especially susceptible. The disease is caused by a heat-resistant virus, passing through pore of 50 nm [1 nm (formerly mμ) = 0.001 micron], and possibly belonging to the *Picorna* virus group.

THROAT TUMOURS IN *MOLLIENISIA*

Schäperclaus[85] investigated peculiar tumour-like growths at the throat of Black Mollies, resembling those found in other positions in *Lymphocystis* and cauliflower diseases. The growth is situated at the ventral side of the head, starting from the border of the operculum. The core of the growth consists of branched strands of connective tissue with black pigment in between. The growth is covered by epithelial tissue, consisting of homologous cells and containing numerous slime cells. Schäperclaus suggests that this condition, too, may be due to a virus infection.

ULCERATIVE DERMAL NECROSIS[86]

This is a condition affecting the skin of mature wild *Salmonidæ* when they are returning from the sea for spawning. In Scotland, losses of fish caused by it in 1967 were estimated in excess of 51 000 and, in 1968, in excess of 38 000. It is thought likely that the disease is due to a virus as the primary cause, with a secondary fungus infection.

REFERENCES

1 WOOD, E. M., YASUTAKE, W. T. and SNIESZKO, S. F., 'Sulfonamide toxicity in Brook Trout', *Trans. Amer. Fish. Soc.* **84**, 155–60 [1954 (1955)]
2 SNIESZKO, S. F. and WOOD, E. M., 'The effect of some sulfonamides on the growth of Brook Trout, Brown Trout and Rainbow Trout', *Trans. Amer. Fish. Soc.* **84**, 86–92 [1954 (1955)]
3 AMEND, D. F., FRYER, J. L. and PILCHER, K. S., 'Studies of certain sulfonamide drugs for use in juvenile Chinook Salmon', *Progr. Fish-Cult.* 31, 202–06 (1969)
4 COWMEADOW, MARY M., STEEGE, P. T., PANG, P. K. T. and GRANT, F. B., 'A study of the physiological effects of sulfisoxazole on the killifish', *Progr. Fish-Cult.* **31**, 226–28 (1969)
5 NECHIPORENCO, YU. D., OSADCHAYA, E. F., KARPENKO, I. M. and MAREEVA, A. V., 'Primenie levomitsetina diya bor'by krasnukhoi karpa', *Rybnoe Khor.* **38**, 30–31 (1962)
6 AXELROD, H. R., 'Further observations on the use of aureomycin', *Water Life* **VII**, 242 (Oct. 1952)
7 WATER LIFE ANALYST, 'Possible effects of antibiotics and auxiliary growth factors', *Water Life* **VII**, 185–86 (Aug. 1952)
8 WOLD, A., 'Effects and use of aureomycin', *Aquarium Journal* (U.S.A.) **XXIII**, 232–35 (Nov. 1952)
9 VAN DUIJN, Jnr., C., 'Tuberculosis disease in fishes', *The Microscope* **13**, 23–28 (1961)
10 MEYER, F. P., 'Field treatments of *Aeromonas liquefaciens* infections in Golden Shiners (*Notemigonus crysoleucas*)', *Progr. Fish-Cult.* **26**, 33–35 (1964)
11 MITRA, RITA and GHOSH, S. C., 'The effect of Terramycin on the growth of some freshwater food fishes: (*Labeo rohita, Catla catla,* and *Cirrhina mtigala*)', *Proc. Nat. Acad. Sci. India Sect. B. (Biol. Sci.)* **37**, 406–08 (1967)
12 PIPER, R. G., 'Toxic effects of erythromycin thiocyanate on Rainbow Trout', *Progr. Fish-Cult.* **23**, 134–35 (1961)
13 CONROY, D. A., 'Studies on the application of kanamycin to the control and treatment of some bacterial diseases of fish', *J. Appl. Bacteriol* **26**, 182–92 (1963); 'Otras observaciones sobre la putrefaccion de la aleta caudal en los peces', *Microbiol. Españ.* **16**, 63–66 (1963); 'Un caso de *manchas rojas* en peces de acuario', *Microbiol. Españ.* **15**, 95–99 (1962); 'Kanamycin sulphate in the treatment of experimental *Pseudomonas fluorescens* infection in fish', *J. Sci. Technol.* **9 : 4**, 151–53; CONROY, D. A. and HUGHES, M. C., 'Handling of fish for injection', *J. Animal Tech. Assoc.* **11**, 3–4 (1960)
14 COLER, R. A., GUNNER, H. B. and ZUCKERMAN, B. M., 'Tubificid sensitivity to streptomycin', *Trans. Amer. Fish. Soc.* **97**, 502–03 (1968)
15 VOKOUN, P., ZDENEK LUCKY and VACLAV DYK, 'The effect of some antibiotics in food on the reproduction of guppies (*Lebistes reticulatus*)', *Acta. Univ. Agr. Fac. Vet.* **37**, 253–62 (1968)

208   DISEASES CAUSED BY BACTERIA AND VIRUSES

16 GHITTINO, P., 'Piscicoltura e ittipatologia. II. Ittipatologia', *Riv. Zootec.* **42**, 452–68 (1969)
17 BOWERS, C. E., 'Fin-rot cured by phenoxetol', *Water Life* **VIII**, 157 (June 1953); RANKIN, I. M., 'New cure for fin-rot', *Water Life* **VIII**, 251–52 (Oct. 1953)
18 BAGENAL, T. B., 'Propylene phenoxethol as a fish anaesthetic', *Nature (Lond.)* **197**, 1222–23 (1963)
19 POST, G. and KEISS, R. E., 'Further laboratory studies on the use of furazolidone for the control of furunculosis of Trout', *Progr. Fish-Cult.* **24**, 16–21 (1962)
20 VAN HORN, W. M. and KATZ, M., 'Pyridyl mercuric acetate as a prophylactic in fisheries management', *Science* **104**, 557 (1946); RUCKER, R. R., 'New compounds for the control of bacterial gill disease', *Progr. Fish-Cult.* **10**, 166–69 (1948); SNIESZKO, S. F., 'Pyridyl mercuric acetate tech. Its use in control of gill disease and some external parasitic infestations', *Progr. Fish-Cult.* **14**, 153–55 (1949); BURROWS, E. R. and PALMER, D. D., 'Pyridyl mercuric acetate. Its toxicity to fish, efficacy in disease control, and applicability to a simplified treatment technique', *Progr. Fish-Cult.* **11**, 147–51 (1949)
21 SEAMAN, W. R., 'Warning to users of pyridyl mercuric acetate', *Progr. Fish-Cult.* **12**, 126 (1950); RODGERS, E. O., HAZEN, B. H., FRIDDLE, S. B. and SNIESZKO, S. F., 'The toxicity of pyridyl mercuric acetate technical (PMA) to Rainbow Trout (*Salmo gairdneri*)', *Progr. Fish-Cult.* **13**, 71–73 (1951)
22 McFADDEN, T. W., 'Effective disinfection of trout eggs to prevent egg transmission of *Aeromonas liquefaciens*', *J. Fish Res. Board Can.* **26**, 2311–18 (1969)
23 REICHENBACH-KLINKE, H., *Krankheiten und Schädigungen der Fische*, p. 58, Stuttgart (1966)
24 BUTLER, C. H., *The Aquarium* (U.S.A.) **XVII**, 163 (Mar. 1948)
25 CAMPBELL, A. S., *Aquarium Journal* (U.S.A.) **XXI**, 195 (Sept. 1950)
26 SNIESZKO, S. F., 'Therapy of bacterial diseases', *Trans. Am. Fisheries Soc.* **83**, 313–30 [1953 (publ. 1954)]
27 CONROY, D. A., 'La produccion de la putrefaccion de la aleta caudal en los peces por la accion de *Aeromonas punctata*', *Microbiol. Españ.* **14**, 233–38 (1961)
28 SANDER, E., 'Ozone—its application to aquarium-keeping', *Pet Fish Monthly* **I**, 9–10 (1966)
29 BOWERS, C. E., 'Fin-rot cured by phenoxetol', *Water Life* **VIII**, 157 (June 1953)
30 RANKIN, I. M., 'New cure for fin-rot', *Water Life* **VIII**, 215–52 (Oct. 1953)
31 AMLACHER, E., *Taschenbuch der Fischkrankheiten*, VEB Gustav Fischer Verlag, Jena (1961)
32 OPPENHEIMER, CARL H., 'On marine fish diseases', in BORGSTROM, G. (Ed.): *Fish as Food*, Vol. 2, pp. 541ff, Acad. Press, New York and London (1962); CONROY, D. A., 'Un caso de putrefaccion de la aleta caudal observado en la corvina', *Inst. Biol. Marina, Mar del Plata Cien. Invest.* **19**, 333 (1963)
33 FARRIN, A. E., SCATTERGOOD, L. W. and SINDERMANN, C. J., 'Maintenance of immature Sea Herring in captivity', *Progr. Fish-Cult.* **19**, 188–89 (1957)
34 RISELEY, *Tropical Marine Aquaria*, London (1971)
35 SCHÄPERCLAUS, W., '*Pseudomonas punctata* als Krankheitserreger bei Fischen', *Zeitschrift für Fischerei* **XXVIII**, No. 3, 290–370 (July 1930); 'Bakterielle Karpfenseuchen, ihre Bedeutung und Bekämpfung in der Teichwirtschaft', *Fischerei-Zeitung* **36**, Nos 15–17 (1933)
36 WUNDER, W., *Allgemeine Fischereizeitung* **74**, 326–58 (1949); **76**, 159 (1951)
37 SCHÄPERCLAUS, W., 'Beitrag zur Kenntnis der Punctata-Formen und Typen zur Theorie der Entstehung der infektiösen Bauchwassersucht des Karpfens', *Zentr. Bakteriol. Parasitenk.* Abt. II, **105**, Nos 5, 6 (1942)

38 ROEGNER-AUST, S. and SCHLEICH, F., 'Zur Aetiologie einiger Fischkrankheiten', *Z. für Naturf.* **VIb**, 448–51 (1951)
39 GONCAROV, G. D., 'Virusnaya krasnukha ryb v SSR i za rubezhom', *Tr. Soveshch. Ikthiol. Kom. Akad. Nauk. SSSR* **9**, 34–38 (1959)
40 TOMASEC, J., BRUDNJAK, Z., FIJAN, JR., N. and KUNST, L., 'Weiterer Beitrag zur Aetiologie der infektiösen Bauchwassersucht des Karpfens', *Jugoslav. Ak. Znam. Umjetn. Zagreb, Bul. intern.* **16**, 35–44 (1964)
41 HEUSCHMANN-BRUNNER, G., 'Ein Beitrag zur Erregerfrage der infektiösen Bauchwassersucht des Karpfens', in: *Festschrift anl. d. 50 jähr Bestehens d. Teichwirtsch. Abt. Wielenbach d. Bay. Biol. Versuchsanstalt München*, Munich, 41–49 (1965)
42 TETS, V. I., 'O kontagioznosti yazvennoi formy krasnukhi', *Nauchn. Tekh. Byul. Gas. Nauchn. Inst. Ozernogo Rechnigo Rybn. Khoz.* **13–14**, 105–08 (1961); Translation: 'Degree of contagiousness of the ulcerous form of dropsy', *Ref. Zh. Biol.*, No. 7175 (1963)
43 NECHIPORENKO, Y. D., OOSADCHAYA, E. F., KARPENKO, I. M. and MAREEVA, A. V., 'Primenie levomitsetine diya bor "by Krasnukhoi karpa"', *Rybnoe Khor.* **38**, 30–31 (1962)
44 SCHÄPERCLAUS, W., 'Erfolgreiche Bekämpfung der infektiösen Bauchwassersucht des Karpfens mit antiobiotischen Mitteln in 11 Jahren', *Deutsch. Fisch.-Ztg.* **14**, 64–66 (1967)
45 VAN DUIJN, JNR., C., 'Beitrag zur Kenntnis der Schuppensträubung bei Fischen', *Wochenschrift für Aquarien- und Terrarienkunde* **35**, 68–70 (Feb. 1938)
46 VAN DUIJN, JNR., C., 'A contagious disease of labyrinth fishes caused by *Pseudomonas fluorescens*', *The Microscope* **II**, 122–23 (1938)
47 CONROY, D. A., 'Kanamycin sulphate in the treatment of experimental *Pseudomonas fluorescens* infections of fish', *J. Sci. Technol.* **9**, 151–53 (1962); 'Studies on application of kanamycin to the control and treatment of some bacterial diseases of fish', *J. Appl. Bacteriol.* **26**, 182–92 (1963)
48 BRUNNER, G. and REICHENBACH-KLINKE, H., 'Beitrag zur Fleckenseuche des Hechtes', *Allg. Fisch.-Ztg.* **86**, 310–11 (1961)
49 SNIESZKO, S. F., 'Freshwater fish disease caused by bacteria belonging to the Genera *Aeromonas* and *Pseudomonas*', U.S. Dept. of Interior—*Fisheries Leaflet*, No. 459 (1958)
50 AMBRUS, J. L., AMBRUS, C. M. and HARRISON, J. W. E., 'Prevention of *Proteus hydrophilus* infections (red leg disease) in frog colonies', *Am. J. Pharm.* **123**, 129 (1951); SEAMAN, W. R., 'Notes on a bacterial disease of Rainbow Trout in a Colorado hatchery', *Progr. Fish-Cult.* **13**, 139–41 (1951)
51 CONROY, D. A., 'Studies on the application of kanamycin to the control and treatment of some bacterial diseases of fish', *J. Appl. Bacteriol.* **26**, 182–92 (1963)
52 SMITH-ISABEL, W., 'A disease of Finnock due to *Vibrio anquillarum*', *J. Gen.-Microbiol* **24**, 247–52 (1961)
53 KUBOTA, S. S. and HAGITA, K., 'Studies on the diseases of marine-culture fishes. II. Pharmaco-dynamic effects of nitrofurazone for fish diseases', *J. Fac. Fisheries, Prefect. Univ. Mie* **6**, 125–44 (1963); KUSUDA, R., 'Studies on the ulcer disease of marine fishes', *Proc. 1st U.S.–Japan Joint Conference Marine Microbiol.*, Tokyo (1966)
54 CONROY, D. A., 'Un caso de *manchas rojas* en peces de acuario', *Microbiol. Españ.* **15**, 95–99 (1962)
55 REICHENBACH-KLINKE, H., *Krankheiten und Schädigungen der Fische*, Stuttgart (1966)
56 GRIFFIN, P. J. and SNIESZKO, S. F., 'A unique bacterium pathogenic for warm-blooded and cold-blooded animals', *Fish Bull.* **52**, 185–90 (1951)
57 FISH, F. F., 'Ulcer disease of Trout', *Trans. Amer. Fish Soc.* **64**, 252–58 (1934);

WOLF, L. E., 'Observations on ulcer disease in Trout', *Trans. Amer. Fish Soc.* **68**, 136–51 (1938); SNIESZKO, S. F., 'Ulcer disease in Brook Trout (*Salvelinus fontinalis*): Its economic importance, treatment, and prevention', *Progr. Fish-Cult.* **14**, 43–49 (1952); SNIESZKO, S. F., FRIDDLE, S. B. and GRIFFIN, P. S., 'Successful treatment of ulcer disease in Brook Trout (*Salvelinus fontinalis*) with terramycin', *Science* **113**, 717–18 (1951); SNIESZKO, S. F., FRIDDLE, S. B. and GRIFFIN, P. J., 'Antibiotic treatment of ulcer disease and furunculosis in Trout', *Trans. 17th N. Amer. Wildlife Conf.*, 187–213 (1952)

58 SNIESZKO, S. F. and BULLOCK, G. L., 'A massive kill of White Perch (*Roccus americanus*) involving a *Pasteurella*-like bacterium', *Bact. Proc.* G. 154 (1964)

59 VAN DUIJN, Jnr., C., 'Tuberculosis disease in fishes', *The Microscope* **13**, 23–28 (1961)

60 WOOD, J. W. and ORDALE, E. J., 'Tuberculosis in Pacific Salmon and Steelhead Trout', *Contr. Oregon Fish. Comm.* **25**, 1–38 (1958)

61 JAHNEL, J., 'Die Fischtuberkulose', *Wochenschrift f. Aquarien- und Terrarienkunde* **37**, 317–21 (1940); 'Spontaninfektionen mit säurefesten Stäbchen bei Fischen. Neue Beobachtungen über Fischtuberkulose', *Wien. Tieraerztl. Monatsschr.* **27**, 289–302 (1940); REICHENBACH-KLINKE, H., 'Untersuchungen über die bei Fischen durch Parasiten hervorgerufenen Zysten und deren Wirkung auf den Wirtskorper', *Z. f. Fischerei*, N.F. 3, 565–636 (1954), N.F. 4, 1–72 (1955); 'Die Fischtuberkulose', *Die Aquarien- und Terrarienzeitschrift* (DATZ) **8**, 12–17 (1955)

62 BAKER, J. A. and HAGAN, W. A., 'Tuberculosis of the Mexican Platyfish', *J. Infect. Diseases* **70**, 248–52 (1942)

63 BESSE, P., 'Epizootie a bacilles acide-resistants chez de poisson exotique', *Bull. Acad. Vet. France* **23**, 151–54 (1949)

64 NIGRELLI, R. F., 'Two diseases of the Neon Tetra (*Hyphessobrycon innesi*): (A) Tuberculosis, (B) Microsporidiosis', *Aquarium J.* **34**, 203–08 (1953); ROSS, A. J. and BRANCATO, F. P., '*Mycobacterium fortuitum* Cruz from the tropical fish *Hyphessobrycon innesi*', *J. Bact.* **78**, 392–95 (1959)

65 ROSS, A. J., '*Mycobacterium salmoniphilum* n. sp from Salmonid fish', *Amer. Rev. Resp. Dis.* **81**, 241–50 (1960)

66 ARONSON, J. D., 'Spontaneous tuberculosis in salt water fish', *J. Infect. Dis.* **39**, 315–20 (1926); GRIFFITH, A. S., 'Tuberculosis in cold-blooded animals', *A system of Bacteriology in relation to Medicine* **5**, 326–33 (1930)

67 HAUSS, Helga and SIMON, C., 'Über eine Hautinfektion durch *Mycobacterium marinum* sive balnei', *Arch. f. klin. u. exp. Dermatologie* **216**, 334–53 (1963)

68 CONROY, D. A. and VALDEZ, I. E., 'Un caso de tuberculosis on peces tropicales', *Rev. Latinoam. Microbiol.* **5**, 9–16 (1962); CONROY, D. A., 'The study of a tuberculosis condition in Neon Tetras (*Hyphessobrycon innesi*). Symptoms of the disease and preliminary description of the organism isolated', *Microbiol. Españ.* **16**, 47–54 (1963)

69 VAN DUIJN, Jnr., C., 'Tuberculosis disease in fishes', *The Microscope* **13**, 23–28 (1961)

70 VICKERS, K. U. and McCLEAN, R., 'Furunculosis in Lough Neagh Pollan *Coregonus pollan* Thompson', *Nature (Lond.)* **191**, 930 (1961); VAN DUIJN, Jnr., C., 'Taxonomy of the fish furunculosis organism', *Nature (Lond.)* **195**, 1127 (1962)

71 KIMURA, TAKAHISA, 'Studies on a bacterial disease in the adult "Sakuramasu" (*Oncorhynchus masou*) and Pink Salmon (*O. gorbuscha*) rearing for maturity', *Sci. Rep. Hokkaido Salmon Hatchery* **24**, 9–100 (1970) (Japanese with English summary)

72 SNIESZKO, S. F., 'Therapy of bacterial fish diseases', *Trans. Amer. Fish Soc.* **83**, 313–30 [1953 (publ. 1954)]; POST, G. and KEISS, R. E., 'Further laboratory studies on the use of furazolidone for the control of furunculosis of Trout', *Progr. Fish-Cult.* **24**, 16–21 (1962)

73 FLAKAS, K. G., 'Sulfonamide therapy of furunculosis in Brown Trout', *Trans. Amer. Fish Soc.* **78**, 117–27 (1948)
74 RUCKER, R. R., 'A Streptomycete pathogenic to fish', *J. Bact.* **58**, 659–64 (1949)
75 WALKER, R., 'The structure of Lymphocystis virus of fish', *Virology* **18**, 503–05 (1962)
76 ROEGNER-AUST, S. and SCHLEICH, F., 'Zur Aetiologie einiger Fischkrankheiten', *Z. f. Naturforschung* **VIb**, 448–49 (1951)
77 ROEGNER-AUST, S. and DEUBNER, B., 'Weitere Untersuchungen über die Pockenkrankheit des Karpfens', *Z. f. Naturforschung* **VIIb**, 572 (1952); ROEGNER-AUST, S., 'Zur-Frage einer Virus-ätiologie bei verschiedenen Fischkrankheiten', *Müncher Beiträge zur Abwässer-, Fischerei-u-Flussbiologie*, Munich **1**, 120–45 (1953)
78 SCHUBERT, G. and MEYER, G., *Verhandl. Deut. Zool. Ges.*, Münster (1959); SCHUBERT, G., 'Elektronenmikroskopische Untersuchungen zur Pockenkrankheit des Karpfens', *Zeitschr. Naturforsch. B.* **19**, 675–82 (1964)
79 PACHECO, G. and GUIMARAES, J. R., 'Ichthyozooties dans les eaux fluviales de l'Etat de Saõ Paolo', *Compt. Rend. de la Soc. Biol.* **III**, 1401 (1933)
80 LIEBMANN, H. and REICHENBACH-KLINKE, H., 'Untersuchungen zur Epidemiologie und Ökologie der Forellenseuche', *Arch. Fischereiwiss.* **15**, 94–113 (1964)
81 ZWILLENBERG, L. O., 'Elektronenmikroskopische Untersuchungen an Regenbogenforellen mit infektiöser Nierenschwellung und Leberdegeneration', *Arch. ges. Virusforsch.* **14**, 319–31 (1964); ZWILLENBERG, L. O., JENSEN, M. H. and ZWILLENBERG, H. H. L., 'Electron microscopy of the virus of viral haemorrhagic septicaemia of Rainbow Trout (Egtved virus)', *Arch. ges. Virusforsch* **17**, 1–19 (1965)
82 SNIESZKO, S. F. and GRIFFIN, P. J., with assistance of DELISLE, H. A., DUNBAR, C. E., FRIDDLE, S. B. and SANDERSON, A. G., 'Kidney disease in Brook Trout', *Progr. Fish-Cult.*, 3–13 (Jan. 1955); SNIESZKO, S. F., 'Therapy of fish diseases', *Trans. Amer. Fish. Soc.* **83**, 313–30 [1953 (publ. 1954)]
83 TACK, E., 'Beiträge zur Erforschung der Forellenseuche', *Arch. Fischereiwiss* **10**, 20–30 (1959); 'Beiträge zur Erforschung der Forellenseuche', *Allg. Fischereiztg.* **85**, 634–35 (1960)
84 WOOD, E. M., SNIESZKO, S. F. and YASUTAKE, W. T., 'Infectious necrosis in Brook Trout', *A.M.A. Arch. Path.* **60**, 26–28 (1955); SNIESZKO, S. F., WOOD, E. M. and YASUTAKE, W. T., 'Infectious pancreatic necrosis in Trout', *A.M.A. Arch. Path.* **62**, 229–33 (1957); WOLF, K., DUNBAR, C. E. and SNIESZKO, S. F., 'Infectious pancreatic necrosis of Trout', *Progr. Fish-Cult.*, 64–68 (1960); WOLF, K., SNIESZKO, S. F., DUNBAR, C. E. and PYLE, E., 'Virus nature of infectious pancreatic necrosis in Trout', *Proc. Soc. Exp. Biol. Med.* **104**, 105–08 (1960); WOLF, K., QUIMBY, M. C. and BRADFORD, A. D., 'Egg-associated transmission of IPN virus of Trouts', *Virology* **21**, 317–21 (1963)
85 SCHÄPERCLAUS, W., *Fischkrankheiten*, 536, 3rd ed., Berlin (1954); *also see* SINDERMANN, CARL J., *Principal Diseases of Marine Fish and Shellfish*, New York and London (1970)
86 MUNRO, A. L. S., 'Ulcerative dermal necrosis, a disease of migratory salmonid fishes in the rivers of the British Isles', *Biol. Conserv.* **2**, 129–32 (1970)

6

DISEASES OF THE EYE

The eye of a fish (Fig. 6.1) is made up of the same elements as the human eye, with one important difference. In the human eye accommodation takes place by changes in the shape of the lens, but the lens of a fish eye has a fixed shape and cannot be changed. Accommodation is possible, however, by displacement of the lens and this is effected by means of a sickle-shaped appendix which is fastened to the choroid. Thus accommodation in the fish eye resembles the focusing of a camera, which is done by changing the distance between the lens and the photographic plate.

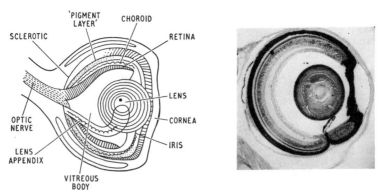

Fig. 6.1. Section of a fish's eye showing its structure

In judging the general health of a fish, a simple test may be made in which the eye plays an important rôle. If a completely healthy fish is taken in the hand (although still kept under the water) and turned on its side, the eye will not share in this movement, but will remain in the same position, so that from above the pupil of the eye remains invisible. But if a fish is very sick, the eye will follow the turning of the body and then the pupil may be seen when the fish is turned on its side. This simple experiment is a valuable aid to diagnosis in cases where more characteristic symptoms are lacking. Another symptom of general disease is a sinking of the eyes into the orbits. The eyes of a healthy fish are always a little raised above the surface of the head. The symptom of sunken eyes occurs in serious afflictions of the internal organs, dropsy, starvation, disorders of metabolism and in some intoxications, especially with chlorine.

There are a few diseases which attack the eye directly and we may now consider these.

EYE FUNGUS

If the cornea of the eye has been damaged, either by mechanical or chemical influences, fungus infections will soon occur. A fungus infection of the eye is much more dangerous than one of the skin, since disease originating on the eye may easily penetrate into the brain, and, in such a case, nothing can save the victim. Consequently it is very important that treatment should start as soon as possible after fungus threads become visible on the eye of a fish.

Eye fungus is characterised by the formation of a tuft of white or grey-white threads, resembling cotton-wool, hanging out of the eye. These fungus threads adhere very firmly to the cornea so that it is impossible to remove them mechanically without destroying parts of the eye. Without any treatment the complete destruction of the eye occurs in a few days, followed by a penetration of the fungus mycelium to the brain and this causes death.

Although there is more likelihood of the fungus developing if the eye has been injured, and consequently only single cases of eye fungus should be expected, I was once able to investigate an epidemic of this disease among Livebearing Tooth-carps. The fishes developed fungus in one eye only, but one fish after another became affected and died. No other parasites that could have opened the way to the fungus infection were found, although there is a possibility that there was bacterial infection, since no bacteriological investigations were made. Another possible cause was the chemical composition of the water but, if this were unsatisfactory, it is difficult to understand why, in each case, only one eye was affected.

Generally speaking, however, we may regard eye fungus as a secondary infection, following either mechanical or chemical injuries to the eye or damage caused by other parasites, mostly worms. Since the disease called worm cataract can occur epidemically, in such cases eye fungus may appear in several fishes at around the same time.

Eye fungus is a most serious disease, but when treated at its commencement, it is possible to cure the fish, although in most cases the eye will be lost. Since it is most important that the fungus is killed as soon as possible, methods described in cases of fungus of the skin are insufficient. The best way of treatment is effected by touching all parts of the fungus and the infected eye with a pencil or brush, dipped in a 1–2% solution of silver nitrate ($AgNO_3$) in distilled water (this chemical is made inactive by tap-water). After this, the eye is touched with a tuft of cotton-wool, dipped in a 1% solution of potassium dichromate. This will neutralise the silver nitrate so that the eye is protected from exposure to excessive influence from this chemical. To avoid new infections after treatment, the fish is placed in a solution of potassium dichromate, 1 : 25 000–1 : 20 000 (1 g in 5 or 6 Imp. gal), till complete recovery is achieved but not exceeding a period of 10 days. If necessary, treatment with the silver nitrate may be repeated at intervals in the meantime.

It might be expected that treatment with phenoxethol, as advocated by Ian M. Rankin for treatment of fungus diseases of the skin and which has also been proved to be effective against some bacteria, would furnish a good cure, too. Details of this treatment are described on page 85.

Eye fungus may also occur in marine fishes kept in sea-water aquaria. Riseley found that in these cases treatment with chlortetracycline (Aureomycin), as described for tail- and fin-rot in marine fishes (see p. 165), is often effective.[1]

EXOPHTHALMUS OR EYE PROTRUSION

Sometimes a disease can occur in fish in which the eye swells and, becoming too large for the orbit, protrudes (Fig. 6.2).

Further developments of the disease may differ in individual cases. Sometimes there are no further symptoms and the fish does

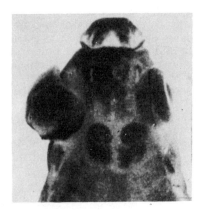

Fig. 6.2. Head of a fish with one-sided Exophthalmus. *This case was found to be due to fish tuberculosis (after Amlacher)*

not seem to suffer much hardship from its illness. It may still live quite happily, but, in other cases, the fish dies after a while. I once observed a very interesting case of *Exophthalmus* in a double-tailed Goldfish. This animal developed an *Exophthalmus* of one of its eyes which gradually increased until the swelling became so great that the eye was pushed out of the orbit and was lost. The

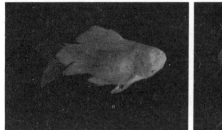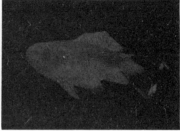

Fig. 6.3. Right and left views of a double-tail Goldfish which had lost both eyes due to Exophthalmus. *The wounds had healed without any infection developing*

yawning wound healed very well and no infection occurred (Fig. 6.3). After some time the remaining eye began to swell and develop *Exophthalmus* in the same way as the other. This eye was also pushed out of the orbit and lost, whilst the socket of the eye healed without any infection. This healing was very remarkable since fungus growth usually develops in such cases. The Goldfish, now completely

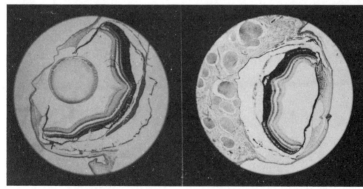

Fig. 6.4. Section through the eye of a Guppy afflicted with Exophthalmus. *It shows considerable swelling and enlargement but no pathological change in the tissues. Magnification* × 21 *(approx.)*

Fig. 6.5. Section from the unaffected eye of the same Guppy as in Fig. 6.4, for comparison (lens was lost during preparation). Magnification × 21 *(approx.)*

blind, lived for several years without suffering and appeared to be in quite good health. Since the fish had obviously no difficulty in seeking food it may be presumed that it made good use of its remaining senses of smell, touch and taste.

Microscopical examination of thin sections cut through the eye of a fish with a well-developed *Exophthalmus* (Figs 6.4, 6.5) often does not contribute very much to the understanding of the causes of this disease. The protruding eye is enlarged, but generally no pathological changes in the tissues can be seen, neither can any parasites be found. However, in Atlantic Herring (*Clupea harengus harengus*) two-sided eye-protrusion, induced by the larval Trematode (sucking worm) *Cryptocotyle lingua*, has been observed.[2] In literature, several statements about *Exophthalmus* have been made, but a complete solution of the problem has not yet been obtained. The late Bruno Hofer stated that it may be caused experimentally by blows or pressure on the head, but it can hardly be likely that such is a natural cause of this disease. Schäperclaus has found *Exophthalmus* occurring after mechanical injury to the eye by a wood splinter and also by attacks

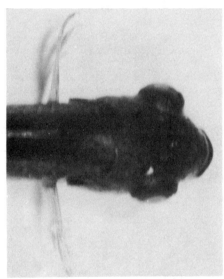

Fig. 6.6. Head of a Pelmato-chromis pulcher *with double-sided* Exophthalmus, *produced by tuberculosis infection. Photograph by the author*

of fish-eating water birds trying to catch a fish with their claws. Mechanical injury has also been reported to induce (generally temporarily) *Exophthalmus* in marine aquarium fishes by Riseley,[1] who also observed its occurrence where the fishes were exposed to a too-bright lighting. In the latter condition they could be cured by moving them to a darker tank or by providing more shade.

About the year 1930, Schäperclaus investigated several cases of *Exophthalmus* in fishes living in ponds and found that these were caused by *Aeromonas punctata* and a variety which he distinguished as *forma sacrowiensis*. Later, however, it has become uncertain whether this variety of bacteria, as a quite distinct variety, does exist. Details of other diseases in which *Aeromonas punctata* has been found are given in Chapter 4.

In most cases which Schäperclaus investigated, the eye protrusion was not a single complaint, but a secondary effect, occurring in cases of scale protrusion, dropsy and other diseases in which the

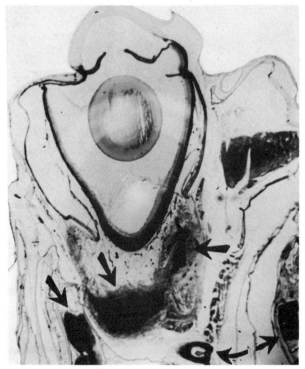

Fig. 6.7. Horizontal transversal section through the head of a Pelmatochromis pulcher, *showing* Exophthalmus *due to tuberculous lesions (indicated by arrows). However, the primary sites of the disease were found in the liver and other internal organs. Gram-staining*

same or other varieties of *Aeromonas punctata* can be found. Such cases of disease were of an epidemic character but most cases that occur in aquaria are non-infectious, as I described previously.

However, it has been shown that *Exophthalmus* may also be produced by tuberculosis infection (see page 184) and by infection with the unicellular parasite *Ichthyophonus*, which belongs to the *Chytridiaceæ*, a group of organisms verging both to *Algæ* and *Fungi* (see page 250), if cysts are formed in or near the orbit of the eye. Occasionally the sporozoan *Glugea pseudotumefaciens* (discovered by Pflugfelder in 1952) has been found as the causative organism in exotic aquarium fishes. This parasite also produces skin ulcers and knots in several internal organs—see p. 138. According to Schäperclaus the condition could also be produced as a secondary symptom

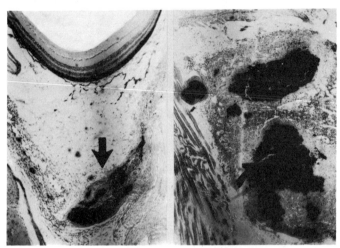

Fig. 6.8. Left: *Part of a section as in Fig. 6.7. at higher magnification (× 50).* Iron-haematoxyline stain. Right: *Darkly stained tuberculous lesions in the liver region of the same fish. Iron-haematoxyline stain. × 50 (photomicrographs by the author)*

of afflictions of internal organs, such as the pancreas, kidneys and liver, of supposed viral origin. It is also observed in cases of fatty necrosis of the pancreas (see p. 231). In large marine aquaria *Exophthalmus* seems to occur quite often, especially in Gurnets (*Trigla* species) and members of the *Gadidæ*, such as Cod, Haddock a.o. Schäperclaus suggests—again without any direct evidence— that these cases could be due to infection of the eye bulb with gas-producing bacteria or with *Vibrio anguillarum*.

At one time I myself investigated a contagious form of eye protrusion in aquarium fishes. It affected full-grown Angel Fish (*Pterophyllum*) and death occurred in a comparatively short time. Unfortunately, however, at that time I had no opportunity for a thorough bacteriological investigation, so that I am unable to tell whether this epidemic could have been caused by bacteria.

In epidemical double-sided *Exophthalmus* in *Pelmatochromis pulcher*, large populations of Mycobacteria of at least two types (long slender rods and short, nearly coccoid forms, see Fig. 6.9) have been found in smear preparations from the eyes. However, similar bacterial populations were found in the eyes of unaffected Pulchers as well as in *Nothobranchus guntheri* (Buenos Aires Tetra). Therefore it is not yet clear whether the infection is dormant for a longer period of time before specific symptoms arise or that they should be secondary invaders to some other infection. Primary tuberculosis occurred in the liver and kidneys of the victims, however.

In *Fundulus heteroclitus, Sparisoma squalidum* and *Bathystoma aurolineatus, Exophthalmus* should have been produced experimentally by injection of testosterone (male sex hormone) or one of the thyroid hormones triiodothyronine and I-thyroxine by Matty, Menzel and Bardach,[3] but this could not be confirmed in experiments with Carp by der Kinderen.[4] However, injection of blood serum from human patients suffering from *Exophthalmus* (as occurring in Basedow's disease, Cushing's syndrome, acromegalia and other

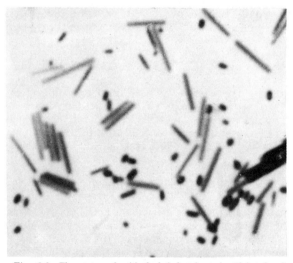

Fig. 6.9. *Two types of acid-alcohol fast bacteria (fish tubercle bacteria) in a smear preparation of the eye of a* Pelmatochromis pulcher *suffering from double-sided* Exophthalmus. *Ziehl-Neelsen staining.* × 4000 (photomicrograph by the author)

conditions) definitely produces eye protrusion in *Fundulus heteroclitus*, Goldfish and Carp. Sensitivity is highly dependent on the season of the year in *Fundulus*,[5] but not in Goldfish or Carp.

Dr. der Kinderen could demonstrate that the causative agent, which had already been provisionally called EPS ('*Exophthalmus* Producing Substance') in medical literature, is produced by the hypophysis. He developed quantitative methods of using Mirror Carp as a test animal for aid in diagnosis of exophthalmic conditions in humans.

Normal human urine also contains EPS, but this cannot be used in experiments with fish, owing to the toxicity of urine injections to fish.

There are indications that another substance exists which has an antagonistic effect to EPS; in normal individuals this substance and EPS should balance each other.

Eye protrusion induced by excess EPS is most probably due to increased liquid content in the orbit, whereas secondary effects are changes of the connective, fat and muscle tissues. It is suggested that changes in the permeability of the walls of the blood vessels may play a rôle in the development of those conditions.

From these investigations it may be inferred that at least part of non-parasitic cases of *Exophthalmus* in fish are due to disturbances of the hormonal equilibrium of the hypophysis. In human medicine severe cases of *Exophthalmus* with acute danger of blindness have been successfully treated by surgery or X-ray irradiation of the hypophysis, but in fish such methods are out of the question.

GREY CATARACT (*CATARACTA TRAUMATICA*)

This disease is characterised by a whitish condition of the lens of the eye, so that it resembles that of a fish which has been boiled. Generally only one eye is affected. Grey cataract occurs particularly in varieties of Goldfish. The cause of this disease is not yet known and details of treatments are also lacking.

WORM CATARACT (*CATARACTA PARASITICA*)

This disease may resemble grey cataract, but it can be distinguished by observation with the aid of a magnifying glass. Then it will be seen that the whitish condition of the eye is not homogeneous, but is due to the presence of small white dots which show clearly against the black background of the pupil. These white dots are, in reality, little worms that are situated between the lens and the lens capsule. They feed on the lens, destroying it and thus causing trouble. When the disease develops, the eye becomes completely white, like that of boiled fish, and, at this stage, it is difficult to observe the worms, even with a magnifying glass, unless the fish is killed and the dissected contents of the eye are examined with a microscope or magnifying glass. Since the worms may reach a length of about 0.5 mm only very low magnifications are required; about × 20 is sufficient even for identifying the species.

Generally it is possible to make the diagnosis of worm cataract, even in such advanced cases, without dissection, merely by following the course of the disease. A watery liquid accumulates in the eye, pressing against the cornea and vaulting it to the outside. In this way a so-called keratoglobus or keratokonus (Fig. 6.10) is produced (from Greek: *keratos* = cornea; *globus* = globe or sphere; *konos* = cone). Finally, the pressure becomes so great that the cornea bursts and the contents of the eye run out. After this, fungus infection will occur, which soon causes the death of the victim.

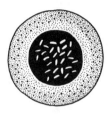 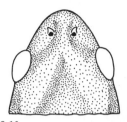

Fig. 6.10.
WORM CATARACT
Left: *Eye of a fish with worm cataract (after Hofer).*
Right: *Head of a fish with worm cataract and a kerato-globus (redrawn after Hofer)*

Worm cataract is due to larvae of several species of sucking worms (*Trematoda*), such as *Proalaria (Hemistomum) spathaceum* (Fig. 6.11). The adult parasite lives in water birds, where eggs are produced that are discharged into the water with the excrements of the birds. The eggs hatch in the water, producing larvae which are taken into the body of a fish.

Fig. 6.11. Young larvae of Proalaria (Hemistomum) spathaceum *(after Nordmann)*

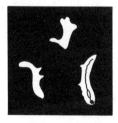

The eggs have a size of only 0.1 mm × 0.06 mm. The period of development before hatching is not known, but a reasonable estimate may be about three weeks. From the eggs, ciliated larvae, called miracidia, appear. The miracidia swim through the water till they find a suitable snail belonging to the Family *Lymnæidae*, generally the great pond snail or fresh-water whelk *Lymnæa stagnalis*, or *Galba (Lymnæa) palustris*, *Radix (Lymnæa) ovata* or *Radix (Lymnæa) auricularia* (Fig. 6.12). The miracidia penetrate into the liver of the snail, where they change shape, losing their cilia, and become sporocysts. These reproduce for three generations, taking about six weeks. The resulting larvae leave the liver of the snail and move into the water. They have a typical forked tail and are called cercariae. Their movement takes place in the direction of higher water temperature, but otherwise it is random; they do not actively seek to make contact with a fish, but are only prepared to attach as soon as such contact is made incidentally. The cercariae have a size of 265 µm × 85 µm for the main body and 240 µm × 40 µm for the tail. They can survive for two days only, so they must contact a fish within this short period of time. Below 9–10°C (48–50°F) the cercariae are unable to maintain their typical 'waiting for attack' position.

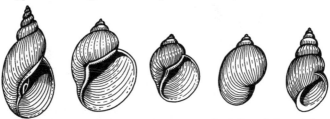

Fig. 6.12. Snail hosts of worm cataract organisms. From left *to* right: Lymnæa stagnalis, Radix auricularia, Radix ovata *(two specimens),* Galba palustris. *Natural size (all after Dorsman and De Wilde)*

When a cercaria contacts a fish, it penetrates *via* the skin or the gills, dropping its tail before penetration has been completed (in this condition it is called *Cercariæum*). The infection of the eye of the fish is accomplished by migration of the parasite inside the fish, or alternatively, the eye may be penetrated directly from the outside. At a temperature of 15–16°C (about 60°F) the cercariae develop inside the fish in about 45 days into another larval form, which was described under the name of *Diplostomum* before it was known that it was not a separate species but merely the larval stage of *Proalaria* (*Hemistomum*). Consequently they are still referred to in some literature as *Diplostomum volvens, Diplostomum annuligerum,* etc. (Fig. 6.13). The *Diplostomum* forms have a size of about 0.4 mm. Inside the

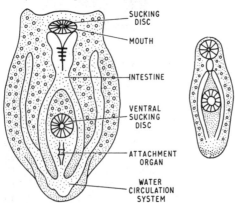

SUCKING DISC
MOUTH
INTESTINE
VENTRAL SUCKING DISC
ATTACHMENT ORGAN
WATER CIRCULATION SYSTEM

Fig. 6.13.
TWO
WORM CATARACT
ORGANISMS
Worm cataract is caused by the larvae of several sucking worms (Trematoda) *such as* Diplostomum volvens (left) *(after Roth) and* D. annuligerum (right) *(after Nordmann). Infection cannot occur from fish to fish but only through an intermediate water-bird host*

eye they may keep alive, meanwhile destroying the eye lens, for eight months or even longer. Spreading of the disease from fish to fish is not possible. The fish must first be eaten by a bird, where the larvae develop into adults, eliminated by quarantining plants for three days and snails for eight weeks. Of course, such quarantining is only necessary if plants and snails are taken from free waters or ponds. Since ramshorn snails (*Planorbis*) are no host for this parasite, members of this genus need not be subjected to this policy.

Diplostomum volvens may keep alive in the lens of dead fishes for 10 days. In ponds it is therefore necessary to remove dead fishes as soon as possible, since eating of such a dead fish by a water bird would spread the infection again.

Amphibians are also susceptible to worm cataract. Adult frogs and newts can only be penetrated by cercariae *via* the cornea of the eye itself, whereas in tadpoles infection may occur over the entire body surface, reproducing themselves with the production of eggs so that the cycle starts again. In an aquarium this disease can only occur if larvae of the parasite are introduced with snails, plants or live food.

Methods of curing fishes with this disease are still in an experimental stage. The following treatments have been suggested: (a) Potassium antimonyl tartrate (Tartar Emetic). Dosage 1.5 mg/l (1 gr/Imp. gal or 0.8 gr/U.S. gal). Since this drug is poisonous, it should be used with caution. Dosage has to be very accurate, while treatment should not be extended for a longer period than strictly necessary. This treatment has been suggested by Dr. C. van Dommelen.[6] (b) Phenoxethol. Infected fish are fed with dried food soaked in a 1% solution. Further, 10 cm³ of this 1% stock solution per litre (or 45 cm³/Imp. gal; 37 cm³/U.S. gal) or water are added. This treatment has been used by Mr. Ian M. Rankin against intestinal worms with success and it might be expected to be effective against worm cataract, too, if this has not advanced too far. (c) Sulphamerazine sodium has been reported to be effective[7] in a dosage of 1 g/l for 2–3 weeks. According to more recent experience it should be given orally (mixed with the food) in the same way as described for treatment of bacterial infections (see pages 152 and 351).

Since worm cataract is not infectious from fish to fish, it would be unwise to apply any treatment to all inhabitants of the tank in which some fish are affected. The diseased fish should be removed from the community tank and treated separately. In advanced cases of the disease, where already a keratoglobus or keratokonus has been produced, no medicament is capable of curing the victim. The only way of dealing with this advanced condition is a surgical treatment. It may be tried (but only by qualified persons) by opening the diseased eye with a sharp needle, so that the contents run out and, after that, disinfecting the wound thoroughly by bathing it with a tuft of cotton-wool dipped in a 1% solution of potassium dichromate. After this treatment the fish is placed in a solution of potassium dichromate (1 : 25 000) until the wound has been healed. Use fresh, clean water to prepare this bath and give the fish good, nourishing food. In this way it will be possible to rescue some fishes from death, although the diseased eye will be lost. In cases where both eyes are attacked, however, it is better to kill the fish.

OTHER WORM INFECTIONS OF THE EYE

Tylodelphys clavata Diesing (Fig. 6.14a). In the vitreous body of *Cyprinidæ*, *Cobitidæ* and *Percidæ*. Occasionally also in the scales. Herons are the final hosts.

Diplostomulum scheutingi Hughes. In the vitreous body of *Cyprinidæ*, *Esocidæ*, *Percidæ*, *Siluridæ*, *Centrarchidæ* and *Salmonidæ* in North America.

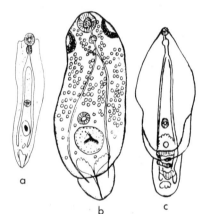

Fig. 6.14. Metacercariae of sucking worms found in fish eyes. (a) Tylodelphys clavata *Diesing (after Ciurea).* (b) Diplostomulum truttæ *Lacépède (after Hoffmann).* (c) Posthodiplostomum cuticola *Dubois (after Ciurea)*

Diplostomulum truttæ Lacépède (Fig. 6.14b). In the eyes of Scottish Trout.

Posthodiplostomum cuticola Dubois (Fig. 6.14c). Occasionally in or on the cornea, see pages 32–34 (black spot).

Posthodiplostomum brevicaudatum (Nordmann). In the vitreous body, the cornea and brains of *Cyprinidæ*, *Esocidæ*, *Percidæ* and Eelpout (*Lota lota*).

REFERENCES

1 RISELEY, R. A., *Tropical Marine Aquaria*, London (1971)
2 SINDERMANN, CARL J., *Principal Diseases of Marine Fish and Shellfish*, Academic Press, New York and London (1970)

3 MATTY, A. J., MENZEL, D. and BARDACH, J. E., *J. Clin. Endocrinol* **17**, 314 (1958)
4 DER KINDEREN, P. J., 'Onderzoekingen betreffende EPS (Een *Exophthalmus Producerende Stof)' M.D. Thesis*, Utrecht University (1965)
5 DOBYNE, B. M., WRIGHT, A. and WILSON, L., *J. Clin. Endocrinol* **21**, 648 (1961)
6 VAN DOMMELEN, C., 'Chemotherapie', *Het Aquarium* **18**, 215–16 (1948–49)
7 EBELS, E., 'Onderzoek naar een geneesmiddel voor wormstaar', *Het Aquarium* **27**, 113 (1946–47)

7

DISEASES OF THE INTERNAL ORGANS

In this chapter the diseases of the internal organs will be considered under two headings, the first being non-parasitic disorders and the second (page 236), parasitic diseases. Among the former are suffocation, inflammation, constipation, catarrh, degeneration, cysts, petrifaction, infertility and swim bladder trouble.

INFLAMMATION OF THE STOMACH AND INTESTINES

Most cases of inflammation of the stomach (stomachitis) and/or the intestines (enteritis) in fish are due to incorrect feeding. No fish can live on dried foods alone for a long period, and continuous feeding with only one kind of live food may also have bad results. Such diseases can consequently be completely avoided by giving fishes a suitably mixed diet. In times when no supplies of live food are available, do not use only one kind of dried food, but give different types in rotation.

Signs of any intestinal inflammation cannot be seen externally, although general symptoms may give a warning that fishes are not healthy; these may be lack of appetite, darkening of colours, etc. From a section of a fish that has died from the disease, the condition may be easily recognised. Healthy intestines of most fishes have a whitish or pink colour, whilst an inflamed intestine is red (Fig. 7.1). This is due to a widening of the blood vessels. The exterior of the intestinal wall will swell so that the organs appear enlarged and may be one and a half times their normal size. Inside the intestine a bloody pus-like liquid is usually present, which flows from the anal opening when light pressure is applied to the belly wall. Bloody or

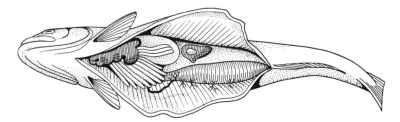

Fig. 7.1. Dissected Trout showing inflammation of the intestine. The intestine is swollen and blood-coloured instead of whitish pink (redrawn after colour-plate by Hofer)

yellowish-coloured slimy excrements are therefore a certain sign of inflammation of the intestine.

The remedy is simple. If blood-flecked excrements have been found in a tank, feeding must cease immediately and the fishes be subjected to four or five days of fast and, after that, gradually fed with increasing quantities of another kind of food than was given before the disease occurred. Complete recovery will be effected if these recommendations are observed. In severe cases, the period of fast must be increased—this may even be extended to a period of weeks, if necessary. Feeding may be recommenced when no more bloody excrements are found.

Inflammation of the stomach is generally due to excessive amounts of salt contained in the food, and thus, when live food is given, this disease will not often occur. All salted artificial foods should be soaked in water to remove the salt. Smoked beef, which is sometimes used as a nourishing food rich in proteins, must be dried thoroughly; during this process most of the salt will crystallise and form a white layer on the surface which can be removed easily. The beef should not be used until no more salt crystallises; it may then be rasped and used for feeding, although it is not satisfactory to use it as the sole food for a long period. A better policy is to mix the rasped beef with other kinds of food which contain fats and carbohydrates.

The chief symptom of inflammation of the stomach is a reddening of the mucous coat of this organ, but naturally this can only be recognised by examining sections. Treatment is the same as that recommended for inflammation of the intestines.

Afflictions of the stomach and the intestines may also result from feeding only one kind of live food such as *enchytræ* or red mosquito larvae ('blood worms') for a prolonged period, whereas even simple overfeeding may cause an acute outbreak of inflammations of the internal organs. Of course, inflammations can be produced in the course of bacterial or other internal infections, too.

Severe inflammations of the intestine may be caused by infections with *Sporozoa*, such as *Eimeria cyprini* Plehn and *E. subepithelialis*

Moroff & Fiebiger in Carp. Apart from the other symptoms already mentioned, the affected fishes are characterised by emaciation and gaunt eyes, whereas post-mortem examination will reveal yellow knobs of about 2 mm in size. Such cases cannot easily be cured. See Chapter 4.

CONSTIPATION

Constipation is another complaint that may result from incorrect feeding. Some fishes are more susceptible to it than others and in aquaria it will be met mostly in Veiltails and other varieties that possess a compressed body.

Symptoms are lack of appetite and some swelling of the belly. Constipation may be cured by giving the fish some dried food which has been soaked in medicinal paraffin oil. If it will not take this, some drops of paraffin oil may be applied directly into the mouth by means of a small syringe. In obstinate cases, the laxative can be applied into the anal opening but this must only be done with large fishes and great care is necessary to avoid perforation of the intestinal wall. In fact, this operation should only be done by a qualified person. The syringe must not be inserted farther into the anal opening than is absolutely necessary. The fish is held in the left hand, with its head to the left, and so firmly that it cannot sprawl. Then the syringe is introduced into the anal opening, making an angle of about 45° with the horizontal axis of the body. It should not be inserted more than a few millimetres. The amount of laxative that is to be injected must be chosen in relation to the size of the fish and may vary from one drop to 0.5–1 cm^3. Paraffin oil, glycerol or castor oil may be used. The laxative activity increases from the first mentioned to the last.

Constipation particularly occurs after long periods in which only dried foods or enchytrae have been fed. If sufficient *Daphnia*, mosquito larvae and other natural foods are given in addition, fishes will not become affected.

CATARRH OF THE INTESTINE

Catarrh of the intestine may occur when fishes have eaten decaying food. Symptoms are lack of appetite and thinness, whilst thin, slimy excretions are produced, and these sometimes dissolve in water. The disease occurs more often in young fishes than adults. Fishes showing such symptoms should be fasted for a few days and then fed with dried food only until the abnormal excretions have disappeared.

JAUNDICE (*ICTERUS*)

Long periods of lack of food may not only result in wasting, but these may interfere with normal bile production as well. Bile is produced in the liver and stored temporarily in the gall bladder. When no food is taken in, no bile flows out of the gall bladder into the intestine, thus increasing the internal pressure in the gall bladder. Now bile is pressed back into the liver and taken up by the blood vessels. Owing to the circulation of bile pigments in the blood the fish may show a yellowish or yellow-green colour, provided that it does not contain a highly pigmented skin (as in Bettas, Black Mollies a.s.o.) preventing such external observation.

Further symptoms are excessive paleness of the skin and the gills (apart from the yellow-green discoloration), and internally a heavily filled gall bladder, small bile stones in the intestine and sometimes a green colour of the liver.

The remedy is simple. Just supply food, at first in small quantities and of an easily digestible kind, otherwise the starved fishes would overeat themselves and die from acute inflammation of the stomach, intestines and liver. Thus, only small quantities of food should be given at a time, but the intervals between feedings should be much shorter than for healthy fish.

The condition is observed most often in cold-water fishes that have hibernated through a cold and long winter in free waters or ponds.

FATTY DEGENERATION OF INTERNAL ORGANS

Fatty degeneration of the internal organs is one of the commonest causes of death in aquarium fishes, as has been proved by examining sections from many fishes which have died without external signs of disease. This disease may also be caused by incorrect feeding. If too many materials containing fats and carbohydrates, in comparison with proteins, are given (as would be the case when enchytrae are fed continuously without varying the diet with other foods which are poor in fat content) fatty degeneration of several internal organs will take place. The disease takes a very slow course and will not give many indications, but it finally causes death of the fish. Old fishes are more susceptible than younger ones. The liver, spleen, kidneys, heart and swim bladder may all be embedded in heavy amounts of fatty tissue. Often crystals of fatty acids may be observed in the belly, sometimes surrounding fat droplets that show optical birefringence between crossed polarisers under a polarising microscope.

Liver fatty degeneration can be recognised by the presence of white portions between the normal liver tissue, which is of a reddish-brown colour. This condition may also be produced by lack of vitamin A, which in fish is not very likely to occur unless the level of illumination is insufficient (see p. 293).

If the process develops to a great extent, dropsy may occur (dropsy may also be due to a combined virus and bacterial infection; see page 166). In the spleen and the kidneys fatty degeneration is

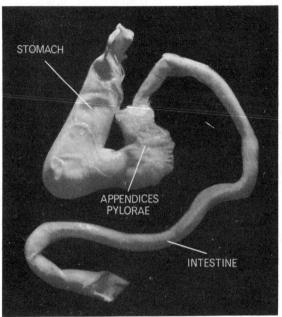

Fig. 7.2. Part of the alimentary canal of the Haddock,
showing relative positions of the several organs includ-
ing stomach, appendices pylorae and intestine

recognisable by small yellow bodies lying in the tissue. In fishes having a very compact liver, a lipoid degeneration of the liver may occur, in which case this organ becomes yellowish-grey, yellowish or spotted. Since these organs are all of vital importance, too large an extent of fatty degeneration will cause death. In Goldfish and other *Cyprinidæ* the normal liver tissue may be substituted nearly completely by fatty tissue before death occurs.

Veiltails are especially liable to fatty degeneration of the spleen, the kidneys and the ovaries.

In fatty degeneration of the ovaries the ova become affected and are whitish-grey in colour; when normal they are translucent and pink or reddish. In further development of the disease the ovary may harden so that it is visible as a swelling from the outside, or at least may be felt when the fish is taken between the fingers.

Chemical investigations would show that such ovaries consist to a large extent of cholesterol esters and other pathological lipoid substances. From this description it will be obvious that fatty degeneration of these organs will produce infertility. A cure is impossible. The fish may live for a relatively long period, but cannot be used for breeding.

Knowing the causes of this disease it will be easy to avoid it by choosing a varied diet, but it should be borne in mind that not only may unsuitable foods cause distress, but also overfeeding of fishes may have bad reactions. Breeders of fish often subject fish to a few days' fast prior to mating and this policy may prove very beneficial.

FATTY NECROSIS OF THE PANCREAS

This disease has been observed in Golden Carp (Hi-Goi, *Cyprinus auratus*). External symptoms are a swelling of the belly with protruding scales and some *Exophthalmus*, often combined with paleness, due to anaemia, of the gill sheets. Internally, there are heavy amounts of fat tissue as in fatty degeneration described previously.

It has been found that the origin of the disease is due to the occurrence of small parts of pancreas tissue or small amounts of pancreas cells, in places outside the pancreas proper. This condition is essentially an anomaly of the preceding embryological development of the individual, to which Golden Carp appears to be more liable than other species.

The secretion of the isolated pancreas tissue destroys the surrounding tissues, especially where bile is present, too. Lipolytic pancreas enzymes are activated by bile, so lipids are split into fatty acids and glycerol. Between the normal fat tissue crystals of fatty acids or derivatives are found. Inflammatory processes may often develop later on, resulting in peritonitis. Other complications are uptake of the pancreatic enzymes in the blood and lymph, producing lipomatosis (pathological deposition of fat) of the heart, the mesentery, lymphatic cavities and at other places. Death may arise from the high fat content of the blood itself, but the enzyme (pancreas lipase) may also attack the lining of the blood vessels, causing release of the destroyed epithelial tissue with consequent obstruction of the vessels as in thrombosis.

It is thought that certain granulation tumours and even some cases of carcinoma (cancer) may have developed from the initial conditions of the disease.

Life in captivity and overfeeding are considered to stimulate the development of the anomaly of the viscera into a dangerous disease. No cures are known.

OVARY DISORDERS

DEGENERATION OF THE OVARIES

The ovaries of different groups of fish may show much variety in structure. In egg-laying fish there are two ovaries, while in live-bearing species the ovary at first consists of two parts, but during development these soon merge, thus forming a single ovary. The ovaries are essentially sac-like organs, lined by the so-called germ-epithelium, which produces the ova by a process of cell division. At the posterior end of the ovary there is a tube (the Fallopian tube or oviduct) through which the eggs can be discharged if the fish is an egg layer, while in livebearing fish the youngsters are expelled this way on being born.

The surroundings of the germ-epithelium contain a large number of blood vessels. If, for some reason, the blood supply to it becomes insufficient, the germ-epithelium may lose its capability for ova production, the fish becoming sterile in consequence. If the condition of insufficient blood supply exists, degeneration of the ova (and of the embryos in livebearing fishes) and of the ovary itself may occur (Fig. 7.3). Generally, this disease does not give rise to

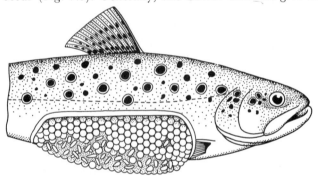

Fig. 7.3. Degeneration of the eggs in a Trout

special symptoms. Post-mortem examination may reveal that the ovaries are enlarged and show some spottiness; they are most likely to consist mainly of a large number of degenerated ova (ova and embryos in the case of a livebearer). In some parts, a small residue of intact germ-epithelium may be found.

If part of the germ-epithelium is preserved, the sterility may not prove permanent, since the remaining part is capable of regeneration and may even produce an entirely new ovary to replace the degenerated one. Degeneration of the ovaries is most likely to be caused by incorrect feeding, especially overfeeding in the period when the ova are produced, at the beginning of the spawning season.

OVARY CYSTS

In this complaint the ovaries are swollen to a bladder-like extent and are filled with a yellowish or reddish liquid. Histological examinations show a degeneration of the follicles of the ova. Generally, both ovaries have grown together and with the peritoneum also. The intestines are pressed together and the body swells, so that one must be careful not to confuse this disease with dropsy. With ovary cysts, the swelling will be very much nearer the hind part of the belly, which is generally not rounded, whilst in dropsy the greater swelling will be near the centre of the belly and it will show a gradual rounding.

Under aquarium conditions I have found the disease only in Veiltails (Fig. 7.4) which are always very susceptible to diseases of

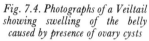

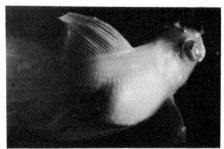

Fig. 7.4. Photographs of a Veiltail showing swelling of the belly caused by presence of ovary cysts

the internal organs. However, there is no reason why it should not occur in other fish. Stolk has observed it in *Ephippicharax orbicularis* and in the Dwarf Gourami (*Colisa lalia*).[1] The exact cause is not known although it seems that not allowing the fish to breed may sometimes be responsible to a greater or lesser extent.

PETRIFACTION OF THE OVARIES

In this disease the ovaries show degeneration with an extensive formation of connective tissue in which they become very hard. From the outside a swelling of the belly may be seen, resembling that described in ovary cysts, but not reaching such proportions. Whilst the belly of a fish with ovary cysts feels soft, in petrifaction of the ovaries the belly feels hard and the swelling cannot be pressed in. Sometimes parts of the ovary may be affected by this condition whilst in other parts ovary cysts are present.

In aquaria the disease occurs mainly in egg-laying Tooth-carps, and members of the *Characidæ*. It occurs generally when spawning has not been possible, but the way in which it is caused is not yet known. Diseased fishes may live for a long period but they are infertile. To avoid this disease, give the fishes an opportunity for spawning if they show ripeness, and do not overfeed.

This may result from many diseases, such as degeneration of the ovaries, fatty degeneration, ovary cysts, petrifaction of the ovaries, swim bladder trouble, dropsy or internal parasites. Many cases are due to either incorrect feeding or overfeeding. Too fatty foods, given for a long time, will produce all kinds of fatty degenerations in the internal organs and in the reproductive organs as well. Overfeeding has a bad effect, since more blood will flow to the digestive organs, so that the reproductive organs get less oxygen and other necessary substances which they must receive through the blood. Therefore it is always wise to feed fish less abundantly when the breeding season approaches and to give them 3–5 days of fast before the spawning. This is particularly important with fish which produce large numbers of eggs at a single spawning. Livebearers will never give trouble and the *Labyrinthici* are not easily overfed.

Lack of vitamins may also result in infertility, especially if vitamin E is not present. In females, the adverse effects of lack of vitamins can be completely overcome as soon as the required substances are supplied, but in males permanent changes in the reproductive organs may occur if they have suffered from avitaminosis for some period. A varied diet will prevent the occurrence of avitaminosis.

A temporary sterility may be produced by certain drugs employed for curing infectious diseases, namely, quinine derivatives, acriflavine and malachite green or brilliant green.

SWIM BLADDER TROUBLES

SWIM BLADDER DISEASE

In transit, tropical fishes are sometimes kept at low temperatures and afterwards swim bladder complaints may occur; these are recognisable by the behaviour of the fishes. Specimens thus afflicted have difficulty in maintaining their equilibrium and sometimes fall 'head over heels', making tumbling movements. Finally they rest at the bottom or, in other cases, they float at the surface. In such cases the disease is obviously due to chilling, which may cause inflammation of the bladder wall.

Other non-parasitic causes of swim bladder troubles are due to pressure from some of the internal organs, such as may result from constipation or other afflictions in which the volume of the internal organs increases. Alternatively, it may be due to a fatty degeneration of the tissues of the bladder itself. Swim bladder disease is not fatal and under good conditions fishes suffering from it may live for long periods.

These swim bladder troubles are best prevented by giving fishes a varied diet with sufficient supplies of fresh foods. Sudden changes of temperature must be avoided as should subjecting the fish to too low temperatures for long periods.

BURSTING OF THE SWIM BLADDER

This may occur when fishes living in deep waters are caught in a net and brought to the surface too rapidly. The pressure in the bladder increases with increasing depth of the water where the fishes are living, to make equilibrium with the increasing water pressure. When the external water pressure is suddenly released, this equilibrium is destroyed and the high internal pressure not being balanced by the external pressure any more, the bladder wall may burst. The same effect can be caused by explosions. Depending on the position of the fish relative to the site of an explosion, and on the type of explosion, the victims may either sink to the bottom or rise to the surface at once, where they keep floating.

Whatever the cause, bursting of the swim bladder kills the fish.

CAISSON DISEASE

Essentially this is a mild form of the condition causing bursting of the swim bladder. In the practice of fish-keeping it has become of some interest, too, since the introduction of transporting fishes in plastic bags or closed vessels with compressed air or oxygen above the water, intended to last for a long journey. The internal pressure in the swim bladder will balance the gas pressure above, so if the bags or vessels are opened and the external pressure is released, the fishes get into trouble, especially those species which either have an undivided swim bladder or in which the course connecting the two parts of the bladder is very narrow. Such conditions exist in Perch, Pike-Perch, *Coregonidæ* and others.

Fishes suffering from caisson disease float helpless at the surface of the water. If they have sufficient resistance and are not damaged too much, they will recover spontaneously; more delicate and young fishes may die unless special measures are taken in time, consisting of bringing the fish back in a closed container and connecting this to an air-pump to restore the excessive initial pressure. After some time the pressure is released very gradually *via* a reducing valve or a diffuser.

INFECTIOUS DISEASES OF THE SWIM BLADDER

COCCIDIOSIS

Some *Sporozoa* occur as parasites of the swim bladder (Fig. 7.5). Diseased fishes show an emaciated tail part of their body and skin lesions. In the swim bladder a white or brown mass of slimy to crumbled consistence may be observed which may fill the bladder

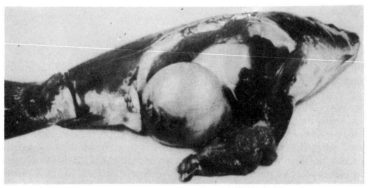

Fig. 7.5. Dissected Carp showing pathologically enlarged swim bladder. Photograph Bayerische Biologische Versuchsanstalt, *taken from Reichenbach-Klinke (1966)*

nearly completely. Microscopical examinations of smears made from this substance at the post-mortem investigation reveals that the peripherous parts consist almost entirely of sporozoan spores. Development of the spores takes place in the layer of connective tissue of the bladder wall. Reproduction in the deeper layers of connective tissue is asexual, whereas in the surface layers sporogonia are found. Ripe sporocysts fall into the cavity of the swim bladder where they may open to release the sporozoites that may again penetrate into the bladder wall.

Sporozoans that have been identified as causative agents of this disease thus far are *Myxobolus ellipsoides* Thélohan (see page 133) in Tench (*Tinca tinca*), *Myxobolus physophilus* Reuss in Rudd (*Scardinius erythrophthalmus*) and *Eimeria gadi* Fiebiger in Cod, Haddock and other *Gadidæ* (all marine fishes). No cures are known.

INFLAMMATION OF THE SWIM BLADDER

External symptoms of this condition are generally similar to those of non-parasitic swim bladder disease (see page 234). In translucent fishes the swim bladder will appear more or less opaque instead of silvery, owing to its being filled with a purulent bloody exudate.

The exudate contains large amounts of lymphocytes (a type of white blood corpuscle characterised by hyaline cytoplasm, which stains with basic dyes, and having slight phagocytic activity).

Epithelial cells are destroyed and the lesions are filled up by proliferation of connective tissue cells (fibroblasts), producing granulation tissue, i.e. newly formed vascular connective tissue growing to fill the gap of a wound or other lesion, producing a white scar as the final result. Granulation tissue is not elastic; consequently its formation will reduce the ability of the swim bladder to inflate or narrow as required for regulating the specific gravity of the fish in accordance with that of the water. This leads to the symptoms of swim bladder trouble.

Inflammation of the swim bladder is caused by several bacteria, in particular species of the Family *Pseudomonadaceæ* such as *Aeromonas* (formerly *Pseudomonas*) *punctata*. It also occurs in infectious virus-septicaemia in Trout (INul, Egtved-disease, see p. 202), whereas a non-contagious form may be due to certain disturbances of metabolism.

For treatment chloramphenicol and kanamycin may be employed, as described in Chapter 4 (pages 154 and 155). However, unless the elasticity of the swim bladder wall has not yet been impaired too much by the formation of granulation tissue in the lesions, the fish will remain a cripple with chronic swim bladder trouble.

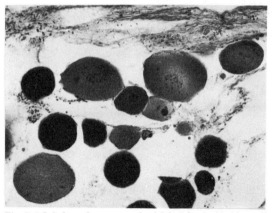

Fig. 7.6. Ichthyophonus *cysts in vicinity of swim bladder wall (upper part of picture) found in* Hyphessobrycon flammeus *with severe swim bladder trouble.* × 250 *(photomicrograph by the author)*

SWIM BLADDER TROUBLE OWING TO ICHTHYOPHONUS INFECTION

In cases of infection with *Ichthyophonus* (see Fig. 7.6, page 237) where cysts are produced in the vicinity of the swim bladder, proper functioning of the latter may be impaired, external pressure preventing full inflation of the bladder. The victims will lie at the bottom of the water and are not capable of rising for more than short moments. (See also pages 250–259.)

PARASITIC DISEASES OF THE INTERNAL ORGANS

WORM INFECTIONS

*SUCKING WORMS (TREMATODA)**

Parasites that belong to the *Trematoda* (sucking worms) are often to be found in fish (Fig. 7.7). They have more or less flattened bodies, are not membered, and are equipped with sucking discs or hooks for

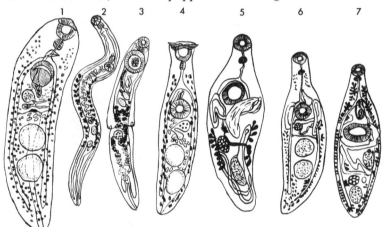

Fig. 7.7. Sucking worms of the intestinal tract of fishes. 1, Crepidostomum farionis *Müller.* 2, Azygia lucii *Müller.* 3, Hemiurus appendiculatus *(Rud.).* 4, Bunodera luciopercæ *Müller (1–4 after Dawes).* 5, Asymphylodora tincæ *(Modeer).* 6, Allocreadium isosporum *Looss.* 7, Sphærostoma bramæ *Müller (5–7 after Lühe)*

fastening themselves to their hosts. As a rule, sucking worms that are parasitic in the internal organs of fish have one or two sucking discs. The intestines of the creature have no anal opening and are generally forked. Reproductive organs have a complicated structure.

* Detailed descriptions of a larger number of species occurring as fish parasites are given in more specialised literature.[2]

These sucking worms are hermaphrodites, i.e. each contains both male and female reproductive organs. Some sucking worms produce eggs, whilst others are livebearing. Larvae which hatch from the eggs often show a complicated metamorphosis.

Most species of *Trematoda* that have been found in the intestines of fish are egg-producing worms. An example of these parasites is *Bucephalus (Gasterostomum) polymorphus* Baer., represented on page 115. Its metacercaria stage is known as ox-head worm and parasitises on the gills of fishes. It belongs to the *Digeneæ*. Larvae hatch from the ova and they swim freely through the water by means of cilia which cover the body. This first larval stage is called miracidium. The miracidium attacks its first host which is a snail or mussel and then it develops into a band-like shape, called sporocyst, which produces a large number of new sporocysts by simple division. Finally, the sporocysts change into a new stage, consisting of an oval or ellipsoidal body with a tail, called cercaria (from Latin 'tail stage'). The cercariae leave their host and swim freely through the water until they find a second host, which may also be a mollusc, or fish or other animal living in the water. Then the parasite produces a cyst and rests until its host is eaten by the definite host of the sucking worm. When this happens the cyst is freed and the young cercaria ripens to an adult sucking worm which produces eggs and starts the complicated life cycle again.

From this description it can be seen that the introduction of these parasites into the aquarium may occur when infected snails or mussels are brought into the tank. Theoretically it would be possible to introduce them with other materials from free waters but that risk is very small. To avoid infection, it is advisable to introduce to your tanks only snails from waters in which no fish are present, if this is possible. If not, the snails can be kept in quarantine for some weeks in a small container where no fish are present before putting them in the tank. Then the parasites will leave the host and die. A few specimens of sucking worms in the intestine of a fish will not do much harm. If there are a number, or if the fish is small, the victim may become thin, but these parasites will not cause death.

In the same Order worms are found that in their adult stage live in the pancreatic ducts and the bile ducts of dogs, cats and humans. The cat liver fluke *Opistorchis felineus* Rivolta (Fig. 7.8) is found abundantly in the Baltic region and in Eastern Europe. The eggs of this worm are taken in by the snail *Bythinia leachi*, where they develop into cercariae that infect whitefish in which they live in the muscles. Human beings are infected if they eat infected fish without sufficient heat treatment. Related Genera of these worms are *Pseudoamphistomum*, *Metorchis*, *Haplorchis* and *Pachytrema*.

In the blood of fishes several species of the real bloodworm *Sanguinicola* may be found as parasites. The adult worms as living in the fish do not possess suckers. Instead they swim actively through the blood by waving movements of their body. They occur most abundantly in the heart and in the larger blood vessels of the gills.

The infected fishes show pale or even translucent gill sheets; their movements are often sluggish.

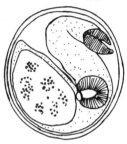

Fig. 7.8. Metacercarian cyst of the cat liver fluke Opistorchis felineus *Rivolta (after Vogel)*

In the period from May to November triangular eggs are produced, one at a time, that after having left the body of the female increase in size up to 45–75 μm length and 30–45 μm width (depending on species). Each embryo contains a peculiar black pigment spot, a drilling sting and several highly refractive bar-shaped particles near the anterior edge.

The eggs are transported by the bloodstream and may settle in the capillaries of the gills, the kidneys, the heart, the liver and other organs. Generally the larvae (miracidia) hatch from the eggs situated in the gills. They bore through the wall of the capillary and enter the water, where they have to find a snail for further development. Most common snail hosts are the great pond snail *Lymnæa stagnalis*, further *Radix* (*Lymnæa*) *ovata*, *Valvata piscinalis* and *Bythinia leachi* (see Figs 7.9 and 7.10).

Fig. 7.9. Valvata piscinalis *Müll., one of the snail hosts of the bloodworm* Sanguinicola *(after Dorsman and De Wilde)*

Fig. 7.10. Bithynia leachi *Shepp. Snail host of the cat liver fluke* Opistorchis felineus. *The next intermediate host is a fish (after Dorsman and De Wilde)*

In the snail each miracidium develops into a sporocyst, from which after two generations forked cercariae are produced. These cercariae possess a waving membrane and have been known as *Cercaria cristata*. They swarm out into the water until they meet a fish, where they penetrate through the gill sheets and weaker parts of the skin, throwing off their hind part with the forked tail, which is left behind on the surface of the fish.

A few adult worms do not harm the fish very much, but the penetration of a large number of cercariae may kill it. Large numbers of eggs circulating in the bloodstream may cause thrombosis and clotting, especially in the capillaries of the gills, which will also cause death. Eggs and miracidium larvae may be found in scrapings or smear preparations from the gill sheets.

At present no cures are known, but from the natural history of the parasites it is obvious that the infection can be prevented by not introducing snails from free waters, where fishes are present.

Species of bloodworms known thus far are: *Sanguinicola inermis* Plehn, up to 1 mm, without prickles on their body (Fig. 7.11); in

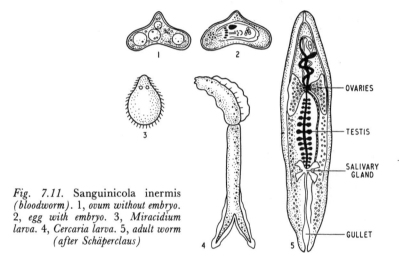

Fig. 7.11. Sanguinicola inermis *(bloodworm).* 1, *ovum without embryo.* 2, *egg with embryo.* 3, *Miracidium larva.* 4, *Cercaria larva.* 5, *adult worm (after Schäperclaus)*

OVARIES

TESTIS

SALIVARY GLAND

GULLET

Carp (*Cyprinus carpio*); *S. intermedia* Ejsmont, less than 1 mm, main part of the body covered with prickles, in Prussian Carp (*Carassius carassius*), *S. armata* Plehn, up to 1.5 mm, with heavy prickles; in Tench (*Tinca tinca*); *S. chalmersi* Odhner, in Egyptian Catfish of the River Nile.

TAPE WORMS (CESTOIDEA)

Tape worms do much more harm to fishes than the sucking worms, but they are seldom found in aquarium fish. A tape worm has a so-called 'head', or scolex, bearing sucking discs, hooks, or both, for fastening it to the organs of the victim. Except in the *Cestodaria*, the body of an adult tape worm consists of a number of members, called proglottides, in each of which all the important organs are present, including those for reproduction. The scolex of the tape worm

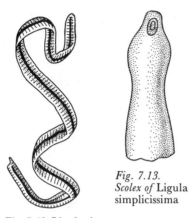

Fig. 7.13.
Scolex of Ligula
simplicissima

Fig. 7.12. Ligula sim-
plicissima   *(redrawn
after Hofer)*

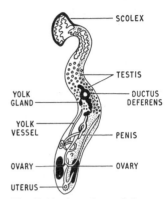

*Fig. 7.14. A specimen of the tape
worm species* Caryophyllæus
mutabilis *(redrawn after M.
Schultze), indicating position of the
reproductive organs and scolex. With
this Genus the fish is the final host of
the worm*

produces the proglottides which in turn produce eggs. From these
the larvae hatch out and they must be taken up by a suitable host.
If this host is eaten by the definite host the larvae develop into the
adult tape worms. Some tape worms of fish differ from this general
scheme by having a simpler structure, e.g. *Ligula simplicissima*,
which is not membered (Figs 7.12, 7.13).

For practical purposes the tape worms to be found in fish may be
classified into four groups. The first which will be discussed are those
living in the intestine. To these parasites the fish is the final host in
which the worm reaches the adult stage. One of the commonest
members of this group is the clove worm, *Caryophyllæus laticeps*
(Pallas), or other species (Fig. 7.14) of the same Genus, belonging
to the Order *Caryphyllæidea* of the *Cestodaria*. This species may reach
a length of 3 cm. The larvae live in tubifex and fishes may thus be
infected with this parasite by eating infected tubifex worms. This
risk does not arise if tubifex which have been obtained from waters
where no fish are present, or which have been cultured, are offered.

Another worm of this group is *Proteocephalus* (*Ichthyotænia*), belonging to the Order *Proteocephalidea* of the *Cestoda*. These organisms
have a membered body and a scolex with four sucking discs without
hooks. The larvae live in *Cyclops* and *Diaptomus*. These species will
not do much harm.

The second group of tape worms lives in the belly of their
victim and to these the fish is not the final host. Two species must
be described here, namely, *Ligula simplicissima* Creplin, which is
a larval stage of *Ligula intestinalis* Linnaeus and *Schistocephalus gas-*

terostei Fabr. [*Sch. dimorphus* Crepel; *Sch. nodosus* Bloch; *Sch. solidus* Rud.]. They belong to the Order *Pseudophyllidea* of the *Cestoda. Ligula* is not membered and lives free in the water during its first larval stage (coracidium) until it is eaten by a cyclopid (*Diaptomus*) where it develops into its second stage (procercoid). If this organism is eaten by a fish the parasite penetrates from the intestine into the belly and reaches its third stage (plerocercoid). Development into the adult worm takes place in the intestines of water birds after the fish has been eaten by the bird. When in the bird, the creature produces eggs which leave with the excrements and fall into the water, where they hatch and start the cycle anew. Thus infection of fishes can only occur if they are fed with cyclopids that have been obtained from waters where there are fish-eating water birds or where fishes live. Consequently it is not difficult to avoid introducing these parasites into a pond or an aquarium.

Symptom of infection with this type of tape worm is a swelling of the belly of the fish due to the space which is occupied by the parasite. The extent of this swelling depends on the size and the number of worms present. The swelling may be distinguished from enlargements due to dropsy, constipation, or diseases of the ovaries, by the fact that the belly is caved in near the heart. The reproductive organs of the fish will be destroyed completely by these parasites so that they become infertile and finally the victims die. If examined in section, the diagnosis will be certain, for the large worms may be easily recognised.

Ligula may reach a considerable length (a worm of about 2 m was once found); however, the average size is about 20–30 cm, which is large enough to do considerable damage to the fish in which it is living. In cases where very strong fishes are infected, the victim may live until the pressure of the worms in its belly has become so great that it bursts (Fig. 7.15).

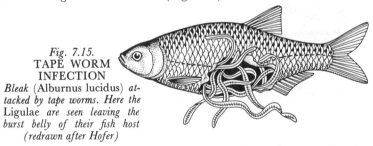

Fig. 7.15.
TAPE WORM
INFECTION
Bleak (Alburnus lucidus) *attacked by tape worms. Here the* Ligulae *are seen leaving the burst belly of their fish host (redrawn after Hofer)*

Then the worms escape into the water, where they may live for ten days. If they are eaten by a water bird, they develop into adult worms in the intestines of the bird. It may be mentioned that *Ligulæ* are eaten by fishermen in some parts of Italy and France. They call them 'maccaroni piatti' or 'vers blancs' (white worms).

Schistocephalus gasterostei has, until now, only been found in Sticklebacks (*Gasterosteus*), where it appears very often (Fig. 7.16). This worm is smaller than *Ligula* and is membered. It may reach a length of up to 30 cm but generally it will be 2–7 cm only. Symptoms are the same as in *Ligula* infections of fishes in the Carp Family. In female

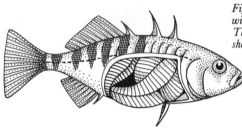

Fig. 7.16. A Stickleback afflicted with Schistocephalus *worms. The belly has been cut open to show these parasitic worms (redrawn after Hofer)*

Sticklebacks the fishes appear to be full of ripe eggs, but in reality such fishes are full of worms and are completely infertile since their reproductive organs have been destroyed by the parasites. *Sch. pungitii* Dubinina is found in Ten-Spined Sticklebacks (*Pygosteus pungitius*).

The third group of tape worms are those which live as larvae in the bellies of some fishes, and as adults in the intestines of others. The most common member of this group is *Triænophorus lucii* (Müller) (= *nodulosus*) Pallas (Order *Pseudophyllidea* of the *Cestoda*) (Figs 7.17,

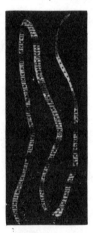

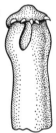

Fig. 7.18 (Right). *Scolex of* T. lucii *worm*

Fig. 7.17. Triænophorus lucii *(Müller) (* T. nodulosus *Pallas) tape worm (after Bremser)*

7.18). The larvae, which hatch from the eggs eight days after they have been produced, are eaten by *Cyclops*, *Diaptomus* or related small *Copepoda*. If the *Cyclops* is eaten by a fish, the larva penetrates from the intestine into the liver, where it encysts. The cysts have a size of some millimetres and can be easily distinguished in section. A few cysts are sufficient to produce serious illnesses, even in big fishes.

Common intermediate fish hosts are Rainbow Trout (*Salmo gaird-neri*), Arctic Char (*Salvelinus alpinus*) and Minnow (*Phoxinus phoxinus*). If such a fish is eaten by another, the cysts open and produce the adult *Triænophorus* worms. In Nature, the adult worm is found mostly in Pike and the larger Salmonid fishes.

The fourth group of tape worms comprises parasites with a multiple change of hosts, the last one being a mammal. To this group belongs the dangerous tape worm *Diphyllobothrium latum* L. (formerly *Dibothriocephalus* = *Bothriocephalus latus*) and related species (also belonging to the Order *Pseudophyllidea*). The adult worm, which reaches a length of 8–10 m or even more (!), lives in the human intestine. The eggs are excreted with the faeces. If they enter any water, they develop into free-swimming, ciliated coracidium larvae, that must be eaten by a *Cyclops* or *Diaptomus* to develop further into procercoid larvae, up to about 0.5 mm in size. After the *Cyclops* has been eaten by a fish, the procercoid changes into the last larval stage, called plerocercoid, which lives in the interstitial space of the muscles or the liver and other internal organs.

The most common fish hosts in Europe are Northern Pike, Lake Perch, Eel, Lake Trout, Ruff (Pope) and Eelpout (Burbot). In North America in Northern Pike, Yellow Perch, Walleye, Sauger and the Trout *Oncorhynchus perryi*. In Madagascar in the Barbel.

The infected fishes do not suffer much, since the parasites in the fish are mainly dormant until the latter is eaten by a human being who has failed to cook or fry the fish properly. In Western Europe this tape worm seems to be nearly extinct now, owing to good hygiene preventing spread of human excreta to fishing waters, and to improved cooking habits as well.

TREATMENT OF TAPE WORM INFECTIONS

Adult tape worms in the intestines of fish can be removed by adding $1\frac{1}{2}$–2% kamala to the food for one week. To ensure complete elimination of the worms it is advised to continue this treatment for another week.[3]

An alternative treatment by the same drug consists in introducing capsules containing 180–220 mg of kamala per pound of fish into the stomach, for three successive days. This treatment was first used by Snieszko and also tried by Albert Powell, Superintendent of Maryland fish hatcheries, as mentioned by Allison.[4] Using this treatment, great masses of the tape worm *Proteocephalus ambloplitis* could be removed from infected Large- and Small-mouth Bass. Of course, this way of application is only suitable for big fishes in ponds and fish-breeding practice. For small fish, as in aquaria, oral application is the only choice.

Di-n-butyl zinc oxide added to the food (0.3%) for one day is a more recent treatment.[5] Addition of 500 mg/kg of body weight of di-n-butyl tin oxide to a commercial pelleted diet, fed over a 3-day period ($\frac{1}{3}$ dose per day) was 100% effective in removing *Eubothrium crassum* from *Salmo gairdneri*.[6]

Evidently treatment of tape worm infections can only be successful if the worms have not yet penetrated into other internal organs.

ROUND- OR THREAD-WORMS (NEMATODA)

Some species of this group of worms (Fig. 7.19) live in fish during their larval stage, whilst the adult form is produced when the fish is eaten by the definite host. The larvae have a size of a few millimetres and live for a short period in the skin or in the internal organs and then they encyst. Generally the cysts are the size of a pinhead, although larger ones may occur. They are formed on the outside of the intestine, or on the peritoneum, pancreas, liver or other internal organs. If there are many cysts, serious inflammation of the internal organs of a fish may occur.

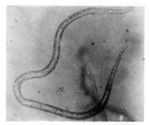

Fig. 7.20. A species of Nematode worm, Camallanus lacustris (Cucullanus elegans) *(after Hofer)*

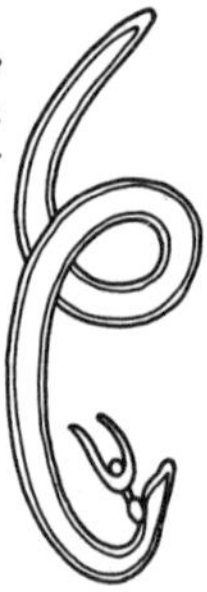

Fig. 7.19. Photomicrograph by Ian M. Rankin of a parasitic Nematode

Other species of *Nematoda* live in fishes in the adult stage. Most of these are found in the intestines, the muscles and the reproductive organs. *Ancyracanthus cystidicola* Rud. is a worm of about 3 cm in length and it lives in the swim bladder; occasionally also in the oesophagus (gullet) and the stomach. It may cause anaemia and wasting. *Philometra abdominalis* Nyb. [*Ichthyonema sanguineum* Rud.] is characterised by its red colour and it lives in the belly; it reaches a length of 4–6 cm. This worm bores into the intestinal wall and induces it to produce an exudate in which the worm lives. This worm does not do much harm to the fish. The capped worm, *Camallanus lacustris* Zoega [*Cucullanus elegans* Zed.] (Fig. 7.20) lives in the intestines, the appendices pylorae and in the eye. It may be found very often in Perch (*Perca fluviatilis*). Females have a size of about 12–18 mm, while the males are only 5–8 mm. The organism is livebearing and produces larvae of about 0.4 mm in length. These swim freely through the water till they are eaten by a *Cyclops*. In the belly of this little animal they grow and develop further, but reproductive organs are not formed. These only develop when the *Cyclops* is eaten by a fish.

Another species of *Nematoda* which may be mentioned here is *Paramermis crassa* (Fig. 7.21). The larvae of this worm have a length of 5–9 mm and width of 0.15–0.25 mm. They live in the body of red mosquito larvae ('bloodworms', larvae of *Chironomus*). If the red mosquito larvae are eaten by a fish the larva develops into the adult

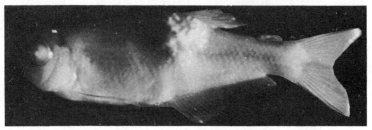

Fig. 7.21. An Australian Rainbow Fish (Melanotænia nigrans) *with an ulcer caused by a* Paramermis crassa *having left its body.* Paramermis *worms are Nematodes*

worm which reaches a length of 3–5 mm and width of 1 mm. When it is full grown, it may leave the fish by boring through the internal organs, the muscles and the skin. In most of these cases a tumour is formed on the dorsal surface of the body which bursts open and the worm emerges. The fish dies afterwards as a result of the damage.

The risk of introducing this parasite into tanks will be eliminated if only mosquito larvae from waters containing no fishes, or that have been cultured, are used for feeding.

THORNY-HEADED OR SPINY-HEADED WORMS (ACANTHOCEPHALA)

This is still another group of worms that may attack the internal organs of fishes and they are typical parasites of the intestine. They are characterised by the possession of a protrusible proboscis, bearing a large number of hooks, by means of which the creatures fasten themselves to the intestinal wall of their victims. The body is not membered. They do not possess a mouth or alimentary canal. The larvae live in the so-called fresh-water shrimp (*Gammarus pulex*), the water louse (*Asellus aquaticus*) or in insect larvae. If the organism is eaten by a fish, the parasite bores into the wall of the intestine with its proboscis, and grows and develops into sexual ripeness. After mating, eggs are produced. In the members of one Genus, namely, *Pomphorhynchus* (Figs 7.22, 7.23), a fish is probably not the definite host, but the secondary host only, and the adult stage of the parasite is reached when the fish is eaten by a water bird or by another species of fish.

248

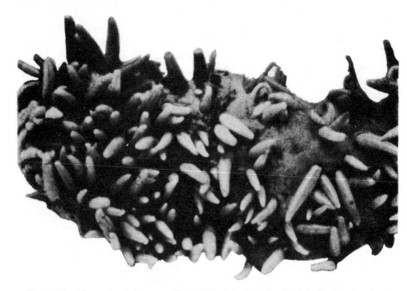

Fig. 7.22. Thorny-headed worms. Part of the intestine of a Barbel (Barbus barbus) *with numerous specimens of* Pomphorhynchus lævis *(after a colour photograph by the* Bayerische Biologische Versuchsanstalt, *published by Reichenbach-Klinke, 1966)*

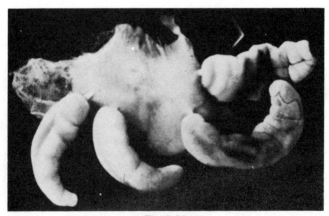

Fig. 7.23.
THORNY-HEADED WORMS
Part of the intestine of a Trout with four specimens of Pomphorhynchus lævis *(after J. Fiebiger)*

Introduction of these parasites into the aquarium may occur with live food but if this is sieved, so that the organisms in which the larvae of *Acanthocephala* may be present are separated, there will be no risk whatsoever. *Gammarus* and *Asellus* are, however, excellent food for large fishes, such as Acaras and other Cichlids, but it is often possible to recognise the presence of worm larvae in these live foods as they appear as dark or coloured (sometimes orange) spots in the grey body of the little animal. Consequently it is possible to feed these organisms without risk, if only they are examined prior to feeding.

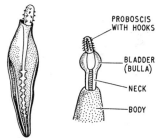

Fig. 7.24. Two members of the Acantho-cephala. *Right:* Echinorhynchus globu-losus *(after Bremser) and,* extreme right: *'head' region of* Echinorhynchus proteus *(after Roth). Both are dangerous species*

PROBOSCIS WITH HOOKS

BLADDER (BULLA)

NECK

BODY

The *Acanthocephala* (Fig. 7.24), of which the most important Genera are *Echinorhynchus, Neoechinorhynchus* and also *Pomphorhynchus, Acanthocephalus, Corynosoma, Bolbosoma, Metechinorhynchus* and *Rhadino-rhynchus*, are very dangerous parasites and will cause death of their victims, due to the perforation of the intestine.

TREATMENT OF WORM INFECTIONS

Generally, prospects of curing fish suffering from worm infections of the internal organs are poor. In most cases, too much damage has been caused to important organs before the disease is recognised.

It is unlikely that any treatment of fish infected with *Acanthocephala* could be successful, but with *Trematoda* and *Nematoda* there is a chance of recovery, provided that the internal organs have not been damaged too severely by the parasite.

Mr. Ian M. Rankin has succeeded in curing Neon Tetras suffer-ing from an infection with *Nematoda* (see Figs 7.19, 7.20) by feeding them with dried food previously soaked with a saturated aqueous solution of *para*-chlorometaxylenol (chloroxylenol) (saturated at 20°C), combined with bathing them for one or two hours in a solution of 10 cm^3 of the stock solution in 1 l of water (45 cm^3/ Imp. gal). Some time after they had been transferred to fresh water, a few worms were observed swimming with a figure-of-eight motion through the water. The fish treated in this way recovered completely. However, for most tropicals, the solution is too strong, so that it is advisable to give it in the food only. (Also see page 339.)

The symptoms of this infection were those of *wasting*, with *collapse of the abdominal region* and general *emaciation*. Later, a white area developed from the centre of the green line, and extended on both sides, until it reached a diameter of about a quarter of an inch. Untreated fish stopped eating some seven days after its incident and died. Later on, Rankin tried phenoxethol for treatment of fish with worm infections, also with good results, and he considers this further treatment preferable to chloroxylenol because it is less toxic. Diseased fish should be fed with dried food soaked with a 1% stock solution of phenoxethol, while 10 cm^3 of this stock solution are added to the aquarium water.

For treatment of tape worm infection see p. 245.

INFECTIONS BY UNICELLULAR ORGANISMS

ICHTHYOPHONUS DISEASE

This is due to *Ichthyophonus* (*Ichthyosporidium*) *hoferi* Plehn-Mulsow or related species belonging to the *Chytridiaceæ* of the Order *Chytridiales*, Class *Phycomycetes* of the *Fungi*. In living fish diagnosis is often difficult since no distinctive symptoms appear. Diseased fishes may swim with sluggish movements as if they were numbed, while their bellies may grow thin and show a concave instead of convex contour. Then the fish lose their equilibrium and finally die, without showing signs of disease. In cases where the parasites have penetrated into the brain, fishes make tumbling movements.

At times, cases of this infection have been investigated in Paradise Fish (*Macropodus*), where the fish showed ulcerous formations in the

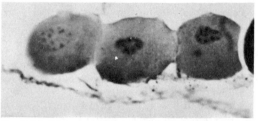

Fig. 7.25. Three cysts of Ichthyophonus, *each containing one parasite.* × 500 *(photomicrograph by the author)*

skin, about the size of a pea. These ulcerous parts contained many cysts of *Ichthyophonus* (Fig. 7.25). In similar cases in Siamese Fighting Fish, a clouding and dulling of the colours are observed where the main body tissues are affected; these may also be accompanied by raw sores or unbroken boils, generally showing a red colour. Such symptoms may also occur in other fishes.

In case of heavy primary infestation of the liver the belly may appear swollen, whereas infection of the orbit of the eye or of the eye itself results in eye protrusion (*Exophthalmus*, see page 214) and destruction of the eye.

The fins of diseased fishes may get torn and folded, they may appear whitish at the ravelled brims and waste away. Often such symptoms are preceded by the appearance of small red elevations at the fin base.

In other cases irregular black spots may occur in the skin, especially in Angel Fish (*Pterophyllum*), or blackening of the whole body is observed, especially in several species of Trout. The parasites are never found in the epidermis (upper layer of the skin), but they occur very often in the cutis. In Angel Fish diseased parts of the skin may often get loose and fall off, leaving ulcerating wounds. Occasionally the gills may be attacked, leading to symptoms of asphyxiation. Secondary fungus or bacterial infections occur often where wounds are present, or where the fins, gills or skin have been weakened.

If cysts of the parasite are produced in the vicinity of the swim bladder, proper functioning of the latter may be impaired. The external pressure exerted by the cysts prevents full inflation of the bladder. The fish will lie at the bottom and appears not to be capable of rising for more than short moments.

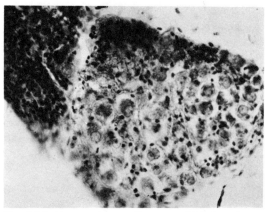

Fig. 7.26. Numerous young yellow cysts of Ichthyophonus *in the spleen of a* Hyphessobrycon flammeus *(photomicrograph by the author)*

Generally, however, the parasites are to be found in the internal organs, i.e. the heart, liver, kidneys, spleen (Fig. 7.26), reproductive organs, stomach and intestines and also in the muscles. In section the cysts may be recognised easily, frequently even with the naked eye, or at least with the aid of a low-power magnifying glass. The cysts

(Figs 7.27, 7.28) appear as whitish-grey granules lying between the tissues of the organs. They may also be present in the organs themselves, when the colour may vary from yellowish to yellowish-brown and brown or sometimes even black. The diameter can vary from

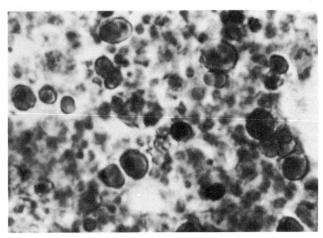

Fig. 7.27. Young cysts of Ichthyophonus (Ichthyosporidium hoferi) *in section of a diseased fish.* × 1000

10 μm to 500 μm, 150 μm being an average size, but old encysted parasites may reach a size of 2 mm or even more. When examined under the microscope they seem to be surrounded by a thick membrane. They contain an amoeboid stage or plasmodium which grows out periodically and penetrates through the whole organ.

The parasite excretes an external membrane, which is surrounded by white blood cells and fibroblasts (connective tissue cells) of the host, producing the cyst wall. Rings of connective tissue are

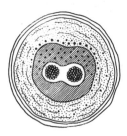

Fig. 7.28. A cyst of Ichthyophonus. *This parasite belongs to the* Chytridaceæ *group*

gradually built up around the parasite. If the wall of the cyst becomes thick enough to prevent its penetration by reproductive stages of the parasite, the latter will become necrotic. This condition is often characterised by increasing black pigmentation of the parasite, starting from the outside, the final product being an opaque black mass (Fig. 7.29). In other cases, however, no blackening occurs, the encysted parasite being gradually dissolved (*lysis*), leaving an empty cyst as the final product. In this way the fish may cope with an

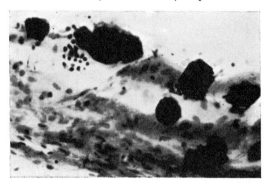

Fig. 7.29. Blackened cysts of Ichthyophonus. × 500

Ichthyophonus infection of only few specimens, but if the development of the parasite proceeds more rapidly than the building up of the cyst wall by the host, the parasite will be able to penetrate the wall and leave the cyst in an amoeboid stage (Fig. 7.30), reproduce and increase the infection.

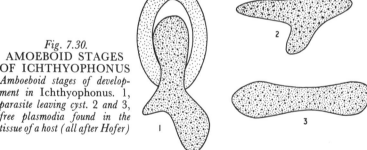

Fig. 7.30.
AMOEBOID STAGES
OF ICHTHYOPHONUS
Amboeboid stages of development in Ichthyophonus. *1, parasite leaving cyst. 2 and 3, free plasmodia found in the tissue of a host (all after Hofer)*

The globules to be found in the internal organs have to be regarded as once having been normal tissue, which has been changed under the influence of the parasites to form the cyst, thus, the more cysts there are present in an organ, the greater the loss of functioning normal tissue. Normal tissue is replaced by scar tissue, which is not elastic, thus resulting in shrinkage of the organs. Remaining normal tissue surrounding the cysts of the parasites is pushed aside and may degenerate.

Organs which contain many cysts feel hard, like stones, and sandy if they are held with forceps. The disease takes a very long course. It may be months, or even years, before the victims die as a result of the gradual destruction of the infected organs. During this period they will slowly become thin and dark-coloured.

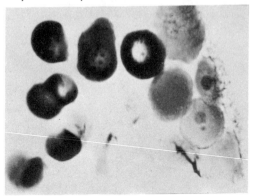

Fig. 7.31. Ichthyophonus *in different stages of development.* × *500*

Infection may take place if a fish eats an infected fish which has died or if it eats the cysts, which have entered the water from the gills or the skin of an infected specimen. In the stomach the cysts open and produce a number of plasmodia, which have a size of 10–20 μm. After a day these penetrate into the mucous coat of the stomach, then into the blood, and finally they are transported by

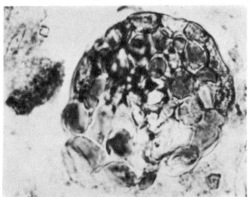

Fig. 7.32. Reproduction of Ichthyophonus. × *1000*

the bloodstream to all internal organs. Ten days after the infection occurs, the cysts may be found in the heart, liver and other internal organs. The parasites reproduce themselves in the organs of their host, if the temperature is sufficiently high (thus in cold-water fishes during the summer and in tropicals the whole year through). In some

cases reproduction (Figs 7.31, 7.32) may be so rapid that in a fortnight an organ can be totally filled with cysts so that, if it is vital to
the creature, death may occur in a very short time.

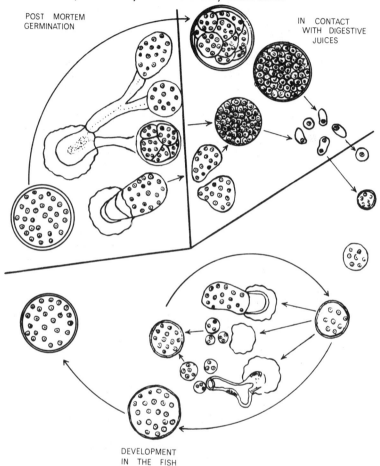

POST MORTEM
GERMINATION

IN CONTACT
WITH DIGESTIVE
JUICES

DEVELOPMENT
IN THE FISH

Fig. 7.33. Life cycle of Ichthyosporidium hoferi *(Plehn and Mulsow) (after Dorier
and Degrange)*

On the Continent, large losses of Trout are due to this parasite.
In *Salmonidæ*, the parasites attack the nervous system, thereby
causing a tumbling sickness, in which the victims are tottering and
tumbling 'head over heels' as if they were either benumbed or drunk.
From this description the seriousness of the disease will be evident.

In female fish, *Ichthyophonus* causes sterility if it attacks the ovaries.
The granules narrow the ovary cavity, while the oviduct is obstructed.

Male fish will also become sterile if their testes (soft-roes) are damaged by the parasites, directly or by enclosure of the *vas deferens* (tube through which seminal fluid is discharged).

SEX REVERSAL AND PARTHENOGENESIS CAUSED. In female Guppies (*Lebistes reticulatus*) sex reversal has been observed.[7] The infection of the ovaries resulted in death of the ova and embryos, although the latter two were not penetrated themselves. The ova were resorbed by the follicular epithelium and the embryos by the epithelial cells of the oviduct in which phagocytosis was induced. The remaining degenerated organs now changed into male function and started to produce spermatozoa (male germ cells), while the fish took the shape and colours of a male, although preserving female size. Such pathological sex reversal can be explained as follows: Every individual animal produces both male and female sex hormones, the amount of one of them normally greatly exceeding that of the other, so that a normal individual will function either as a male or as a female. If the production of the dominating hormone is disturbed or even entirely stopped by destruction of the hormone-producing cells or tissue, whereas the production of the antagonistic hormone is not, the equilibrium is broken and the animal will now be under the unrestricted influence of the remaining hormone of the opposite sex, leading to sex reversal. In most animals this is only partial, but in the case of Guppies it is apparently nearly complete, the only remnant deviation being body size.

An even more striking phenomenon which may be caused by *Ichthyophonus* infection of the ovaries in Livebearing Tooth-carps is parthenogenesis, i.e. development of ova into embryos without fertilisation. It has been observed in Guppies (*Lebistes reticulatus*), Swordtails (*Xiphophorus helleri*) and in Mosquito Fish (*Heterandria formosa*).[8] The case of Mosquito Fish, described by Stolk in 1961, concerned a female isolated immediately after birth. When the animal had reached a size of 27 mm, it gave birth to four young females. Later on, two further pregnancies followed, resulting in six and ten female youngsters, respectively. Microscopical investigation of the internal organs did not reveal any spermatozoa or male tissue, thus excluding the theoretical possibility of bisexuality, which has also been observed in *Pœciliidæ*. However, in the cranial part of the ovary and in the adjacent regions an infection process caused by *Ichthyophonus* was found. Birth of the young could take place undisturbed because no extensive process was present in the caudal part of the ovary and the oviduct; if this should have occurred, normal birth would have been impossible. Since in fish, as in most animals, sex of the offspring is determined by the spermatozoa (birds are an exception), parthenogenetically produced youngsters could only be females. This origin was further proved by counting of the chromosomes of the cell nuclei. All youngsters were found to have only half the normal number of chromosomes, owing to their lacking the paternal contribution.

WATER FLEAS AS CARRIERS OF ICHTHYOPHONUS. Elaborate experiments have been performed by J. Lewer to find out whether *Ichthyophonus* could be introduced with live food.[9] The parasite could be cultured on blood serum and used for infection experiments. Tubifex remained completely unaffected and did not transmit the parasite, but water fleas (*Daphnia*) soon showed traces of it and all became infected. When these infected water fleas were fed to fishes, all of those showed *Ichthyophonus* infection within 5–12 weeks. Some of the specimens were used for histological sectioning and were found to contain typical cysts in the brain and liver. These experiments seem to prove that water fleas can transmit *Ichthyophonus* parasites.

Investigations by others make it probable that *Copepoda* (to which the *Cyclopides* belong) can also be carriers of *Ichthyophonus*.

ICHTHYOPHONUS FOUND IN MANY SPECIES. *Ichthyophonus* infections are extremely widespread among fishes in aquaria and in free waters, both fresh-water and marine. Schäperclaus (Berlin) found *Ichthyophonus* as the causative organism of disease in aquarium fishes in 59% of all cases in 1949 and in 24% of 161 cases investigated in the period 1945–1950, whereas Reichenbach-Klinke reported in 1950 to have found this parasite in 50% of cases investigated in Munich.

In 1954 Reichenbach-Klinke listed 52 different species of fresh-water fishes and 21 of marine fishes in which *Ichthyophonus* had been found.[10] This list includes the Shark *Scyllium canicula* as well as nearly all families of fishes that are regularly represented in fresh water and in marine aquaria, whether tropical or cold-water tanks. The number of species in which the parasite has been found has since that time increased considerably, especially with marine species. Widespread epidemics with high mortalities have been observed in such important marine food fishes of man as Herring, Mackerel, Haddock, Cod and Plaice.

In acute infections of Atlantic Herring, massive invasions of the tissues leading to necrosis were observed and death occurred within 30 days, whereas in chronic infections cell infiltration and progressive encapsulation of spores by fibroblasts (connective tissue cells), followed by black pigmentation due to accumulation of melanophores, as described previously (p. 252), prevailed. However, even in those cases most of the infected fishes died within six months. During recent epidemics, about 25% of all Herring sampled was infected.[11]

There is evidence that *Ichthyophonus* also occurs in amphibians.[12]

TAXONOMY OF ICHTHYOPHONUS PARASITES. Although these parasites had already been detected by Bruno Hofer as early as 1893[13] as the causative organisms of the tumbling disease of Trout, he did not investigate them completely, but thought it probable that they should belong to the *Sporozoa*. A satisfactory biological description and naming of the parasite was given by Marianne

Plehn and Mulsow in 1911.[14] However, in the meantime a similar
parasite had been observed in the marine fishes *Onos mustela* and
Liparis vulgaris by M. Caullery and F. Mesnil. They named it *Ichthyosporidium gasterophilum*. Consequently, the Genus name *Ichthyosporidium*
has priority over that of *Ichthyophonus*. *I. gasterophilum* has also been
described to occur in Sea Trout (*Salmo trutta*) by A. Alexeieff (1914),
but this species has not been specifically mentioned in new
investigations, so it has been supposed to be identical with *I. hoferi*.
These questions of nomenclature have been surveyed by Reichenbach-Klinke in 1954 *loc. cit.* It appears now that *Ichthyophonus hoferi*
Plehn and Mulsow should be properly named *Ichthyosporidium hoferi*
(Plehn and Mulsow), whereas the related species *Ichthyophonus
intestinalis* Léger and Hesse and *I. lotæ* Léger are incorporated in a
different Genus, namely *Basidiobolus*, owing to differences in the
process of germination and reproduction. The Genus *Basidiobolus*
was already known to contain several parasites of frogs and lizards.

However, since the parasites have become widely known by now
under the name of *Ichthyophonus*, whereas the splitting of the Genus
does not coincide with specific differences in the disease, it is
considered reasonable to maintain the general name *Ichthyophonus*
as a practical fancy name in the field of fish diseases, although when
dealing with any special parasite as such, the revised nomenclature
should be followed.

Some other parasitic organisms have been described as belonging
to this group, but could be shown later on to be in reality *Sporozoa*.
A so-called '*Ichthyosporidium phymogenes*' Caullery and Mesnil, found
in *Crenilabrus ocellatus*, is identical with *Glugea gigantea* (Thélohan),
whereas '*Ichthyosporidium hertwigi*' Swarczewsky, found in *Crenilabrus
pavo*, is in reality a sporozoan, belonging to the *Microsporidia*.

TREATMENT OF ICHTHYOPHONUS DISEASE

For a long time it has been utterly impossible to heal fishes infected
with this parasite. While it is still difficult to cure this disease, some
cases, where the disease had not proceeded too far, have been cured
by the phenoxethol treatment after Rankin, applied in the same way
as described for treatment of intestinal worms. The infected fishes are
fed with dried food soaked in a 1% solution of phenoxethol, while 10
cm^3 of this stock solution are added per litre aquarium water (45 cm^3/
Imp. gal or 38 cm^3/U.S. gal). For success, all depends on early
treatment and this will often be difficult owing to the symptoms being
not easily recognisable in the early stages of the infection. Generally,
at least one fish has to die before a certain diagnosis can be given,
based on the post-mortem examination of its internal organs.

Lewer (see reference 9 on page 267) found that cultures of *Ichthyophonus* were killed by penicillin, but adding this antibiotic to the
water of an infected tank had no effect, which is not surprising

since penicillin is rapidly destroyed and will not reach the internal organs of the fishes under these conditions. However, by a series of intramuscular injections of penicillin on consecutive days all infected fishes but one could be cured. From this result it may be inferred that other antibiotics probably will be equally well or even more effective and it is suggested to use Chloromycetin (chloramphenicol), mixed with the food, as described at pages 154 and 323, or to try the specific fungicides griseofulvin and nystatin (see last chapter).

According to Reichenbach-Klinke[15] antibiotics act only on the penetrating and migrating stages of the parasite in the intestinal wall, but not on those that are already developing in the other organs or have encysted. This stresses the importance of early treatment. If spreading of the parasites is prevented by antibiotics, this may in itself already be sufficient to enable the fish to cope with the encysted parasites as described before (pages 252–253).

FUNGUS INFECTIONS

Several species of true moulds have been found in the internal organs of fishes not showing specific external symptoms of disease:

Penicillium piscium Reichenbach-Klinke, in the ovary and the body cavity of European as well as tropical fishes. It may be identical with *Nephromyces piscium* Plehn, detected in 1916 in whitish foci in the kidneys of Carps, characterised by dull swimming.

Unidentified moulds have been observed in the eye of Pike-Perch, in kidneys of Carp and in Trout and *Trichogaster leeri*.

A mould incorporated in the Genus *Pullularia* has been detected in the liver of the Ray *Trigon pastinacea* with indefinite symptoms of disease. Pure cultures proved highly infectious to Carp; these died after 28–32 days. Symptoms had been the same as in the Rays.

Members of the Genus *Aphanomyces* may be highly pathogenic to fishes. A case has been described of such infection of the dorsal muscles of tropical aquarium fishes. Death occurred when the skin was perforated.

For treatment, feeding minced meat mixed with a specific antifungal antibiotic is suggested. As such, griseofulvin and nystatin could be tried.

SLEEPING SICKNESS

In fish, a sleeping sickness may occur which is related to the sleeping sickness of men and cattle. The skin and the gills are pale. The eyes appear deeply sunken in the orbits. Often fishes may lie on their side for weeks, slowly breathing and showing very little movement. If they are placed in an upright position they will swim for a while, but then they fall on their sides again. Gradually they grow thin, since no food is taken, and finally die from weakness and exhaustion.

Microscopical examination of the blood of such diseased fishes will show the presence of small unicellular parasites, belonging to the *Mastigophora*. Although in sleeping sickness of men and cattle, species of the Genus *Trypanosoma* of the Family *Trypanosomidæ* (characterised by the possession of one flagellum only) are found, most cases of this disease in fish are due to members of the Genus *Cryptobia* (*Trypanoplasma*, incorporated in the Family *Bodonidæ*) which have two flagella. Infection takes place if a fish is attacked by a leech which has sucked blood from another infected fish. Direct infection from fish to fish cannot occur and therefore the disease will not often be met with in aquaria, since leeches are not introduced into a tank intentionally. When such organisms are present on plants or other materials they may be seen easily and removed. In ponds it will be more difficult, whilst in free waters nothing at all can be done.

ORGANISMS RESPONSIBLE FOR SLEEPING SICKNESS (Fig. 7.34)

Species of the Family *Trypanosomidæ* which are found in the blood of fish, are: *Trypanosoma remaki* Laveran and Mesnil, *forma parva*—length 15–20 μm, breadth 1.4 μm, length of flagellum 14 μm. *Trypanosoma remaki, forma magna*—length 26–28 μm, breadth 2–2.5 μm, length of flagellum 17–19 μm. Both varieties live in the blood of Pike (*Esox lucius*); *Trypanosoma granulosum* Laveran and Mesnil—

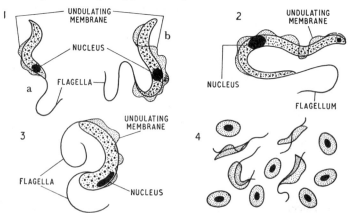

Fig. 7.34. Organisms responsible for sleeping sickness in fish. 1, Trypanosoma remaki. (a) forma parva *and* (b) forma magna. 2, Trypanosoma granulosum. 3, Cryptobia borelli. *All after Laveran and Mesnil.* 4, *Specimens of* Cryptobia cyprini *between the red blood corpuscles of an infected Carp (after Marianne Plehn)*

length up to 55 μm, breadth 2.5–3 μm, length of flagellum 25 μm. This parasite has been found in the blood of Eels (*Anguilla anguilla*); further *T. abramidis* Laveran and Mesnil and *T. bliccæ* Nikitin, in Silver Bream (*Blicca bjoerkna*); *T. barbi* Brumpt, in Barbel (*Barbus barbus*); *T. percæ* Brumpt, in Perch (*Perca fluviatilis*); *T. acerinæ* Brumpt and *T. phoxini* Brumpt, in Minnow (*Phoxinus phoxinus*); *T. danilewski* Laveran and Mesnil, in Carp (*Cyprinus carpio*); *T. scardinii* Brumpt, in Rudd; *T. cobitis* (Mitrophanow), in Weather Fish; *T. tincæ* Laveran and Mesnil, in Tench; *T. carassii* (Mitrophanow), in Prussian Carp; *T. leucisci* Brumpt, in *Leuciscus* species.

A large number of species of *Trypanosoma* have been described as parasites of marine fishes, among them are *T. æglefini*, in Haddock; *T. flesi*, in Flounder; *T. platessæ*, in Plaice; *T. soleæ*, in Sole; *T. rajæ*, in several species of Thornback; *T. scyllis*, in several Sharks of the Genus *Scyllium*; *T. caulopsettæ* Laird in *Caulopsetta scapta* (Forster).

Generally, the *Trypanosomidæ* do not cause much harm to the infected fishes. The severe cases of true sleeping sickness are due to *Cryptobia* (*Trypanoplasma*) infections.

Species of *Cryptobia* found in fish are: *Cryptobia borelli* (Laveran and Mesnil)— length to 20 μm, breadth 3–4 μm, length of flagella 15 μm. It has been found in the blood of Rudd (*Scardinius erythrophthalmus*) and Minnow (*Phoxinus phoxinus*); *Cryptobia cyprini* (Plehn)—length 10–30 μm. The flagella are not the same length, one being only half as long as the other. This parasite has been found in the blood of Carps (*Cyprinus carpio*), Prussian Carp (*Carassius carassius*) and Goldfish which become anaemic if large numbers of parasites are present. The gills will become pale and the blood becomes watery. Thus normal respiration is impeded until finally the victims die from anaemia. Similar symptoms, but in an even more serious form, are produced by *Cryptobia tincæ* (Schäperclaus) in Tench (*Tinca tinca*).

In Volga Sturgeon (*Acipenser ruthenus*) *C. acipenseri* (Joff, Lewaschoff and Boschenko) has been found. *C. salmositica* Katz is transferred by the leech *Piscicola salmositica* to North American Salmonids.

A number of other species, described in literature, is considered to be doubtful, according to Schäperclaus. In marine fishes *Cryptobia gurneyorum* Laird has been found.

No cures are known, but experiments with tryparsamide might be worth while (see page 353).

HEXAMITA (OCTOMITUS) INFECTIONS (HEXAMITIASIS)

The organism *Hexamita* (*Octomitus*) (*Urophagus*) *intestinalis* (Dujardin) is an intestinal parasite (Fig. 7.35), belonging to the Family *Bodonidæ* of the *Mastigophora*. It was found for the first time in the intestines of amphibians by Dujardin, in the year 1841, while later on other investigators detected this parasite in the intestines of fresh-water fishes. Members of the Genus *Hexamita* have two groups of three flagella at the broader end of the body, which are used for swimming, while a further two longer flagella are situated at the other end. The parasite has an oval or spindle-shaped body with a length of 12–16 μm and a breadth of 6–7 μm. The nucleus is vesicular. It is situated in the broader part of the body, but it is often difficult to see. *H. intestinalis* has sometimes been found in fish suffering from inflammation of the intestine (enteritis).

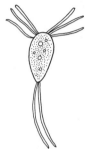

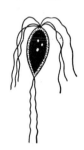

Fig. 7.36. Hexamita truttæ *(after Amlacher, Taschenbuch der Fischkrankheiten, Jena 1961)*

Fig. 7.35. The protozoan Hexamita (Octomitus) (Urophagus) intestinalis *(after Moroff)*

Another closely related species is *Hexamita truttæ* (Fig. 7.36). It also possesses two groups of three flagella and a further two at the other end. Its length is about 10 μm and its breadth 2.9–6.0 μm. It is mainly a parasite of the stomach, but it may also occur in the gall bladder and in the liver as well as sometimes in the intestine. The parasite has been found in Trout. In aquarium fish, it occurs mainly in Angel Fish (*Pterophyllum*), in Mosquito Fish (*Heterandria formosa*) and in *Cichlasoma severum*, but on rare occasions it has been found in Black Widows (*Gymnocorymbus ternetzi*), Goldfish, Shubunkins and Golden Rudd.

In Angel Fish, the black bandings become much more intense and brilliant, provided that the fishes are kept at an appropriate water temperature. Further symptoms are a slight stagger in swimming and spasmodic dippings of the caudal fin.

In Mosquito Fish, the main symptoms are emaciation, the belly showing a concave contour, although they still show appetite. Symptoms may closely resemble those of *Ichthyophonus* disease (see pages 250–259).

Microscopical investigation of histological sections of the internal organs reveals purulent inflammations, especially in the gall bladder, where local shrinkages and dilations may be observed, as well as changes in the structure of the bladder wall.

In the U.S.A. *Hexamita* (*Octomitus*) *salmonis* (Moore) has been found in the intestines of Trout and Salmon. It has caused serious mortalities among fingerling Trout up to 7–10 cm (3–4 in) long,

Brook Trout and Rainbow Trout. *H. salmonis* should be characterised by some sucker-like structure at the anterior end. However, similar observations seem to have been obtained with *H. truttæ*, but then they were interpreted as a *cytostoma* (cell mouth). *H. salmonis* is pear-shaped (Fig. 7.37). The cell body has a length of 7.4–12.3 μm and a width of 3–6 μm. It contains typical dark-coloured basal bodies.

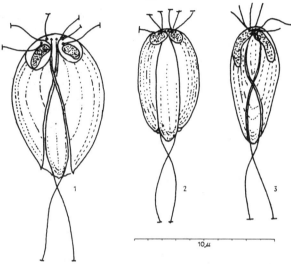

Fig. 7.37. *Organisms causing* Hexamitiasis. *Flagella have only been indicated (compare Fig. 7.36).* 1, Hexamita salmonis *(Moore).* 2, Hexamita intestinalis *(Dujardin).* 3, Spironucleus elegans Lavier *(after Kulda and Lom)*

Schäperclaus thinks it likely that *H. salmonis* could be identical with *H. truttæ*, because the symptoms produced in *Salmonidæ* in Europe and in America are the same.

In Rainbow Trout the main symptoms of *Hexamita* infection are emaciation, some darkening of the skin and finally infection of the gall bladder with thickening of its wall and a jelly-like consistency of its contents. It has also been found in the blood.

Hexamita species reproduce by simple cell division after cyst formation. Each cell may in this way give rise to two new ones. Such cysts are excreted with the faeces. Consequently, a certain diagnosis can be obtained by microscopical examination of freshly dropped faeces of a diseased fish. In fishes that have died some time prior to the post-mortem investigation, the parasites cannot be detected any more.

The infection may remain latent for several periods of time and may break out again suddenly at some change of environmental conditions, such as removal to another pond, tank or container or a change of food. Outbreaks may be provoked by unsuitable food, especially in case of lack of vitamins. Depending on the severity of the attack it may cause death or after some time become latent again.

Amlacher[16] observed *Hexamita* infections in Pompadour Fish (*Symphysodon discus*), differing in some respects from those described thus far. The parasites occurred abundantly in the liver, the heart, gall bladder and the intestine; a few specimens only were found in the spleen, whereas the parasites were never observed in the kidneys. The parasites had a length of 11.5 μm and a width of 4.6 μm. The length of the two long steering flagella was about 12 μm. The parasites showed a spirally rotating movement and were able to remain moving in 40% ethanol for 30 min or more. In only partially coagulated blood smears the organisms were still alive after an hour. Experiments to infect the Dwarf Cichlid (*Nannacara anomala*) were completely negative, even after one month of feeding with infected material. Amlacher designated this parasite as a new species, now bearing the name *Hexamita (Octomitus) symphysodonis* (Amlacher). In Angel Fish (*Pterophyllum scalare*) still another parasite of the same Family has been found, namely *Spironucleus elegans* Lavier.[17] This species also occurs in Carp and in amphibians.

TREATMENT OF HEXAMITA DISEASE

Several drugs have been found effective for curing fish suffering from *Hexamitiasis*. All of these must be administered with the food.

CALOMEL (mercury-I-chloride, mercurous chloride). This is the first chemical introduced for curing this condition.[18] It is added at a rate of 0.2% to the food for several days. Although calomel has been employed with good results for a long time in America, it is not recommended any more, owing to its toxicity to fish, since other less harmful drugs have become available.

CARBARSONE (*para*-ureidobenzenearsonic acid, *para*-carbamido-benzenearsonic acid). 0.2% of this drug is thoroughly mixed with the food and administered during four consecutive days; then treatment is stopped for three days, after which it is repeated once.[19]

FUMAGILLIN (Fumidil, Amebacilin). This is an antibiotic substance, produced by the fungus *Aspergillus fumigatus*. It is also used at a rate of 0.2% in the food, for four days.[20]

In the same way *2-amino-5-nitrothiazole* (Enheptin, Entramin) and a compound, designated as PR-3714 may be employed.[20]

The following drugs were found effective when used at a rate of 1% admixed to the food: *Aureomycin*[R] (chlortetracycline), *ARTHINOL*, and *4,7-PHENANTHROLINE-5,6-DIONE* (*Entobex*, Ciba 11, 925, 4,7-phenanthroline-5,6-quinone).

FURAZOLIDONE, applied as described for treatment of bacterial infections (see page 158), may also be expected to be effective, since it is used against related infections in veterinary practice.

ACRIFLAVINE has been used as a 0.1% solution admixed to minced meat by Amlacher and Steffens (Germany) for treatment of young Trout, but 25% of the fishes refused to take this drugged food, whereas in the others the incidence of the disease was still 16.6% as compared to 50% in the untreated controls.[21]

SPOROZOAN INFECTIONS

A large number of sporozoan parasites may be found in the internal organs of fish. On post-mortem examination, yellow bodies can often be found in the internal organs, which have been produced by the fish itself at places where the parasite has left the tissue and the resulting gap had to be filled. A number of *Coccidia*, mainly belonging to the Genus *Hæmogregarina*, are blood parasites that penetrate into the erythrocytes (red blood corpuscles) and give rise to anaemia. Other symptoms may somewhat resemble those of sleeping sickness (p. 259). For a further description of sporozoan infections, see Chapter 4.

NECROSIS OF THE MUSCLES

Degeneration of the muscles occurs in different diseases, such as neon disease, caused by the sporozoan *Plistophora hyphessobryconis* (see page 141), *Ichthyophonus* infections (page 250) and tuberculosis (page 184), as well as in case of malignant tumours that invade the muscles and destroy them (see page 273).

In red-tailed Guppies a serious epidemic of necrosis of the muscles has been observed by Dr. Richard Pohl in Ames, Iowa, U.S.A. (personal communication, November 1964). The outward symptom was a whitening of the caudal peduncle, especially evident in females. The normally darkish and somewhat translucent flesh became milky and opaque. After some period of time, the fishes weakened and were in danger of losing the use of one or both pectoral fins. The progress of the disease was long and continued over weeks. No external or internal parasites could be found. In histological sections widespread deterioration of the muscles was observed. Having been sent some of the microscopic preparations made for Dr. Pohl by Dr. John Kluge of the Animal Disease Laboratory in Ames, I was able to find large numbers of tiny microbes in the section stained with Weigert's iron-haematoxyline, but not in those stained with Harris's alum-haematoxyline or Gomori's one-step trichrome stain. Their presence was confined to the deteriorated muscles, that appeared as if partly dissolved and showed only weak staining behaviour. From the tiny shape and size the organisms might belong to the Family *Chlamydozoaceæ* of the Order *Rickettsiales*, consisting of microbes which are small, pleomorphic, often coccoid obligate intracytoplasmic parasites, with a diameter of 0.2–0.5 μm or up to 2 μm in length in the rod-shaped forms. The accompanying photomicrograph (Fig. 7.38) shows coccoid forms, but at certain sites clusters of rod-shaped forms could also be found. However, the available evidence is not sufficient to warrant a more definite identification.

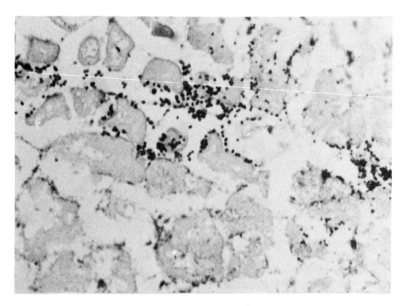

Fig. 7.38. Tiny coccoid microbes possibly belonging to the Family Chlamydo-zoaceæ *of the* Rickettsiales, *in deteriorated muscle in a section of diseased red-tailed Guppy.* × 3000. *Weigert's iron-haematoxyline stain (photomicrograph by the author)*

For treatment of Rickettsia infections in general, administration of chloramphenicol (Chloromycetin) or oxytetracycline (Terramycin) in the food is suggested. For fishes that are big enough for handling, injection therapy with these drugs may be employed.

NECROTIC ULCERS IN *TETRAODON*

In monocytes (one of the several types of white blood cells) and in blood plasma of *Tetraodon fahaka* Hass with necrotic ulcers at the head and the body, Schäperclaus found *Rickettsia pisces* Mohamed as the causative agent.

REFERENCES

1 STOLK, A., 'Visziekten', *Diergeneesk. Memo.* **8**, 173–251 (1961)
2 DAWES, B., *The Trematoda*, Cambridge (1946); SPREHN, C., *Trematoda und Cestoidea*, in: BROHMER, P., *et al.*, *Die Tierwelt Mitteleuropas, Quelle u. Meyer*, Leipzig (1960); YAMAGUTI, S., *Systema Helminthum. I. The Digenetic Trematodes of Vertebrates*, Interscience, London and New York (1958)
3 McKERNAN, D. L., 'A treatment for tape worms in Trout', *Progr. Fish-Cult.*, No. 50, 33–35 (1940)
4 ALLISON, L. N., 'Advancements in prevention and treatment of parasitic diseases of fish', *Trans. Amer. Fish. Soc.* **83**, 1221–28 [1953 (publ. 1954)]
5 REICHENBACH-KLINKE, H., *Krankheiten und Schädigungen der Fische*, p. 335, Stuttgart (1966)
6 HNATH, J. G., 'Di-n-butyl tin oxide as a vermicide on *Eubothrium crassum* (Bloch, 1779) in Rainbow Trout', *Progr. Fish-Cult.* **32**, 47–50 (1970)
7 WURMBACH, H., 'Geschlechtsumkehr bei Weibchen von *Lebistes reticulatus* bei Befall mit *Ichthyophonus hoferi* Plehn-Mulsow', *Roux. Archiv. f. Entwicklungs-Mechanik.* **145**, 109–24 (1951)
8 SPURWAY, H., 'Spontaneous parthenogenesis in a fish', *Nature (Lond.)* **171**, 437 (1953); STOLK, A., 'Pathological parthenogenesis in viviparous Tooth-Carps', *Nature* **181**, 1660 (1958); 'Pathological parthenogenesis in a viviparous Tooth Carp', *Nature* **191**, 507 (1961)
9 LEWER, J., *Die Aquarien- u. Terrarienzeitschr.* (Oct. 1952)
10 REICHENBACH-KLINKE, H., 'Untersuchungen über die bei Fischen durch Parasiten hervorgerufenen Zysten und deren Wirkung auf den Wirtskörper', *Z. Fisch. N.F.* **3**, 565–636 (1954); **4**, 1–52 (1955)
11 SINDERMANN, C. J., *Principal Diseases of Marine Fish and Shellfish*, Academic Press, New York and London (1970)
12 REICHENBACH-KLINKE, H., *Krankheiten der Amphibien*, Stuttgart (1961)
13 HOFER, B., 'Eine Salmonidenerkrankung', *Allg. Fischereizeitung*, No. 11 (1893)
14 PLEHN, M., and MULSOW, K., 'Der Erreger der *Taumelkrankheit* der Salmoniden', *Zentr. Bakteriol. Parasitenk. Abt. I* **59**, 63–68 (1911)
15 REICHENBACH-KLINKE, H., 'Über den Zusammenhang und die ökologische Abhängigkeit zwischen Kiemen- und Lebererkrankungen bei Süsswasserfischen', *Z. Fisch. N.F.* **13**, 747–67 (1964)
16 AMLACHER, E., *Taschenbuch der Fischkrankheiten*, Jena, 157–58 (1961)
17 KULDA, J. and LOM, J., 'Remarks on the diplomastigine flagellates from the intestine of fishes', *Paras.* **54**, 753–62 (1964)
18 TUNISON, A. V. and McCAY, C. M., 'Nutritional requirements of Brook Trout', *Trans. Fish. Soc.* **63**, 167–77 (1933)
19 FISH, F. F. and McKERNAN, D. L., 'Calomel *v.* Carbarsone', *Progr. Fish-Cult.*, No. 51, 7–9 (1940); NELSON, E. C., 'Carbarsone treatments for *Octomitus*', *Progr. Fish-Cult.*, No. 55, 1–4 (1941)
20 YASUTAKE, W. T., BUHLER, D. R. and SHANKS, W. E., 'Chemotherapy of hexamitiasis in fish', *J. Parasitol* **47**, 81–86 (1961)
21 AMLACHER, E., *Taschenbuch der Fischkrankheiten*, p. 157, Gustav Fischer Verlag, Jena (1961)

8

TUMOURS IN FISH

In fish several kinds of real tumours may occur, i.e. pathological growth of tissue cells without previous inflammation and without traceable infectious origin. Most of them are not dangerous, but there are some forms that have a malignant character. Some cases of real carcinoma (malignant epithelium cell tumour; cancer) and sarcoma (malignant connective tissue) have been found.

Benign or simple tumours are of restricted extension; although they may have a large size, they are localised and encapsulated, pressing upon, but not invading, adjacent tissues. When they are removed surgically, there is no recurrence. Generally, a simple tumour grows slowly. It may cause death, but only indirectly when a vital organ is suppressed mechanically to such extent as to be prevented from proper functioning.

Malignant tumours consist of cells that do not correspond to the normal cells of the tissue in which they arise. These tumours are not surrounded by an encapsulating membrane, but their cells grow freely in all directions, spreading between normal tissue and invading it. In tumours of warm-blooded animals the most convincing evidence of malignancy of a tumour is its metastasising tendency, i.e. the transfer of its cells to other parts of the body via the blood or the lymphatics, giving rise to fresh tumours. In fish tumours, however, metastasising is highly exceptional, even in the most malignant tumours. On the other hand, there is no infallible criterion to discriminate between metastases and tumours that have come out independently (multiple tumours), although in some cases the transfer of tumour cells from one tumour to another place can be traced.

However, infiltration and invasive growth into the surrounding tissues and organs, coupled with destruction of these tissues and organs, does occur in all malignant tumours in fish.

The nuclei of tumour cells are generally larger than those of normal cells, whereas they often stain more heavily with certain dyes. The nucleoli (small bodies inside the nucleus) that are normally spherical or oval are often swollen and irregular in shape, whereas their number (normally one to three, depending on the type of cell) may be increased. Many tumour cells contain more than one nucleus (Fig. 8.1). In tumour tissue many cells show mitosis (the process of nuclear duplication preceding cell division, normally providing each daughter cell with exactly the same number of chromosomes as the original one); this is an indication for the rapid multiplication of tumour cells—the more mitotic activity, the higher the malignancy of a tumour. Often the mitosis proceeds aberratic and nuclei with deviating chromosome numbers are produced,

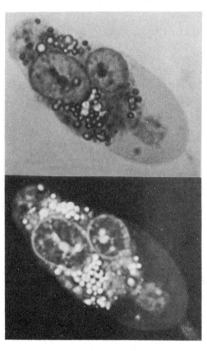

Fig. 8.1. Living malignant cell, grown in tissue culture, photographed with a Baker interference microscope. Upper: *Positive*, Lower: *Negative Interference Contrast. The cell contains two large nuclei in which nucleoles are shown, and heavy granulation. There are many other types of malignant cells, however (photomicrographs by the author)*

sometimes even up to four times the normal amount. Such deviations are also among the characteristics of malignant cells, whereas benign tumour cells more closely resemble those of normal tissue.

In descriptions of tumours some special terms are often encountered:

Hyperplasia is the name for any excessive multiplication of cells in a specific tissue, excluding, however, proliferation as a response to loss of tissue or to increased intensity of function;

Neoplasia is that kind of hyperplasia, which is characterised by persistent uncoordinated growth independently of the stimulus that induced it; the resulting growth is called neoplasm;

Anaplasia is the loss of the distinctive properties of the original normal cells in neoplastic growth, the cells tending to revert to a more primitive and less differentiated form; this is generally the case in malignant growth, the degree of malignancy increasing with increasing dedifferentiation;

Metaplasia is the change of one kind of tissue into another; this may be a normal process, as in ossification of cartilage, or in producing scar tissue from normal fibroblasts of connective tissue, or it may differ from normal transformations.

Black pigment cell tumours (melanoma) often occur in some Swordtail × Platy hybrids and in Black Mollies. Further, there are benign epithelium cell tumours (papillomata) and malign types of these (epithelioma and carcinoma) and tumours consisting of connective tissue (fibroma and the very malignant sarcoma), lymph gland tumours (lymphosarcoma), muscle tumours (myoma; if they consist of unstriped muscle fibres they are called leiomyoma), nerve cell tumours (neuroma), fatty tumours (lipoma), and tumours consisting of glandular tissue (adenoma). Tumours of bone tissue (osteoma) and cartilage (chondroma) have but seldom been observed in fishes. Often a malignant growth may contain more than one type of tumour cells, such as in the adenocarcinoma of the thyroid, sometimes encountered in fish. This is a mixed tumour, consisting of both malignant glandular cells and of malignant epithelium cells.

Proliferation of normal body or tissue cavities may give rise to cyst formation (cystoma). Generally, early stages of cystomata are benign and they may remain so, but often such cysts develop into other types of true tumours and may ultimately form the basis of a highly malignant growth, such as a fibrosarcoma or a carcinoma.

Tumours of fish are often histopathologically strikingly similar to those found in human beings, although it must be emphasised that fish tissues differ from tissues of warm-blooded animals and that the interpretation of tumour structure used in, for instance, human pathology, is not always applicable without modification. In some literature on fish diseases, *benign* epithelium cell tumours are called epitheliomata, which is contradictory to the terminology used in general oncology (= the scientific study of tumours; 'cancer research'); this may give rise to confusion.

Some fish tumours have been grown in tissue culture and others are transplantable. In human beings, tumours are treated surgically or by irradiation (X-rays, radium), while sometimes hormones are administered. For treating fish, such methods are out of the question.

ORIGIN OF TUMOURS

There is not one single cause to be held responsible for the induction of tumour growth, but many different conditions may give rise to it. Among them are prolonged influence of adverse chemical or physical stimuli, including a large amount of known chemicals, ultraviolet irradiation, X-ray irradiation and atomic radiations, presence of certain viruses, hormonal disturbances, but also primary changes induced by the effects of certain parasites. The latter are generally indicated as pseudo-tumours, but a true borderline cannot be drawn. After all, a neoplasm of at present unknown origin may at some later date be found to be due to some microbial or viral infection. In individual cases it is generally useless to seek for a primary cause. The growth of pseudo-tumours is often arrested as soon as the primary cause has been removed or neutralised. Generally these are simple hyperplastic growths.

Tumours with unknown origin are called 'spontaneous', as opposed to 'induced' ones, that have been produced experimentally or under conditions where the primary cause can be traced. Among them are tumours caused by hereditary predisposition.

Expecially in marine fishes many neoplastic or hyperplastic diseases are thought to be of viral origin.[1]

INVESTIGATION

Only some types of tumour will be described in some detail, as examples, since the investigation of tumours requires specialised histological work. Small fish must be fixed as a whole, whereas large fish are dissected first, and suspected organs are fixed and prepared separately. As a general-purpose histological fixative for fish tumours Bouin's fixative is recommended.

After embedding in paraffin wax, sections are cut with a microtome. Several staining techniques may be employed, but as a rule these should always include a haematoxyline and eosin or azophloxin method, and a method especially suited for demonstrating connective tissue, such as Azan or Mallory and its modifications. Further suitable methods are the silver impregnation technique after Laguesse and a Ziehl–Neelsen staining. Details can be found in any textbook of animal histological technique.

Extensive reviews of tumours in fish have been given by Ross F. Nigrelli,[2] by Schlumberger and Lucke,[3] and also by Reichenbach-Klinke.[4]

A CASE OF SPONTANEOUS SARCOMA IN AQUARIUM FISH[5]

The fish (Fig. 8.2) was a half-grown female *Pseudocorynopoma doriæ* Perugia, about $4\frac{1}{2}$ cm in length (adult size up to 8 cm). It was obtained from its aquarist owner for post-mortem examination. The fish showed a large tumour at the left-hand side below the dorsal fin, while additional symptoms were a crooked spine (skoliosis) and a

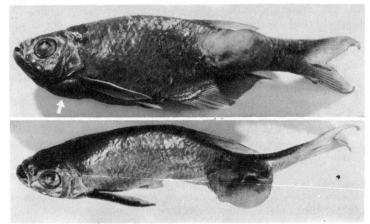

Fig. 8.2. Female Pseudocorynopoma doriæ Perugia, *showing large sarcoma tumour near the tail and a smaller one at the throat (indicated by arrow).* Upper: *side view.* Lower: *same specimen photographed from above, showing tumour and crooked spine (skoliosis).* × 2

swelling at the throat (Fig. 8.3). The symptom of skoliosis may be attributed to the destruction of muscle by the tumour and the necessity of keeping balance against the overthrowing moment caused by the weight of a large tumour; microscopically the spine was found normal. The tumour had developed very rapidly; it took but one week between the appearance of the first externally visible symptoms and the moment of death.

Low-power microscopic examination of a cross-section through

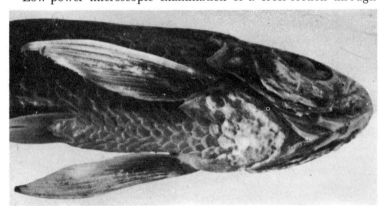

Fig. 8.3. Ventral view of part of same fish as in preceding photographs, showing sarcoma tumour at the throat, which might have developed as a metastasis of the large tumour in the tail region. The throat tumour is also visible as a swelling near the arrow at the first picture of this series. × 5 *(all photographs by the author)*

the middle of the tumour showed that the muscles had been destroyed completely by the rapidly growing tumour cells, while penetration of strands of tumour tissue into the muscles of the other side of the body could be clearly seen (see Figs 8.4–8.9).

The tumour fibrous material stains intensely blue with the Azan staining method, whereas the connective tissue sheath of nerve and

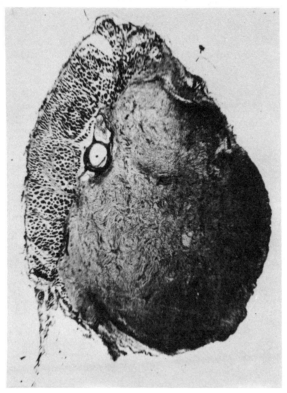

Fig. 8.4. Cross-section through tumour region, stained with haematoxyline-azophloxin. × 15

cells derived from it never stains intense blue, but at the most a very pale blue, which may be clearly distinguished from the intense staining in the sarcoma. This staining behaviour indicates that the tumour is not a neurofibroma (a type of tumour that occurs more often in fish) but a true sarcoma.

Obviously the tumour originated in the muscles and penetrated more and more till at the side of its origin all normal tissue had been destroyed and replaced by tumour cells. Sections from that part of the body that did not yet show external symptoms of tumour showed penetrated tumour tissue inside. Strands of tumour tissue could be observed following the borders of muscle bundles, obviously penetrating along the lines of least resistance investing normal muscle fibres and afterwards destroying them completely.

Whereas the peripheral parts of the tumour tissue have still some residual regularity, the older it becomes, the more irregular and wilder the growth is seen to be. In the interior of the tumour no trace of normal tissue structure can be found, the whole mass consisting of strands of cells that have grown without any regulating mechanism (Fig. 8.5). The swelling at the throat, visible in Fig. 8.3, was found to contain strands of tumour tissue penetrating into the

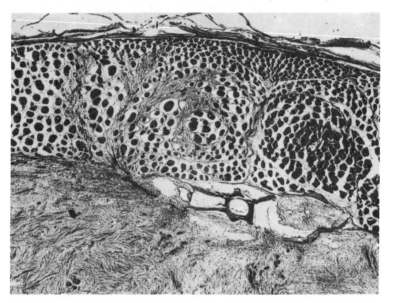

Fig. 8.5. Strands of sarcoma tumour tissue penetrating between the normal muscles at the other side. × 37

muscles in a similar manner to that shown in Fig. 8.5; although an infallible proof cannot be given, this may be considered to be a metastasis of the large primary tumour. All nerve sheaths recognisable in the sections appeared completely normal.

For a fish tumour, the present tumour has to be considered of the highest degree of malignancy, since it is highly destructive and rapidly infiltrating into normal tissue, tends to metastasising, rapidly growing and causing death of the fish within one week, although organs that are indispensable for life had not yet been damaged. The immediate cause of death must therefore have been exhaustion and/or intoxication by the products of tissue destruction.

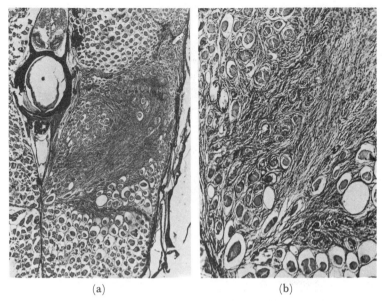

(a)   (b)

Fig. 8.6. (a) *Section of tail behind main tumour region, showing penetration of tumour.* × 50. (b) *Part of the same region as preceding photomicrograph, at higher magnification.* × 120

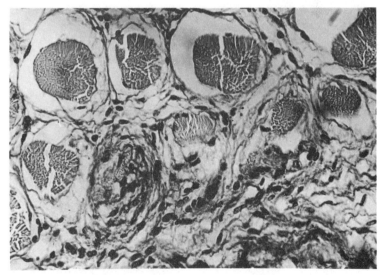

Fig. 8.7. Border region of sarcoma tumour and normal tissue, showing penetration of tumour cells between the muscle fibres. × 600

276

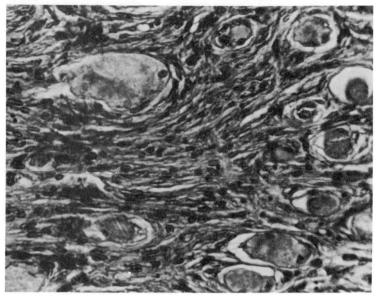

Fig. 8.8. Further morbid growth of sarcoma tumour cells. Destructive effects on the inverted muscle fibres are already visible. × 600

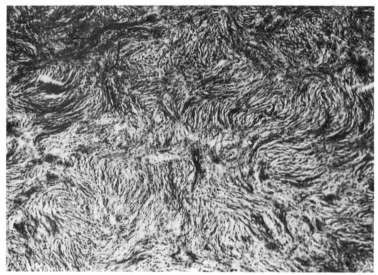

Fig. 8.9. Interior part of sarcoma tumour of Pseudocorynopoma doriæ, showing wild irregular growth. × 140

Cytologically, two main types of sarcoma are distinguished, namely the spindle-cell type and the round-cell type. This tumour is a spindle-cell sarcoma, as is demonstrated most clearly by Figs 8.7 and 8.8.

A CASE OF CARCINOMA (CANCER) IN PERCH

The fish to be described here was caught by N. M. Bailey in the reservoir of one of the many mills near Bury, Lancashire, in December 1953. The fish had a length of 14 cm and showed a tumour on the upper and left lateral part of the head. The tumour was 2.2 cm across the widest diameter, and little less than this in other diameters. The tumour was of a firm consistency and moved freely on the underlying bone of the head. It was partially covered by a thin membraneous epithelium, and in part a necrotic white ulcer, 1.5 cm dia. The tumour did not affect the left eye, but displaced it laterally quite considerably. Otherwise the fish, which on dissection proved to be a female, appeared quite normal, the skin was lustrous, and the gills and mouth quite clean.

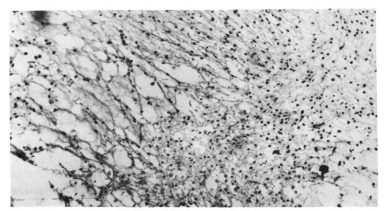

Fig. 8.10. Carcinoma *(cancer) in Perch. The tumour is penetrating from right to left upwards along the diagonal. Haematoxyline-eosin stain*

On bisection the tumour was found to be of a uniform whiteness and firmness throughout; it encircled the left eye and was continuous around the left optic nerve. There was no macroscopic abnormality of the abdominal contents; microscopical investigation of fresh smears from a small part of the tumour did not reveal any parasites.

The remaining part of the tumour was preserved in ethanol and sent to me, together with the description quoted above. The tumour was now embedded in paraffin wax and sections cut with a microtome. Although tissue structure was not preserved very well, owing to bad

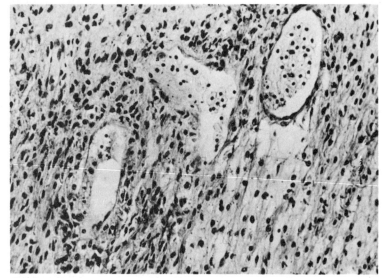

Fig. 8.11. Cancer of Perch at higher magnification than Fig. 8.10. Notice large number of nuclei

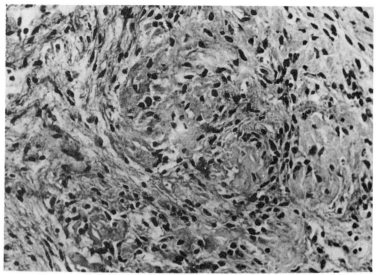

Fig. 8.12. Cancer of Perch. Part of tumour with highly irregular growth

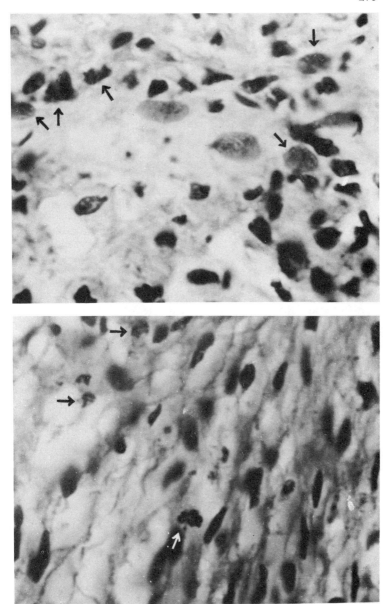

Fig. 8.13. Small detail of section of carcinoma of Perch at high magnification, showing highly irregular shapes and sizes of nuclei, staining anomalies and mitoses (indicated by arrows). × 1200 (all photomicrographs by the author)

fixation (ethanol alone is no good fixative for histological purposes), a certain diagnosis could still be obtained. This tumour consisted of a highly malignant growth of epithelium tissue, in fact a real carcinoma (cancer) with strong invasive power. The eye itself was not yet penetrated, but the surrounding parts showed only occasionally some small piece of normal tissue, which was already becoming invaded by malignant cells. The accompanying photomicrographs (Figs 8.10–8.13) further demonstrate a big difference in cell structure of this carcinoma and those of the sarcoma mentioned previously.

A MALIGNANT KIDNEY TUMOUR INDUCED BY VIRUS INFECTION

In 1956 an epidemic tumour disease was observed in Guppies (*Lebistes reticulatus*) (see Fig. 8.14) and *Pristella riddlei* in the Aquarium of the Zoological Institute of the University in Bonn, Germany.[6] Most of the victims died within a period of 23–111 days, but young Guppies up to four weeks of age showed resistance and embryos were never affected either.

Diseased fishes nearly always showed kidney tumours from which malignant cells invaded the adjacent organs and destroyed them. Invasive growth was observed in the kidneys, the muscles (Fig. 8.15) and the heart, the intestines, as well as the soft roes (testes). In the liver, spleen, ovaries, bones and cartilage and the nervous system no tumour growth was observed. There were indications of formation of metastases, spreading of tumour cells being accomplished via the bloodstream.

The individual tumour cells were either round or spindle-shaped and completely dedifferentiated so that their true origin remained obscure. Although this tumour is as invasive as the sarcoma described on page 271, the photomicrographs demonstrate clearly that they consist of entirely different cells and the kind of invasion is obviously all but strand-like, as in the sarcoma.

From investigations with ultracentrifugation of cell-free extracts of such tumours followed by infection experiments, it could be shown that this type of tumour is due to infection with a relatively small kind of virus.

MALIGNANT PIGMENT CELL TUMOURS

Most of the tumours in this group arise from the black pigment cells whence they are called melanoma. They occur most often in darkly coloured fishes. In Tench (*Tinca tinca*) melanomata have been observed on many occasions (Fig. 8.16). These were situated above and on the pectoral and ventral fins. The tumours consist mainly of proliferating epithelial cells of the epidermis, with a large number of blood-vessels penetrating into it from the cutis, together

281

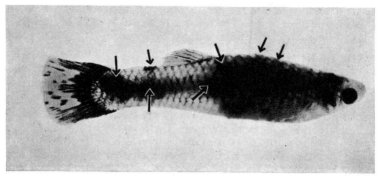

Fig. 8.14. Guppy with numerous muscle tumours (indicated by arrows) of viral origin (photograph by courtesy Dr. A. Wessing, Bonn)

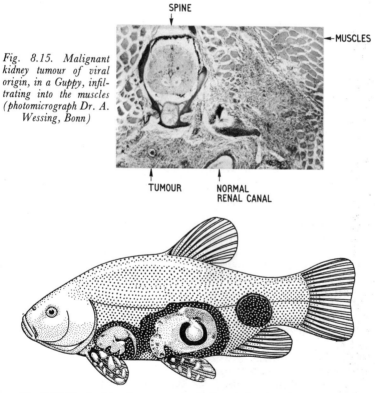

Fig. 8.15. Malignant kidney tumour of viral origin, in a Guppy, infiltrating into the muscles (photomicrograph Dr. A. Wessing, Bonn)

SPINE

MUSCLES

TUMOUR

NORMAL RENAL CANAL

Fig. 8.16. Tench with melanoma tumours (schematic drawing after colour-plate by Hofer)

with strands of connective tissue. Along the latter a large amount of black pigment is found. The luxurious growth appears to start from the epithelium, whereas permeation with blood-vessels and connective tissue occurs at a later stage. The tumour could thus be considered to be a true epithelioma (malignant epithelial tissue).[7]

Other types of melanomata are often encountered in Black Mollies and in certain Swordtail × Platy hybrids. A so-called 'Berlin hybrid' is obtained by crossing of a wild-type Swordtail (*Xiphophorus helleri*) female with a red-spotted (Rsp) male Platyfish (*Xiphophorus maculatus*). These hybrids appear nearly black at a red background. When these hybrids are crossed back with normal Swordtails, a type of fish is produced which is highly predisposed to the occurrence of spontaneous black pigment tumours at the base of the dorsal and caudal fins, on the head or at the belly. Similar tumours are encountered in the 'Hamburger hybrids', obtained by crossing of a wild-type Swordtail female with a Nigra (black) Platy male, especially in the next generation obtained on back crossing with an ordinary Swordtail. It is entirely clear that in these cases the tumour growth depends on certain adverse genetic combinations leading to uncontrolled luxuriation of one type of tissue or cells.

These tumours are not of epithelial, but of fibroblastic origin; they are highly malignant melanosarcomata. The fins of the fish get lost, the eyes may get lost, too, the brains may be destroyed and the abdominal wall may burst open.[8] In all cases of melanosarcomata and other malignant melanomata the macromelanophores are the primary proliferating and infiltrating pigment cells. Stolk has also described cases where a primary proliferation of macromelanophores led to the induction of an epidermis carcinoma in a Swordtail variety.[9]

Swordtails and their hybrids are also susceptible to tumours in which other types of pigment cells are involved, such as the yellow and red ones (xanthophores and erythrophores, respectively), called xanthophoromata and erythrophoromata, or a mixture of both (xanthoerythrophoromata), or even combinations with melanomata.[10] An erythrophoroma in the skin of a European Trout was described by Thomas[11] in 1931; it showed an orange colour and had invaded the anal fin, whereas another orange tumour was found in the peritoneal wall of the stomach, suspected to be a metastasis of the fin tumour.

Iridocytomata are tumours composed of malignant iridocytes, these being the reflecting guanine-containing cells which give white fishes their iridescent appearance. These are the rarest of pigment cell tumours. They have been observed by Dr. E. S. Schmidt of the Biological Research Institute, Hamburg, Germany, in certain albino strains of the Siamese Fighting Fish (*Betta splendens*).

In marine fishes pigment cell tumours seem to be encountered more often than in fresh-water fish.[12]

TUMOURS OF NERVE TISSUE

A neurofibroma is a tumour composed of fibrous tissue derived from the connective tissue sheath of a nerve-fibre fascicule. It consists of soft nodules and appears on the skin and elsewhere in the body. A related type of tumour is called neurolemmona or neurinoma; it is produced from the nerve sheath proper (neurolemma). Occasionally a neurolemmona may be pigmented with melanin.[13] True nerve cell tumours (neuromata) are extremely rare in fish.

Neurofibromata and neurolemmonata occur quite often in Goldfish and other species. They appear often in greater numbers (multiple tumours) as in the human condition known as von Recklinghausen's Disease (neurofibromatosis or *molluscum fibrosum*). Most of these tumours are benign, but some were shown to be malignant on histological examination.

Some tumours of the eye start with proliferation of the cells of the cornea or its surrounding tissues. The cornea is thickened and infiltrated with other cells, whereas cavities (cysts) are produced. Occasionally this condition develops further into a true tumour with massive hyperplasia and sometimes neoplasmic growths at the eyelid as well. These are true neurofibromata. The eye may be destroyed completely.[14]

TERATOMATA

These are tumours consisting of tissues derived from all three germ layers of the embryonic stage of an animal. They may show some degree of uncoordinated growth, but as a rule they appear like different kinds of tissue combined to form an organ. In human beings teratomata often occur in or about the uterus or other female organs and may contain rudimentary organs.

In Tooth-carps ovarial teratomas seem to be not uncommon. According to investigations by A. Stolk these may arise from pathological parthenogenesis (development of embryos from unfertilised eggs).[15] It is assumed that toxic substances produced by *Ichthyophonus* could provide the artificial stimulus for such development of unfertilised ova (see page 256).

An extensive review of this type of tumours was given by Gemmill as early as 1912.[16]

The presence of a big teratoma may show externally as a swelling or bump, but since such symptoms may also occur in other diseases, such as ovary cysts, obstipation, internal worm infections and others, this phenomenon is not characteristic. A correct diagnosis is only possible on microscopical examination of histological sections.

Teratomata have not necessarily the feature of indefinite autonomous proliferation characteristic for true tumours. Some may remain in a stationary condition after having developed to a certain extent and then the main consequence will be sterility of the fish. Such growths are essentially benign. Generally speaking, two main types of teratoma may be distinguished, namely the cystic type, characterised by a low degree of differentiation of tissues, enlargement of the ovary being mainly due to accumulation of secretion within cysts, and the solid type, which generally forms irregular mass, containing a great variety of tissues with no or only few cysts of small dimension in it. In connection with a solid teratoma malignant growth may develop, usually a carcinoma.

The accompanying photomicrographs have been made after stained histological sections of a solid teratoma of the ovary in a young Blue Gourami (*Trichogaster trichopterus* var. *sumatranus*) (Figs 8.17–8.22). The fish had a length of about 3 cm when it died. The only symptoms of disease prior to death were lack of appetite and the fish hiding itself. Coloration was normal. The tumour contains some cysts, large masses of epithelial tissue with some mitoses, muscle, cartilage, pigment, nerve tissue and connective tissue. In one region the growth has developed into a granulosa-cell tumour (folliculoma or *carcinoma folliculoides*), which has malignant properties, although of a low degree as compared with other forms of cancer. Whether there was a direct causal relationship between the tumour growth and death of the fish or that it died as a result of other conditions could not be ascertained.

Granulosa-cell tumours of the ovary are generally believed to arise from granulosa cell rests which have not been used up in the formation of follicles. Their histological structure is rather variable. The cells may be round or polyhedral and arranged in solid masses as in a carcinoma, or they may appear cubical or columnar and show an acinous or follicle-like arrangement, although even a diffuse, sarcoma-resembling structure may sometimes be observed.

PAPILLOMATA

These are (generally benign) tumours resulting from new growth of cells of the skin or the mucous membranes. These appear as small round, warty nodules or as large cauliflower-like masses. In a papilloma, both the epidermis and the underlying connective tissue are extremely hyperplasmic.

Often multiple wart-like papillomata occur in a number of fishes living in the same water. Although this might suggest an infectious origin (virus),[17] there have also been observations where this kind of tumour developed after mechanical injury of a fish.

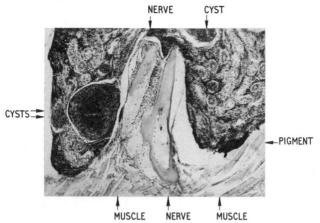

NERVE   CYST

CYSTS

PIGMENT

MUSCLE   NERVE   MUSCLE

Fig. 8.17. Part of histological section of teratoma of the ovary of Blue Gourami, showing different kinds of tissues and organ development. Haematoxyline-eosin stain. × 40

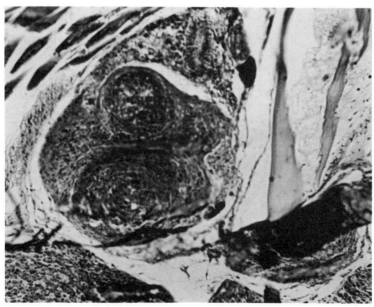

Fig. 8.18. Other part of teratoma tumour, showing double cyst (middle), *nerve tissue* (upper right) *and pigment* (lower right). × 200

286

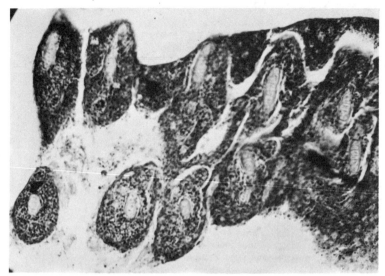

Fig. 8.19. Part of teratoma, consisting of a large number of separate units, each of which contains a centre of cartilage. × 200

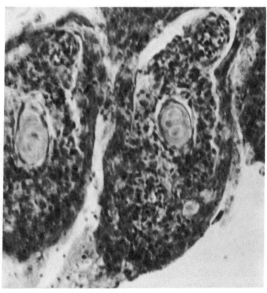

Fig. 8.20. Detail of preceding tissue section, at higher magnification. × 500

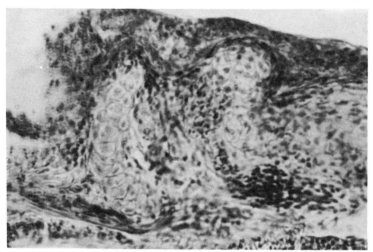

Fig. 8.21. Detail of teratoma tumour, showing development of cartilage and pigment.
× 500

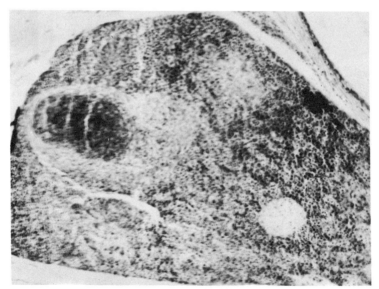

Fig. 8.22. Granulosa-cell tumour of ovary, developed from solid teratoma. A cyst is shown to the left. This tumour has malignant properties. × 200

ADENOMATA

These benign epithelial tumours with a gland-like structure have been observed in the kidney of Pike, in the liver of Trout and in the ovary and kidneys of Goldfish and Catfish.

SWELLINGS AND TUMOURS OF THE THYROID

Swellings of the thyroid (goitre) can sometimes be recognised by the formation of red spots on the throat. They may be due to a lack of iodine and occur mostly in young fishes, especially of *Salmonidæ*. Healing is possible by mixing some iodine with the dried food; 1 part of a solution of 1 g iodine and 3 g potassium iodide in 100 cm^3 of water mixed with 2500 parts of dried food. Too much iodine is harmful. True tumours of the thyroid may be benign adenomata, but often they start as, or develop into, highly malignant adenocarcinomata (cancer) (Fig. 8.23).

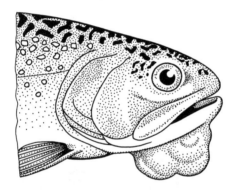

Fig. 8.23. Head of Salmo fontinalis *showing malignant tumour of the thyroid gland (modified drawing after Hofer)*

The histological structure of the thyroid in fish is a rather loose assembly of follicles. This facilitates proliferation and spreading of small parts of follicular tissue into surrounding organs and into the bloodstream, which may transport them to widely separated parts of the body, where they may settle and develop into a tumour *in situ* (benign) or into an invasive growth (malignant). Malignant thyroid tumours occur often in the gills and the mouth fundus. Generally these are or become carcinomata. If thyroid tumours are produced in the kidneys, the fish will develop oedema, leading to heavy swelling of its body. These symptoms may easily be confused with those of dropsy (see p. 166) or kidney cysts.

An endemic outbreak of thyroid tumours in four-year-old Brook Trout has been reported from Roumania.[18] These were thyroid adenomata. The condition occurred in a region where human goitres are endemic, too. 27% of Trout were affected and 70% of these died within two months. Death was attributed to destruction of the respiratory parenchyma, nutritional deficiency due to obstruction of the pharynx, and impairment of the circulation.

Early stages of thyroid tumours may be successfully treated with iodine and potassium iodide in the food, as mentioned before, or by adding potassium iodide (KI) to the water at a rate of 0.25 mg KI per litre. Treatment must be continued over long periods of time.

Berg and Gordon have reported successful treatments of Xiphophorid fishes suffering from goitre by a combined addition of iodide to the water and of thyroid tablets. They also applied injection therapy with the thyroid hormone thyroxin. One weekly injection of 30 µg thyroxin (dissolved in 0.05 cm^3 of a 0.65% sodium chloride solution) cured some of the affected fishes in three months.[19]

Advanced malignant thyroid tumours cannot be cured.

REFERENCES

1 SINDERMANN, C. J., *Principal Diseases of Marine Fish and Shellfish*, New York and London (1970)
2 NIGRELLI, R. F., 'Tumors and other atypical cell growths in temperate freshwater fishes of North America', *Trans. Amer. Fish. Soc.* **83**, 262–96 [1953 (publ. 1954)]
3 SCHLUMBERGER, H. G. and LUCKE, B., 'Tumors of fishes, amphibians and reptiles', *Cancer Research* **8**, 657–754 (1948)
4 REICHENBACH-KLINKE, H., *Krankheiten und Schädigungen der Fische*, Stuttgart (1966)
5 VAN DUIJN, Jnr., C., 'A case of spontaneous sarcoma in fish', *The Microscope* **11**, 133–38 (1957)
6 WESSING, A., 'Ueber einen bösartigen virusbedingten Tumor bei tropischen Zierfischen', *Die Naturwissenschafften* **46**, 517–18 (1959), and personal communication.
7 HOFER, B., *Handbuch der Fischkrankheiten*, Munich (1904)
8 SCHÄPERCLAUS, W., *Fischkrankheiten*, 3rd ed., Berlin (1954); GORDON, M., 'Genetic and correlated studies of normal and atypical pigment cell growth', *Growth* **15**, 153–219 (1951 Suppl.)
9 STOLK, A., 'Tumors of fishes I–IV', *Proc. Kon. Ned. Akad. Wetensch.* C**56**, 28–33, 34–78, 143–48, 149–56 (1953); C**57**, 652–58 (1954)
10 NIGRELLI, R. F., JAKOWSKA, S. and GORDON, M., 'The invasion and cell replacement of one pigmented neoplastic growth by a second and more malignant type in experimental fishes', *Brit. J. Cancer.* **5**, 54–68 (1951); BREIDER, H. and SCHMIDT, E., 'Melanosarkome durch Artkreuzung und Spontantumoren bei Fischen', *Strahlentherapie* **84**, 498–523 (1951); BREIDER, H., 'Über Melanome, Melanosarkome und homologe Zellmechanismen', *Strahlentherapie* **88**, 619–39 (1952); 'Farbgene und Melanosarkomhäufigkeit', *Zool. Anz.* **156**, 129–40 (1956)
11 THOMAS, L., 'Les tumeurs des poissons. Étude anatomique et pathogenique', *Bull de l'Assoc. Franc. pour l'Etude Cancer* **20**, 703–60 (1931)
12 NIGRELLI, R. F. and GORDON, M., 'A melanotic tumor in the Silverside *Menidia beryllina peninsulæ* (Goode and Bean)', *Zoologica* **24**, 45–47 (1944); SCHLUMBERGER, H. G. and LUCKE, B., 'Tumors of fishes, amphibians and reptiles', *Cancer Research* **8**, 657–754 (1948)

13 SCHLUMBERGER, H. G., 'Krankheiten der Fische, Amphibien and Reptilien', in: COHRS, JAFFÉ and MEESEN (Eds): *Pathologie der Laboratoriumstiere*, II, Springer Verlag (1958)

14 SCHLUMBERGER, H. G., 'Limbus tumors as a manifestation of Von Recklinghausen's neurofibromatosis in goldfish', *Amer. J. Ophthalm.* **34**, 415–22

15 STOLK, A., *Enige gevallen van gezwellen en ontstekingen bij poikilotherme Vertebraten*, Thesis, Utrecht (1950); 'Pathological parthenogenesis in viviparous Tooth-Carps', *Nature (Lond.)* **181**, 1660 (1958); 'Development of ovarial teratomas in viviparous Tooth-Carps by pathological parthenogenesis', *Nature* **183**, 763–64 (1959); 'Pathological parthenogenesis in a viviparous Tooth-Carp', *Nature* **191**, 507 (1961)

16 GEMMILL, J. F., *The Teratology of Fishes*, Univ. of Glasgow Press, J. Maclehose & Sons (1912)

17 NIGRELLI, R. F., 'Virus and tumors in fishes', *Amer. N.Y. Acad. Sci.* **54**, 1076–92 (1952)

18 RADULESCU, I., VASILIU, D. G., ILIC, E. and SNIESZKO, S. F., 'Thyroid hyperplasia of the Eastern Brook Trout (*S. fontinalis*), in Romania', *Trans. Amer. Fish. Soc.* **97**, 486–88 (1968)

19 BERG, O. and GORDON, M., 'Thyroid drugs that control growth of goiters in Xiphophorin fishes', *Proc. Amer. Assoc. Cancer Research* **1**, Abstr. 5 (1953)

9

MISCELLANEOUS COMPLAINTS

SUFFOCATION

In several instances I have observed suffocation caused through fish swallowing too large food particles. This occurred when comparatively large living food was given to small fishes. The fish tried to swallow a worm or a midge larva ('bloodworm', larva of *Chironomus* sp.) that was too big to pass their gullet. After swallowing it partially, they could neither swallow it completely nor spit it out; consequently the fishes died (Fig. 9.1).

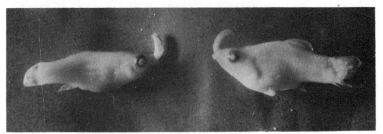

Fig. 9.1. Two female Platies which died as a result of their trying to swallow bloodworms that were too large, illustrating the importance of grading food

Although this cannot be called a disease (it is more in the nature of an accident) it is sufficiently important to mention here in order to warn fish-keepers not to feed such large food to their very small fishes.

RETARDED GROWTH

Where this occurs in spite of absence of specific diseases, water pollution or insufficient oxygen supply, the most probable cause will be insufficiency of the food with respect to essential vitamins and/or proteins. Preliminary investigations have shown that Eels need the amino-acids valine, methionine, tryptophan and threonine, whereas proline could be dispensed with.[1] Glycine was not tested. Fish fed deficient diets failed to grow until the missing amino-acid was supplied.

Good sources of proteins of all kinds needed by fishes are baker's yeast and soya beans.

LACK OF VITAMINS (AVITAMINOSES)

For fish nutrition a number of vitamins are necessary.[2]

Among these are biotin ('vitamin H'), choline, folic acid ('vitamin M'), inositol ('bios I'), pyridoxine ('vitamin B_6'), riboflavine ('vitamin B_2', 'vitamin G'; lactoflavine), thiamine ('vitamin B_1'; aneurine), pantothenic acid ('vitamin B_5') and nicotinic acid (niacin, 'anti-pellagra vitamin').

Vitamin requirements may vary among different species of fish and depend on environmental conditions.

Although no definite conclusions could be obtained from feeding experiments with respect to vitamin K (phyllochinon), vitamin B_{12} (cyanocobalamin) and vitamin E (tocopherol), definite deficiency syndromes could be produced by treatments with the antibiotic Aureomycin[R] (chlortetracycline), which affects the intestinal flora. Therefore, if Aureomycin is incorporated in fish food, as is sometimes done in order to increase growth rate, vitamins E, K, B_{12} and folic acid should also be included in relatively large amounts. The related antibiotic Chloromycetin[R] (chloramphenicol), on the other hand, does not produce avitaminoses and is therefore to be preferred for treatment of bacterial infections in fish (see page 154).

Fish embryos should require tocopherol (vitamin E) for normal development and hatching.

Nicotinic acid deficiency leads to large numbers of grey spots appearing at the back of the fish. This condition shows a fortnight after total lack or blocking of nicotinic acid has begun. If no treatment is given (feeding sources of this vitamin: liver, white meat, wholewheat flour) casualties will follow.

Formerly the condition has been thought to be due to the effect of intense sunlight, whence it was called 'Sunburn'.[3]

Avitaminoses may also play a rôle in infectious diseases by lowering the resistance of fishes to pathogenic bacteria. Susceptibility to fin-rot (see page 160) is increased by lack of inositol. The occurrence of blue slime patch disease is furthered by lack of biotin, whereas folic acid deficiency lowers resistance of fishes to infections by *Myxobacteria*, such as *Chondrococcus columnaris*, causing cotton wool disease (see page 159).

Lack of pyridoxine produces specific symptoms in certain fishes. Angel Fish (*Pterophyllum*) gets a greenish colour all over its body, it refuses to take tubifex as food and generally it stays in one corner of the tank. This condition could be cured by addition of $2\frac{1}{2}$ tablets of medical pyridoxine per 2 U.S. qt of water,[4] which is roughly equivalent to 6 tablets per Imp. gal or 4 tablets per 3 litres (since a vitamin is essentially a food substance, dosage need not be very accurate).

In young fishes lack of 'B' vitamins (thiamine, riboflavine and pyridoxine) and biotin will retard growth. Lack of vitamin B_{12}, together with protein deficiency, makes Carp more susceptible to pox disease, which is of viral origin (see page 198).

In *Barbus tetrazona* var. *sumatranus* B-vitamins deficiency induces gradually increasing languor, lack of appetite, head-down inclination and finally swimming on the back, combined with heavy emaciation. The condition takes a lethal course. Occasionally red swellings at the body can be observed.[5] A complete cure has been obtained by application of a vitamin-B-complex medication and adding yeast to the food. First signs of recovery could be observed two hours after the first application, whereas after some days nearly all symptoms had vanished.

Lack of pantothenic acid is the probable cause of dietary gill disease (see page 106).

Some other vitamins are not required in fish food, because fishes can make them themselves. This is the case with vitamin A_1 (retinol; axerophtol), which is produced from carotenoids in the liver, and vitamin D_3 (cholecalciferol) which is synthesised in the liver. Cod liver oil is a well-known example of the high concentration of these natural vitamins in fish liver. Ascorbic acid (vitamin C) is probably not needed by fish, either.

However, if some disturbance of vitamin synthesis occurs, symptoms of deficiencies of these vitamins may nevertheless be produced. Insufficient illumination may interfere with the synthesis of vitamin A. Lack of vitamin A may then give rise to fatty degeneration of the liver.

Further, avitaminoses may be induced by inactivation of vitamins by certain substances that may be present in the food or in the water. The flesh of sea fishes contains a substance that inactivates thiamine (vitamin B_1); if this is used as the main food given to fresh-water fishes, these may emaciate and even die. Biotin becomes inactive when it combines with the protein-like substance avidin that is present in raw egg-*white*, whereas egg-*yolk* is an important source of this vitamin (other ones are liver, kidney, pancreas, yeast and milk).

INTOXICATIONS

Many adverse conditions of a chemical nature can affect the health of fish.[6] Industrial waste disposals often contain heavy fish poisons, such as phenolic and chlorine compounds, heavy metal compounds, arsenicals and all kinds of other toxic substances, which are a real threat to fish population in industrial countries like those of Western Europe. However, discharge of uncleaned sewage from human populations may be an even greater threat than that of industrial waste, since microbial breakdown of the organic material contained in them consumes large amounts of oxygen, thus reducing the oxygen content of the water to or even below critical values, whereas on the other hand, poisonous substances are produced, such as ammonia, hydrogen sulphide, methane and nitrites. Only when there is plenty of oxygen available can such substances be converted further to non-toxic compounds (also see 'autumn sickness', pages 303–307).

The toxicity of poisons may also depend on other environmental conditions, such as temperature, pH value, oxygen content and presence of certain other substances. The toxicity of most poisons is increased by increase of temperature. Ammonia is less toxic at lower than at higher pH values, because then it is converted into ammonium salts. At low oxygen concentrations toxicity of ammonia and of cyanides increases with increasing oxygen content of the water, but this condition is reversed at oxygen contents of more than 50% of the air-saturation value.[7]

Carbon dioxide up to 15–60 p.p.m. reduces the toxicity of ammonia, but higher concentrations are themselves toxic.[8]

Toxicity of chemical substances differs between different species of fish and also with age and size. The lowest concentration of ammonia (NH_3) causing symptoms of acute poisoning in Chub (*Squalius cephalus*) is 1.0–1.2 mg/l, whereas for Rainbow Trout (*Salmo iridæus*) fry it is as low as 0.3–0.4 mg/l.[9]

Symptoms of ammonia poisoning are irritation of the nervous system, producing spasms and jumps above the water surface. Later on, haemolysis occurs, i.e. solution of the red blood corpuscles. At higher concentrations or more prolonged contact the distal parts of the fins lose colour and appear abnormally white or transparent, whereas the ends of the fins get frayed.

Ammonium salts produce excessive excretion of slime on the skin by irritation of the slime cells, which is in itself almost harmless, but there is a highly destructive effect on the epithelium of the gill sheets, which is caused to swell and get loose of its substratum. The tips of the secondary gill sheets may be destroyed. Later on trembling spasms occur suddenly and the fishes may dart wildly around with all fins stretched and with their mouth and gill coverings (opercula) wide open. Blood may ooze through the gill sheets. Concentrations of only 0.05% of ammonium chloride kill fishes within 6 h.

Detergents, phenolic compounds and malachite green may affect spermatozoa and the development of fish eggs; in the case of malachite green this depends on photosensitisation, so apart from the dye concentration itself it is highly dependent on the illumination level.

Phenolic compounds induce anaemia, in which the number of red blood corpuscles (erythrocytes) decreases, but their area is increased.

Extensive information on toxic compounds that may enter natural waters from waste disposals, agriculture (fungicides, herbicides, pesticides) a.s.o., together with toxic and lethal concentrations, has been compiled by Reichenbach-Klinke.[10]

Whereas in free waters all kinds of toxic substances may be introduced with industrial waste and sanitation sewage, in aquarium- and pond-keeping there are generally but few of such adverse conditions that need special consideration.

New tanks and ponds made of cement or concrete cannot be used safely until they have undergone a special process of maturation. On setting and hardening, calcium hydroxide is formed, which dissolves in the water, giving it a highly alkaline reaction. When fishes are introduced in such tanks or ponds, they will be killed with symptoms of severe damage to their skin and gills. This can be prevented by thorough maturation of the cement, which is accomplished by plain soaking and frequently repeated changes of water. The process has to be continued till the pH value of the water is not changed any more on standing for a few days in the tank or pond.

TOXICITY OF METALS

IRON

Iron and manganese may act toxic either in the form of ionised salts, or as coagulated hydroxides that settle on the gills of the fish and damage them. Since the gills of fish have an alkaline surface reaction themselves, toxic activity of iron and manganese ions may also depend on precipitation of their insoluble hydroxides on the gill sheets. Proper exchange of oxygen and carbon dioxide is hampered, whereas the epithelium is irritated and gets a reddish colour resulting from inflammation. In case of iron, filamentous iron bacteria (most often *Leptothrix ochracea*) may settle on the gills where ferric hydroxide is present. By the growth of these bacteria, which in themselves are harmless, further mechanical injury is produced. In iron intoxication in the ferric (Fe^{3+}) form the number of erythrocytes in the blood is increased as well as their surface area.[11]

According to Bandt[12] iron concentrations exceeding 0.9 mg/l at a pH of 6.5–7.5 should cause death of fish, but Schäperclaus[13] states that at pH 6.7, an acid-neutralising power of 0.9 cm^3 of N hydrochloric acid per litre, and an oxygen content of 10.4 mg/l, casualties in Pike and Tench did not occur unless the iron content was in excess of 1.9 mg/l.

MANGANESE

This metal is much less toxic to fish than iron.[14] Symptoms of this poisoning are restlessness, followed after many hours by disturbances of equilibrium, fading of colours, white discoloration of the edges of the fins, the tip of the snout, the barbels and the nostrils. Sometimes further symptoms may appear in addition, namely, folding of the fins, turbidity of the cornea of the eye and occurrence of slimy threads on the skin. Then increasing symptoms of paralysis show and a few hours afterwards the victims die.

According to Lüdemann, the toxic concentration is about 0.5 g/l of manganese when added as manganese sulphate or 0.33 g Mn/l as the chloride. The lethal concentrations are given as 1 g/l of manganese as the sulphate or 0.8 g Mn/l as the chloride. However, the true figures vary with the species of fish. The lethal concentrations have been given as 1.5 g/l for Tench, 0.65 g/l for Carp and 0.1 g/l for yearling Rainbow Trout.[15]

COPPER

This metal is extremely toxic to fish when dissolved in the water, an amount as small as 0.5 mg/l killing large Trout within a few hours. Further details have already been given at pages 56 and 57.

The toxicity of copper is greatly enhanced when zinc or cadmium are present at the same time. This means that the toxic effects of brass (which is an alloy of copper and zinc) dissolving in water are much more pronounced than those of pure copper, not only because brass is corroded by water more easily than copper, but even at the same concentration of dissolved copper. The total effect is higher than the sum of the effects of copper and zinc (or cadmium) separately.

Copper poisoning can occur in tanks with a copper, brass or bronze frame, if the water is slightly acid and has a low amount of carbonates, or when objects made of these metals are introduced in a tank. All objects, such as heaters, made of these metals should be nickel-chromium plated. Nickel is toxic, too, but the final chromium finish is safe.

LEAD

Soluble lead compounds are highly toxic. The solid metal, however, is generally safe in aquarium practice, owing to it becoming passive by formation of a protective insoluble coating on its surface in waters containing sufficient amounts of carbonates. These are neutral and alkaline waters.

In acid waters, however, with low pH value, as may often be used for breeding certain species of tropical fishes, lead may be attacked and then it will be dangerous, too. 0.33 mg/l of dissolved lead has been found lethal to Trout.

ZINC

Dissolved zinc is extremely toxic to fish. Big Trout are killed in a few hours at a concentration of only 2–2.5 mg/l, whereas even 1 mg/l may produce poisoning effects on prolonged contact. Water fleas of the species *Daphnia magna* are killed within 5–10 days at 0.01 mg/l. Although fishes absorb zinc in the intestine and accumulate it in the liver, the only immediate symptom of zinc poisoning consists of a gradually increasing destruction of the tissues of the gills. Early stages may heal spontaneously if the fishes are transferred to fresh zinc-free water.[16]

Because galvanised iron is commonly used for aquarium bottoms, buckets and other containers, zinc poisoning is not an uncommon cause of unexplained casualties in fish-keeping practice. The solubility of zinc in water depends very much on specific conditions, such as salt content, pH, aeration, but tap-waters conducted through galvanised iron pipes commonly carry up to 5 mg/l of zinc and rather frequently even 10–15 mg/l. Since concentrations up to 40 mg/l are completely harmless for human consumption there may be water supplies delivering water safe for human drinking but killing fish.

Toxicity of zinc is highly increased if copper or nickel are present at the same time.

Even with completely safe tap-water, lethal concentrations of zinc can be reached on standing for a day in galvanised iron pails. Although such containers may be used just for transporting fresh water from the tap to an aquarium or a garden pond, they should never be used for transporting fish.

Aquaria with galvanised iron bottoms should not be used without at least a thick layer of sand.

Aquatic plants absorb zinc from the water and accumulate it even at very low concentrations in the surrounding water. In consequence plants having been kept in contact with zinc-containing water may get toxic properties to fish and other aquatic animals that eat them. Therefore it is advisable not to use galvanised iron containers for transporting aquatic plants, either.

Many dyestuffs are manufactured as double salts with zinc chloride or other zinc compounds; for treatment of fish diseases it is of utmost importance that only zinc-free brands of dyestuffs are used. This applies to such dyes as methylene blue, malachite green and brilliant green.

NICKEL

This is toxic to fish. Toxicity is further increased in presence of zinc. Lethal concentrations for nickel only are given as 60 mg/l for Tench, 50 mg/l for Carp and 30 mg/l for yearling Rainbow Trout.

CADMIUM

Highly toxic. Cadmium-plated iron must not be used for any object containing water where fishes are kept. The same holds true for cadmium-containing paints. Toxicity is further increased in presence of copper. Lethal concentrations for dissolved cadmium only are 20 mg/l for Tench, 15 mg/l for Carp and 4 mg/l for yearling Rainbow Trout.

ALUMINIUM

Normally harmless. Only in some acid waters with very low lime content (calcium salts) a slight toxicity might be observed. Generally, however, aluminium paints are about the best to protect galvanised iron frames of aquaria against corrosion as well as to protect fish from zinc or iron poisoning. Dissolved aluminium salts are highly toxic, however; 5 mg/l of dissolved aluminium kills Trout.

INTOXICATION BY CHLORINATED TAP-WATER

For hygienic reasons most municipal tap-waters in the world are chlorinated. The amounts added may vary considerably, from a so-called 'negative chlorine content', meaning that less chlorine is added than can be bound by organic and other substances present in the water, to such excess that its presence can be tasted or even smelt, although generally it is not chlorine itself, but hypochloric acid or chlorophenols and chlorocresols produced from it.

Chlorine amounts exceeding 4 mg/l kill fishes in 7–8 h. Concentrations of free chlorine as low as 0.1–0.2 mg/l at a water temperature of 4–5°C (39–41°F) were found to kill 25% of Carp in a period of 19 days (Schäperclaus); at 10–15°C (50–60°F), however, no casualties occurred. Schäperclaus found toxicity under aquarium conditions always greater than in ponds. 4 mg/l kills Carp within 8 h.

The main symptom of chlorine poisoning in fish is destruction of the gills.[17] The gill sheets appear paled and show a whitish discoloration of their tips. At higher concentrations and/or prolonged contact the epithelium of the gills may be completely destroyed and the cartilage laid bare. The skin may get a whitish appearance, too. The eyes get sunken in the orbits. At first the fishes show restlessness and irritation, but then their activity slows down, breathing frequency decreases and in the next stage the victims will fall aside and die slowly. Only in the very first stage may the victims recover when transferred to fresh water.

Susceptibility of fishes to chlorine differs amongst different species.

According to Schäperclaus susceptibility decreases in the following order: Pike (least resistance), Trout, Rudd, Carp, Perch, Tench, Eel (highest resistance).

Chlorinated tap-water can be made safe by thorough filtration over activated charcoal.

INTOXICATION BY NITRITES AND NITRATES

These substances may accumulate in water either by heavy pollution or by addition of fertilisers to the soil or the water intended to promote plant growth. Nitrites will accumulate only under anaerobic conditions in the soil and low oxygen content of the water (also see p. 305). Normally the amount of nitrites must not exceed the range of 0.001 up to 0.01 g/l, calculated as nitrite ion (NO_2^-). For nitrate ion (NO_3^-) this critical value is of the order of 0.1–0.3 g/l.

Dissolved nitrites and nitrates increase the solubility of many heavy metals, such as copper and lead, that are highly toxic to fish, too.

Symptoms and susceptibility to nitrite and nitrate poisoning differ amongst different species of fish. At concentrations normally encountered under bad aquarium conditions, Guppies, Swordtails, Platyfish and *Colisa labiosa* do not show specific symptoms, where *Barbus nigrofasciatus*, *B. semifasciolatus*, *Badis badis*, *Chanda lala*, *Rasbora heteromorpha* and *Hyphessobrycon scholzei* lose their colours, and *Mollienisia velifera*, *Hyphessobrycon flammeus*, *Barbus sumatranus* and *Melanotænia maccullochi* are killed.[18]

Complete recovery can be accomplished by timely transfer of the fishes to clean, fresh, well-aerated water.

INTOXICATION BY HYDROGEN SULPHIDE

Hydrogen sulphide (H_2S) and sulphides may be produced by anaerobic breakdown of sulphur-containing organic material, mainly proteins. Sulphide ions combine chemically with the iron of the blood haemoglobin, thereby blocking respiration. The first symptoms in fishes are a violet-reddish discoloration of the gills, followed by bloody infiltrations. Then the fishes die from suffocation. Symptoms of lack of oxygen will always precede those of sulphide poisoning. Dead fishes generally show faded colours, stretched opercula and pectoral fins, whereas their bellies may appear swollen. Most often they are either floating near the surface or hovering in the water. 0.5 mg/l of hydrogen sulphide may be lethal for some fishes, whereas Carp may tolerate up to 6 mg/l. White fishes and Pike are among the most susceptible species. 10 mg/l kills all fishes within 4 h.[19]

In aquaria and ponds the condition should be treated as soon as possible before big mortality occurs, by a rapid change of the water, a maximum aeration and addition of methylene blue (see p. 334). At least the upper layers of the compost have to be removed and replaced with well-washed sand.

Hydrogen sulphide increases the respiration process of algae and development of sulphur bacteria that oxidise it; both processes lead to rapid decrease of the oxygen content.

INTOXICATIONS DUE TO LIVING ORGANISMS (BIOTOXICATIONS)

POISONING BY SNAILS

The water snail *Radix (Lymnæa) peregra* (Müller) produces a substance of high toxicity to fish.[20] 25 g of snail in 1 l of water may be sufficient to cause symptoms of poisoning. Fishes are restless and show heavy spasms, followed by turning upon their back, want for breath, immobility and spasmatic quivering. Finally they die lying at the bottom. If fishes showing the earlier symptoms are transferred to fresh water they will recover.

The poison may be isolated as an 'extract' by flooding the snails with either diluted hydrochloric acid or a weak solution of sodium hydroxide and neutralising the excretion afterwards with weak alkali or acid solution, respectively. Excretion of the poison is also induced by temporary drying of the snails. It is not destroyed by boiling, but protein-splitting soil bacteria will break it down. The poison does not act when given to a fish by mouth, which also points to a protein character of it, since the stomach contains the protein-splitting enzyme pepsase ('pepsin'), acting in acid environment, and the intestine the enzyme trypsase ('trypsin') splitting proteins in an alkaline environment, whereas the toxic substance is not attacked by either diluted acids or alkalis.

The toxic effect of the excretion of *Radix peregra* has been observed in many species of fish and it appeared to increase with the oxygen requirements of the species (see pp. 94–96). However, Eel proved immune. No other species of water snail has ever been found to produce intoxications of fish. Therefore it is advised not to introduce specimens of *Radix peregra* in an aquarium, but other species are safe in this respect, although they, too, may carry a risk, namely that of transmitting worm infections (see pp. 185 and 240).

FISH POISONING INDUCED BY WATER BLOOMS

Water bloom is the name given to a sudden mass development of unicellular algae, the water getting a green appearance like vegetable soup. When occurring in clean waters, water blooms are generally harmless, the only risk to fish being that of supersaturation with oxygen with the possibility of embolism (see pp. 98–103) if the water is stagnant, but cases are also known where through a water bloom, ammonia is released from an excess of available ammonium salts, thus reaching toxic concentrations, with a mass death of fish ensuing. This is reported from Germany where sewage-treatment plants have released water with a high mineral content.[21] The unicellular algae *Chlorella* and *Ankistrodesmus* are main constituents of such blooms.

BLUE-GREEN ALGAE

Fresh-water blue-green algae (*Oscillatoriaceæ*) may occur either as bluish-green slimy masses on water plants, stones and on the bottom, or free floating. They may form a scum on the surface of the water as well as giving the water itself a blue appearance (blue water blooms). In tanks and ponds where such conditions are found, casualties may occur. Some *Oscillatoriaceæ* are taken up by fish, as proved by the presence of certain highly unsaturated fatty acids, that are characteristic for these algae, in the body fat of fishes having lived in contact with them. The palatability of edible fish may be affected by such substances. Especially, the species *Oscillatoria agardhii* and *O. princeps* have been found as originators of this condition.[22] When kept in fresh, clean water for some time the muddy taste of such fish is restored to normal.

Since many blue-green algae thrive best in water that is highly contaminated with decaying organic matter, the true cause of casualties generally is the primary condition of the water, of which the appearance of the algae is only a symptom. On the other hand, if a scum is formed on the surface, as by *Microcystis ichthyoblabe*, and normal functioning of the green plants is prevented by the slimy growth covering their leaves, proper oxygen replenishment of the water is interfered with and this in itself may induce death of fish.

However, recent investigations in Russia have shown that some blue-green algae exert high toxicity on Carp.[23] These are members of the Genera *Anabæna* and *Aphanizomenon* (Fig. 9.2), and *Microcystis aeruginosa*. These plants produce toxic substances that act directly via water and sediment, as well as indirectly when fishes eat red mosquito larvae (*Chironomus*) that have fed on these algae.

Fishes should be removed from affected tanks and kept in clean fresh water that is either filtered continuously, or changed several times. The tanks without fish should be treated with copper sulphate

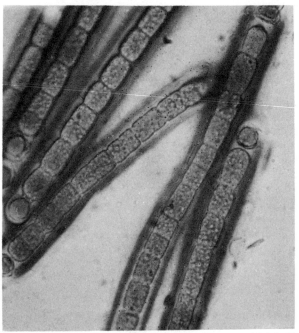

Fig. 9.2. Blue-green algae, Aphanizomenon *flos-aquæ (L.) Ralfs.*
× *750. The slime capsules surrounding the threads are clearly shown (photomicrograph by the author)*

at a rate of 0.3 mg/l for at least four days (0.022 gr/Imp. gal or 0.017 gr/U.S. gal). Then the water is changed several times and the sediment at the bottom as well as the upper layer of the sand is removed, too, prior to reintroducing the fishes.

INTOXICATION BY THE INFUSORIAN STENTOR POLYMORPHUS

Casualties of Trout have been described[24] in ponds where the water level dropped so low that fishes came into contact with water plants on which large amounts of this infusorian had settled. Intoxication effects increased when the infusorians were spread through the water by stirring. Symptoms resembled those caused by the snail *Radix peregra* (see p. 300).

The true cause is not known. Artificial cultures of *Stentor polymorphus* and those of its symbiotic alga *Chlorella* had no adverse effect at all.

AUTUMN SICKNESS

Sometimes mysterious deaths of fish occur in tanks without the victims showing pertinent signs of disease other than a general fading of colours. In some species of fish there may be differences in the speed of swimming as compared with their normal behaviour, whilst in addition some signs of lack of oxygen are generally shown. Thorough investigations do not reveal any parasites. Although this condition can occur at any time of the year, it is observed more often in autumn, particularly in fully planted tanks which are crowded with fish. The course of the sickness may resemble an acute epidemic, but nevertheless it is more like an intoxication than a real disease. In earlier days, when artificial aeration and filtering of aquarium water was not as commonly employed as today, autumn sickness was more often encountered. It now seems to be celebrating a come-back, however, but by understanding the causes of this undesirable course of events it is possible to see a way to avoid it.

Let us first consider what is happening in a fully planted tank during summer when there is biological equilibrium between all inhabitants. The tank will be well lighted and the plants will be flourishing and producing plenty of oxygen. At the bottom of the tank where excrements of fish and snails have settled, together with dead parts of plants and sometimes other organic matter, a vegetation of bacteria is thriving. These bacteria are occupied in mineralising the dead organic matter by oxidising it, thereby converting the nitrogen compounds into ammonium salts and, finally, into nitrates which can be used as food by the living plants. The sulphur content of the organic matter is converted into sulphates and the phosphorus into phosphates. Both are useful for the plants. All these processes require the presence of a large amount of oxygen in the upper layer of the compost and this oxygen has to be taken from the water.

The oxygen from the water can only get into the planting medium by the slow process of diffusion; if more oxygen is present than the water can hold at a certain temperature, the excess escapes gradually at the surface of the water, while the bottom may still be far from saturated with this life-giving gas. Nevertheless, so long as oxygen content is good and the amount of decaying organic matter at the bottom is not excessive, all processes may be in a fair equilibrium and all is well. The bacteria then keep pace in consuming the organic matter and the plants are able to use the remineralised substances in approximately the same tempo as they are formed by the bacteria so that no accumulation of nitrates, sulphates and phosphates occurs in the water.

What will happen when autumn comes and the hours and intensity of daylight are decreased? When the plants receive a decreasing amount of light, they produce less oxygen and growth slows up as well. There will be a decrease in the oxygen content of the water, but an even greater decrease of the oxygen content in the compost. The oxidation of the organic substances by the bacteria will then slow down and this occurs at a time when the amount of settling organic matter is increased by more dead plant parts and by particles of dried food which, in this season, is being added to the diet of the fish. More plant deaths occur as a direct consequence of the diminishing light. Even if artificial illumination is supplied there will always be parts of the plants near the bottom of a fully planted tank where light penetration is insufficient to keep them all alive. When plant growth slows down, the rate of absorption of nitrates and other mineral salts from the water decreases too, since the plants have no longer such a need for them as in the period when they were thriving. Consequently, the first result is a gradual increase in the amounts of nitrates, sulphates and other substances dissolved in the water.

This is not harmful to the fish at this stage; it is very seldom, if ever, that concentrations of nitrates and sulphates, formed by bacterial activity, become so high as to cause intoxication in the fish. Therefore, if all is well, nothing else occurs than that the state of equilibrium is shifted to other relative values of the components that partake in it. This is the case in all well-balanced tanks that are not overcrowded either with plants or fish, that are sufficiently well lighted (even during winter) and that are kept clean.

CONDITIONS IN OVERCROWDED TANKS

A different state of affairs occurs in overcrowded tanks, which are fully planted but which are receiving insufficient light. The animal inhabitants can thus only be kept alive by means of artificial aeration. Aeration will help the fish, not the plants; the latter can only be kept in good condition by giving them sufficient light. Now we must bear in mind that not every kind of light can be used by the plants for the process of photosynthesis; it is only the red rays that are active. Therefore, some modern fluorescent bulbs and tubes with their high amount of rays of the shorter wavelengths and lack of sufficient rays in the red region are highly inefficient for aquarium lighting. The consequence is that, even in a fully lighted tank, the plants may be starved of the light they need and this must result in a higher death rate of plant growth apart from decreased oxygen production. Fluorescent tubes for aquarium illumination should be of the types designated as 'warm-white' or 'rosy-white'.

On the other hand, low levels of illumination may stimulate development of certain algae that are able to assimilate at very low light intensities.[25] If these are green algae, their thriving helps to maintain a sufficient oxygen supply to the fishes, but if blue-green algae or brown algae (diatoms) are the main organisms developing, the higher plants will be even more hampered in their function and the adverse condition is aggravated.

Furthermore, artificial aeration has far less efficiency than the natural source of oxygen, especially near the bottom of the tank. Consequently, we may have to deal with an increased amount of decaying organic matter and a greatly decreased amount of oxygen in the planting medium, which can amount to a complete absence of oxygen immediately below its surface.

When this happens the aerobic bacteria, which can only live where there is a supply of free oxygen, have to give up the battle and are replaced by anaerobic species. These latter can only live where there is no free oxygen. In addition, facultative species will be present and these possess the ability to thrive equally well in both circumstances by using different types of metabolism. It would be far beyond the scope of this book to deal fully with the details of the changes in the bacterial flora of an oxygen-starved planting medium, or with the details of all chemical processes involved, but we have to consider the main results of these changes.

As has already been put forward, the initial trend in shifting the biochemical equilibrium in the compost is to increase the amount of nitrates and other products of aerobic bacterial metabolism. As the conditions change to anaerobic bacterial growth, species will come into activity that convert nitrates into the much more toxic nitrites. In the course of the normal aerobic breakdown of protein and other organic nitrogen compounds nitrites are formed, too, but then they are further oxidised immediately by other bacteria. Now, with lack of oxygen, the cycle is reversed and an accumulation of the nitrites may occur.

Even worse is the influence of anaerobic conditions with regard to the sulphur compounds. Normally, the proteins are broken down with production of hydrogen sulphide, which is utilised immediately by other bacteria, finally yielding non-toxic sulphates. With lack of oxygen to accomplish this complete oxidation, however, hydrogen sulphide may remain. This substance is highly poisonous to fish and higher plants. If the medium contains iron, the production of hydrogen sulphide will at first show itself by the occurrence of a blackening of the bottom layer, due to formation of iron sulphide. After this, the poisonous substance may enter the free water of the tank and add to the general intoxication of the fish.

The cellulose from the cell walls of the plants is, under anaerobic conditions, fermented with the production of methane, another gaseous substance poisonous to fish. With oxygen it can be oxidised by other bacteria to form carbon dioxide and water, while there are also some species of bacteria that can oxidise methane in the absence of free oxygen but in the presence of an excess of nitrates. Then the processes of denitrification and cellulose fermentation are coupled and an increased amount of nitrites is formed. Whether they accumulate or are reduced further to ammonium salts, or even to gaseous nitrogen, depends on the composition of the further bacterial flora.

Methane production occurs mainly in ditches with a black muddy bottom and evil smell. If such mud is stirred with a rod, bubbles of methane mixed with hydrogen and other gases will rise to the surface. In aquaria methane production is most likely to occur if the bottom layer is made up of humus or garden soil. Although the solubility of methane in water is very low, it is sufficient to cause intoxication of the fish.

Recapitulating we may say that a number of toxic products can be formed if there is such a lack of oxygen in the bottom layer of the tank that the normal aerobic microbial processes are shifted to anaerobic decay. This accumulation leads to an increasing intoxication of the fish and, eventually, a critical concentration of one or more of the substances may be reached and then a number of deaths will occur. There may be differences in susceptibility to the toxic conditions in different species of fish; delicate species will be the first to suffer. Generally, fish that are accustomed to living in water with low oxygen content, like the Labyrinths and some Cat-fishes, will stand the unfavourable conditions better.

Of course, a weakening of the fish will have occurred before casualties appear and this leads to an increased susceptibility to other diseases, such as fungus and bacterial infections.

AVOIDING INCIDENCE OF THE DISEASE

Autumn sickness can be avoided by taking suitable precautions. Do not use humus or garden soil in preparing the bottom layer of a tank. When the darker days are approaching, see that the plant growth is not too abundant and, if necessary, thin out, leaving a smaller number of plants that are not packed too closely together so that each can obtain its full share of the available light. Use the siphon more often than in the summer for removing dirt from the bottom. If the upper layer of the sand shows a dark or even black colour, remove this layer. Do not allow the tank to be overcrowded with fish. If the aquarium is placed where it receives insufficient daylight, artificial lighting by means of ordinary incandescent lamps should be employed. For good plant growth 2 decalumens of luminous flux per square decimetre of water surface area are required with water depths of 40–50 cm.

With regard to artificial aeration, for a given air consumption diffusers giving small bubbles are much more efficient than those producing large bubbles. The rate at which oxygen and other gases dissolve in the water depends on the ratio of the surface area of the bubbles to their volume and this ratio increases rapidly when the size of the bubbles is decreased. It is also advantageous to place the diffuser near the bottom, so that the bubbles travel over a greater distance through the water before reaching the surface.

Installing a jet pump and filter may be advantageous; the siphon should drain at a lower spot where dirt usually accumulates and at such a rate that a continual suction along the bottom surface is effected. The resultant circulation will provide the compost of the tank with a good oxygen supply, while accumulation of decaying matter is avoided. A filter with active coal will remove a number of organic substances, hydrogen sulphide and ammonia, but nitrates are not eliminated. Accumulation of nitrates is only controlled by the mechanical part of the filtration, which takes away the excrements of the fish from which the nitrates are derived, and by the activity of the plants. In crowded tanks one has to depend on the removal of the excrements, since there the plants cannot keep pace with the nitrate production.

Ozone treatment of the water, as described on p. 338, can be very effective in speeding up oxidation of waste material. It should be applied in a circulating filter system, not directly in the main stream of water, to prevent the killing of those micro-organisms that are required for the natural biological processes of purification.

In sea-water tanks, accumulation of nitrates is of still greater importance, since nitrates are toxic to the inhabitants of the sea, whilst in these tanks there are no plants effectively using these salts.

When the so-called autumn disease occurs in our tanks, a rapid change of water is required, whilst at least the upper layers of the compost have to be removed and replaced with well-washed sand. Then, to avoid repetition of the trouble, such measures have to be taken as have been described previously.

DISEASES OF DOUBTFUL ORIGIN

SWINGING SICKNESS (SHIMMIES)

In Tooth-carps (*Cyprinodontidæ*) an anomalous behaviour may sometimes occur. The fishes make peculiar shaking or swinging movements, whilst staying in the same place. The fins are retracted while the gill coverings are closed. No pathological symptoms can be found, either in the skin or in the gills, but the colours are generally faded.

Since this behaviour will often occur when fishes are put in a newly arranged tank, it is possible that it is a reaction to unsuitable water. In such cases it is advisable to change the water as soon as possible with some from another source, or to remove the fishes from the tank and then to test the water for its pH reaction. Corrections of pH can be made by adding carbonate of lime to the water if it is too acid (i.e. pH value below 6.5; 6.8 may be considered a normal value) or phosphoric acid if the water should be too alkaline (pH value above 7.6; the most suitable pH range for many fishes is between 6.8 and 7.2). When adding phosphoric acid care must be taken not to add too much; after putting in some of the acid stir thoroughly and test the pH reaction again; repeat this until the desired value has been reached.

Swinging sickness or shimmies (as this condition is called) may also occur among fishes in tanks where the occupants have been present for a long time and where the water has a suitable composition. In such cases, it is possible that the abnormal behaviour could be due to chilling (if the temperature of the water has been too low) in which case the remedy is simple. Cases of swinging sickness in Tooth-carps may be treated by changing the water and raising the temperature.

FRIGHT PARALYSIS AND PSYCHOSIS

In literature, reports have been made recording cases of sudden paralysis and dying of fish and 'fright psychosis', in which the fish try to bury themselves in the sand or try to hide themselves in other abnormal ways. (It should be remembered, however, that some species of fish normally hide themselves in the sand, e.g. Eels and Loaches.) Such behaviour may result from serious frights or shock caused by sudden changes of temperature, or other influences, but further details of the causes of this disease are not known.

In Guppies (*Lebistes reticulatus*) an anomalous behaviour may occur which is possibly related to that mentioned above. The fish show a peculiar restlessness and, if a person approaches the tank, they dart wildly through the water and even bustle into the sand. Soon afterwards they become exhausted and remain near the surface. If they are disturbed they swim very sluggishly into deeper water. After two or three days they die. Nothing definite is known about the cause of this disease. Sometimes it is possible to cure the fishes by a rapid changing of water.

BALD SPOT DISEASE IN POWAN

Stocks of Powan (*Coregonus lavaretus*) in Loch Lomond (Scotland) have been affected by an acute non-ulcerative inflammatory lesion in the centre of the head. No parasites or pathogenic microbes could be detected in these lesions. Fungus was rarely present as a secondary agent. In the following year the condition disappeared, coinciding with a marked improvement in the quality of the fishes.[26]

DEFORMITIES

In fishes, all kinds of deformities may occur. Very little is known of the causes. It has been presumed that lack of vitamins (especially vitamin D) could play a rôle in such cases, but this has not been proved. From several experiments and other investigations it seems that fishes can make vitamin D themselves in their liver and it is difficult to understand how lack of this vitamin could occur, except in cases where the liver is diseased.

Some deformities may be due to infections with sporozoans or other parasites which damage the skeleton or prevent normal ossification of the bones in young fish. If the fish overcomes the infection, a deformity will remain. Crooked spines may sometimes be caused by *Ichthyophonus* disease (see p. 250), or be due to hereditary factors.

Deformities of the mouth and the cheeks may be due to mechanical injury and these can occur in fish which have been caught by angling.

Head deformities have also been observed where young fishes suffered from a low oxygen content of the water during growth. At an oxygen content less than 6 mg/l Barbel (*Barbus barbus*), Perch (*Perca fluviatilis*) and Pike (*Esox lucius*) showed a decreased growth rate, whereas below 3.5 mg/l casualties started to occur, whilst the surviving specimens developed head deformities, mainly consisting of a shortening of the skull and of mouth deformities, eventually leading to a pug-nose shape, especially in the Russian Sturgeon *Acipenser ruthenus*.[27]

Other deformities may be due to hereditary factors.[28] In fact, most of the special varieties of Goldfish such as Doubletails, Veiltails, Telescope-eyes and Lionheads, have been derived by careful selection and line-breeding of types that originated as hereditary abnormalities.

Certain cases of deformity of the spine have been shown probably to be due to lack of nucleoproteins in the food.[29] These may be either *skoliosis* (abnormal lateral curvature of the spine), *kyphosis* (abnormal dorsal convexity of the spine) or *lordosis* (increase of the forward convexity of the posterior half of the spine). In some cases a shortening of the vertebrae would occur (Fig. 9.4, p. 310). On progress of the disease the sympathetic ganglion that operates on the interspineous bonelets that depress or elevate the fins gets paralysed. Generally this paralysis is confined to the dorsal fin; it is caused by pressure of the vertebrae on the ganglion. Later on definite symptoms of emaciation become apparent and after that stage has been reached death will follow soon.

310

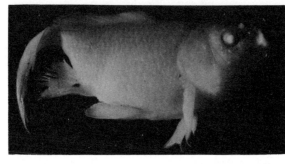

Fig. 9.3.
DEFORMITIES
IN A
GOLDFISH
A Goldfish with deformities to the hindpart of its body and its fins. Original photograph by the author

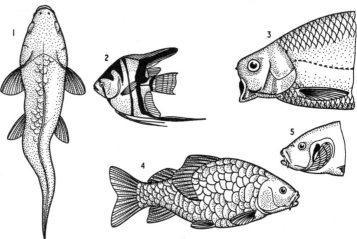

Fig. 9.4. 1, *Carp with crooked spine.* 2, *Angel Fish showing skeletal and fin deform-ities (after Schäperclaus photograph).* 3, *Finta with mouth deformity.* 4, *Carp having deformed dorsal fin and* 5, *Carp with deformed gill covering (1, 4, 5 modified after Hofer)*

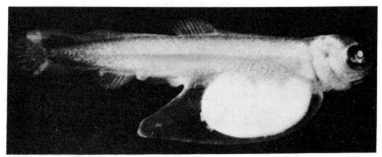

Fig. 9.5. *Trout fry with blue sac disease. After J. Fiebiger*

Don Pavey succeeded in curing this condition by adding shrimp, scrambled egg and lettuce to the diet, combining it with cod-liver oil. The rôle of the latter is not clear, however, since giving it alone did not have any effect whatsoever, whereas it is known that normally vitamin D is not required by fish. The other components of the diet are all rich in nucleoproteins as well as in other proteins, vitamins and lecithins. It was stated that as soon as the nucleoprotein was established definitely in the diet along with vitamin D, the wasting process ceased and in one week's time definite improvement was evident; convalescence immediately ensued.

SOFT EGG DISEASE AND WHITE SPOT DISEASE OF FISH EGGS[30]

In soft egg disease the ova of egg-laying fish become soft and lose their internal pressure (turgor) owing to the occurrence of small holes in the egg membrane. The origin of this condition is unknown.

'White spot' disease of fish eggs occurs in *Salmonidæ* and is characterised by small white spots appearing in the yolk or on the developing embryos. This affliction is thought to be due to mechanical injury.

EMBRYONIC DEFORMITIES

In fish embryos several kinds of deviations of normal development may give rise to monsters, such as an individual with two heads or two tails, or two bodies grown together either with their bellies or with their backs, two complete embryos sharing one yolk sac, a.s.o. In fact these deviations are due to certain cell groups getting loose from each other early in embryological development, so that they do not influence each other's development any more, which leads to duplication of the organs. If, early in development, separation between cell groups is complete, a monozygous twin is produced. The occurrence of monsters seems to be governed at least in part by hereditary factors, since in certain species of fish it is encountered often (Trout), whereas in others it is only very seldom met with.

BLUE SAC DISEASE (HYDROCOELE EMBRYONALIS)

This is essentially a form of dropsy of the yolk sac, in which a blue liquid accumulates between the yolk proper, the intestine and the liver on the one hand, and the membrane of the yolk sac on the other. Anatomically it does not differ from dropsy of the belly in adult fishes (*Ascites*). It is mainly restricted to Trout (Fig. 9.5) and may cause losses of 4–15% of each batch of fry.

It has been believed that there are at least two forms of the condition, one being non-contagious but constitutional, whereas the other one might be of bacterial origin. However, real evidence for either bacterial or viral infections is lacking. From other investigations (Wolf) it has been thought probable that coincidence of several adverse conditions may be involved, such as food factors, premature hatching and toxic chemicals in the water. Fungus growth on or near the eggs may also have some significance, so that egg disinfection and subsequent treatments with malachite green as described on page 331 is recommended as one of the measures for its prevention.[31]

BLUE DISEASE

This so far unidentified disease has been reported by Allan R. Mitchell as occurring in *Hyphessobrycon heterorhabdus*. Harlequin Fish (*Rasbora heteromorpha*) and Angel Fish (*Pterophyllum*). The white flecks on *Hyphessobrycon heterorhabdus* turned blue, while later on the same hue occurred on the body. In Harlequin Fish the symptoms were the development of a blue line on the dorsal side of the body, followed by the occurrence of a blue patch on the head above the eyes, while later on the black of the body became covered with a blue cast. Similar symptoms have been observed in Angel Fish. Nothing is known about the cause of this disease. However, it has been successfully cured by methylene blue, used in twice the strength required for treatment of *Ichthyophthiriasis* (white spot), which is the same strength as is effective against velvet disease. Acriflavine also proved effective, but this may cause a temporary sterility in fish. Quinine hydrochloride proved ineffective.

WASTING DISEASE OF CLOWN FISHES

This is a disease of unknown origin that is apparently confined to Coral fishes of the Genus *Amphiprion* (*Premnas* or *Prochilus*), particularly of the species *percula*. It has been described by Riseley.[32] In the early stages the fish behaves normally, but a little later it will forsake its sea anemone and shimmy miserably, often in a corner of the aquarium. Appetite is lost. Death occurs relatively suddenly. No obvious symptoms of wastage or internal parasites were observed, but the disease appears to be infectious or contagious amongst all Clown fishes, whereas members of other genera are not affected.

No cures are available. Methylene blue, copper sulphate and antibiotics have been tried without any effect. Diseased fish should be removed from the main tank as soon as possible to reduce the risk of infection of any other Clown fishes that are present.

DESTRUCTION OF SMALL FRY BY CYCLOPS

Certain cyclopids, in particular *Acanthocyclops vernalis* Fischer, attack small fry and injure them while swimming. They attack and even ingest them, generally only leaving the spine.[33] Under aquarium conditions ten Silver Carp fry were destroyed every 1.5–2 h at a cyclops concentration of 1500 per litre. A fortnight after fertilisation of the eggs, the fry had reached a stage where they were invulnerable to the attacks.

In the presence of 200 or more *Cyclops vernatis* or *C. bicuspidatus* per litre, mortality of a test group of larval fish was 46.4% after one day, whereas there were no deaths in the control group.[34]

In tropical aquaria I have also often observed cyclopids attacking young fry about 2–3 times their own length. They attacked from the tail or in the belly region. Occasionally they are seen to detach from the victim, which then shows severe damage.

Consequently, it is advised never to introduce cyclops as a live food for small fry in breeding tanks. Youngsters having the size of a new-born livebearer seem to be invulnerable.

REFERENCES

1 NOSE, T., 'A preliminary report on some essential amino acids for the growth of the eel, *Anguilla japonica*', *Bull. Freshwater Fish Res. Lab.* **19**, 31–36 (1969)
2 HALVER, J. E., 'Fish diseases and nutrition', *Trans. Amer. Fish. Soc.*, 254–61 (1953)
3 DE LONG, D. C., HALVER, J. E. and YASUTAKE, W. T., 'A possible cause of "Sunburn" in fish', *Progr. Fish-Cult.* **20**, 111–13 (1958)
4 PARKER, MRS. W. M., 'Pyridoxine', *The Aquarium* **21**, 319–20 (1953)
5 HENRARD, N. A., 'De ziekte van *Barbus tetrazona* var *sumatranus* Bleeker', *Het Aquarium* **20**, 10 (1949–50)
6 JONES, R. E., *Fish and River Pollution*, Butterworths (1964)
7 DOWNING, K. M. and MERKENS, J. C., 'The influence of dissolved-oxygen concentration on the toxicity of un-ionised ammonia to Rainbow Trout (*Salmo gairdnerii* Richardson)', *Ann. Appl. Biol.* **43**, 243–46 (1955); DOWNING, K. M., 'The influence of dissolved-oxygen concentration on the toxicity of potassium cyanide to Rainbow Trout', *J. Exp. Biol.* **31**, 161–64 (1954); HERBERT, D. W. M., 'Measuring the toxicity of effluents to fish', *The Analyst* **80**, 896–98 (1955)
8 ALABASTER, J. S. and HERBERT, D. W. M., 'Influence of carbon dioxide on the toxicity of ammonia', *Nature (Lond.)* **174**, 404 (1954)
9 WUHRMANN, K. and WOKER, H., 'Experimentelle Untersuchungen über die Ammoniak- und Blausäurevergiftung', *Schweiz. Z. Hydrol.* **12**, 210–44 (1949)
10 REICHENBACH-KLINKE, H., *Krankheiten und Schädigungen der Fische*, Stuttgart (1966)
11 HALSBAND, E. and HALSBAND, I., 'Veränderungen des Blutbildes von Fischen infolge toxischer Schäden', *Arch. Fischereiwiss.* **16**, 68–85 (1964)
12 BANDT, H. J., 'Die tödliche Menge an gelöstem Eisen in Fischgewässern', *Fischerei Z.* **41**, 593 (1938)
13 SCHÄPERCLAUS, W., *Fischkrankheiten*, 3rd ed., 564, Berlin (1954)
14 LÜDEMANN, cited after SCHÄPERCLAUS, *loc. cit.*

15 SCHWEIGER, G., 'Die toxikologische Einwirkung von Schwermetallsalzen auf Fische und Fischnährtiere', *Arch. Fischereiwiss.* **8**, 54–78 (1957)
16 SKIDMORE, J. F., 'Toxicity of zinc compounds to aquatic animals, with special reference to fish', *Quart. Rev. Biol.* **39**, 227–48 (1964)
17 EBELING, G. and SCHRADER, T., 'Ueber frees Chlor im Wasser und seine Wirkung auf Fische und andere Wasserorganismen', *Z. Fischerei* **17**, 417–510 (1929)
18 LINSCHOTEN, J. H., *Het Aquarium* **20**, 155–58 (1949–50)
19 VAMOS, R., ZSOLT, J. and RIBIANSKY, M., 'Wasserblüte und Fischsterben', *Acta. Biolog.* **8**, 103–14 (1964)
20 WUNDSCH, H. H., 'Ausscheidungen der Wasserschnecke *Linnaea peregra* (Müll) als rasch wirkendes Fischgift', *Z. Fischerei* **28**, 1–12 (1930)
21 SCHÄPERCLAUS, W., 'Fischerkrankungen und Fischsterben durch Massenentwicklung von Phytoplankton bei Anwesenheit von Ammoniumverbindungen', *Z. Fischerei N.S.* **1**, 29–44 (1952–53)
22 BANDT, H. J., 'Geschmacksbeeinflussung der Fische durch Oscillatorienöl', *Allg. Fisch z.* **60**, 328–30 (1935)
23 KUN, M. S., TEPLYI, D. L. and ASTAKHOVA, T. V., 'O prichinakh rabolevaniya sazana v del'te Volgi', *Vopr. Ikhthiol.* **17**, 159–68
24 OTTERSTRØM, C. V. and LARSEN, K., 'Extensive mortality in Trout caused by infusorian *Stentor polymorphus* Ehrenb', *Rep. Danish Biol. Station* **XLVIII**, 1943–45, Copenhagen (1946)
25 ALBRECHT, M. L., 'Der Einfluss von Licht und Temperatur auf die Sauerstoffproduktion in Wasser unter Eis und Schnee', *Z. Fisch. N.F.* **12**, 167–82 (1964)
26 ROBERTS, R. J., LECKIE, J. and SLACK, H. D., '"Bald Spot" disease in Powan *Coregonus lavaretus* (L.)', *J. Fish. Biol.* **2**, 103–05 (1970)
27 BUSNIŢA, T., 'Ökologische und wirtschaftliche Probleme des Sterlets der unteren Donau', paper read at Langenargen (1964); BUSNIŢA, T. and GHEORGHE, V., 'Die Form des Kopfes und seine Deformationen beim Barsch', *Bul. Ştiinţif. R.P.R.* **1**, 403–13 (1949)
28 GORDON, M., 'The genetics of fish disease', *Trans. Amer. Fish. Soc.* **83**, 229–40 [1953 (publ. 1954)]
29 PAVEY, D., 'Ricketic Brachydanios', *The Aquarium* **6**, 120 (1937)
30 DAVIS, H. S., *Culture and Diseases of Game Fishes*, Berkeley and Los Angeles (1956)
31 SCHÄPERCLAUS, W., *Fischkrankheiten*, 3rd ed., Berlin, 606–10 (1954); WOLF, K., 'Blue-sac disease investigations: Microbiology and laboratory induction', *Progr. Fish-Cult.*, 14–18 (Jan. 1957)
32 RISELEY, R. A., *Tropical Marine Aquaria*, London (1971)
33 SUKHANOVA, E. R., 'Rol'tsiklopov (*Acanthocyclops vernalis* Fisch.) v vyzhivanii lichinok belogo tolstolobika', *Vop. Ikthiol* **8**, 584–86 (1968); VAN IERSEL, R., 'Cyclops, de vernietiger van jongbroed', *Het Aquarium* **25**, 112 (1954–55)
34 FABIAN, M. W., 'Mortality of freshwater and tropical fish fry by cyclopoid copepods', *Ohio Jour. Sci.* **60** (5), 268–70 (1960)

10

THE MEDICINE CHEST

In this chapter brief particulars are given of the chemicals that may be used in treatment of diseased fishes, with particulars of dosage in metric (now S.I.), English and American units. Generally, the S.I. system is the most easy to use, since in this system all units are consistent and have simple relations to each other. In using English units, it is much more easy to use the cubic foot as a unit of volume than the gallon, since the gallon has no direct relation to the unit of length. It must be borne in mind that there is a difference between the English gallon (Imp. gal) and the American gal (U.S. gal). In comparing recipes in English and American literature this must be considered, otherwise considerable errors in dosage could occur.

The S.I. system has the following units:

Length: 1 metre (m) = 100 centimetres = 1000 millimetres.
1 millimetre (mm) = 1000 micrometres (μm, microns) = 1 000 000 nanometres (nm, formerly called 'millimicrons').

Volume: 1 cubic metre (m^3) = 1000 cubic decimetres (dm^3) or litres = 1 000 000 cubic centimetres (cm^3) or millilitres (ml).

Weight: 1 kilogram = 1000 grams = 1 000 000 milligrams (1 kilogram (kg) is the weight of 1 litre of water under specified conditions).

Time: 1 hour (h) = 60 minutes (min) = 3600 seconds (s).

Readers accustomed to the metric system only, should be warned not to confuse the symbol gr (= grain) with g (= gram); 1 grain = $\frac{1}{15}$ gram (approx.).

315

RELATION BETWEEN DIFFERENT UNITS

1 metre (m) = 3.28 feet (ft) = 39.37 inches (in).
1 square metre (m^2) = 10.764 square feet (ft^2) = 1550 sq. inches (in^2).
1 cubic metre (m^3) = 35.314 cubic feet (ft^3) = 61 024 cubic inches (in^3).
1 litre (l) = 1000 millilitres (ml) = 1000 cubic centimetres (cm^3) = 1.7598 pints (pt).
1 cubic inch = 16.387 cubic centimetres.
1 cubic foot = 28.31 litres.
1 pint (pt) = 0.5679 litres.
1 Imp. gal = 4.5459 litres = 0.1605 cubic feet = 277.42 cubic inches.
1 U.S. gal = 3.785 litres = 0.1339 cubic feet = 231 cubic inches.
1 gram (g) = 15.432 grains (gr).
1 kilogram (kg) = 2.205 pounds (lb).
1 pound avoirdupois = 7000 grains = 453.6 grams.

    In the following review of the chemicals used to treat fishes Rp. = recipe and M.D.S. = method of using it; p.p.m. = parts per million; LC_{50} = 50% lethal concentration—concentration which kills 50% of the specimens exposed to it.

DETERMINING THE WEIGHT OF SMALL FISHES

There are a number of drugs that have to be administered orally (by mouth). The only way to do this in fish is to mix it with the food and dosage is often based on 'so much per unit of body weight', which is the only reasonable one, because body size and weight may vary so much. To estimate the weight of small aquarium fish, a plastic beaker with some water may be weighed, e.g. on a letter-balance, then some fish of representative size are put in and it is weighed again. The difference is, of course, the weight of the fish. In this way the total body weight of the fishes that have to be medicated can be calculated with sufficient accuracy for the purpose, without having to handle fishes out of the water, as in the direct weighing method employed with big fishes at fish farms.

ACETARSONE (N-ACETYL-4-HYDROXY-*m*-ARSANILIC ACID; STOVARSOL^R)

For treatment of sporozoan infections, especially by *Myxosoma cerebralis*, administered mixed with the food at a rate of 10 mg per kg fish during 3–4 successive days. Also for treatment of *Hexamitiasis* (*Octomitiasis*).
    Probably useful for treatment of *Leptospira* and certain internal diseases caused by unicellular organisms.

ACRIFLAVINE (NEUTRAL ACRIFLAVINE, TRYPAFLAVINE NEUTRAL)

This is a deep orange, granular powder consisting of a mixture of 2,8-diamino-10-methylacridinium chloride and of 2,8-diamino-acridine. It is recommended that the small commercial tablets which are sold for treatment of sore throats be used. These tablets contain 3 mg (0.046 gr). Aqueous solutions are reddish-orange in colour and fluoresce on dilution. *Be sure to get neutral acriflavine.* There is also an acid compound, acriflavine hydrochloride, which is called 'acriflavine' in the *British Pharmacopœia*, 1932, Add. I. This hydrochloride has a very strong acid reaction and might be dangerous when used in slightly acid water.

The hydrochloride can be distinguished from the neutral acriflavine by its appearance; while the neutral compound is deep orange, the hydrochloride is a deep reddish-brown crystalline powder and its solutions are dark red instead of reddish-orange.

Rp.   Stock solution: One tablet (3 mg) is dissolved in 330 cm^3 of hot water. Keep protected from light.

M.D.S. The following quantities of stock solution are to be added to the aquarium water:

Quantity to be added (in cm^3) per:			
1	ft^3	Imp. gal	U.S. gal
2.2	60	10	8

For very obstinate cases, the strength may be doubled. The water has to be stirred thoroughly while adding the stock solution to the tank. Treatment is extended over a period of three days.

If this should be insufficient (as in the case of velvet disease), the water is changed and a further treatment (2–3 days) is given at the sixth day. The repetition is necessary to avoid reinfections, because encysted parasites are not affected by the treatment. Interrupted treatment is required to decrease the total period that the fishes are in contact with the chemical. Too long a contact of fish with acriflavine should be avoided. Acriflavine produces a temporary sterility in both egg-laying and livebearing fish. However, normal fertility is restored after a period of several months.

Acriflavine is effective against white spot and velvet disease, tail- and fin-rot and fungus. Owing to the harmful effects its use should be confined to stubborn cases of disease where more harmless drugs fail to do the job. Acriflavine should never be used for treatment of fungused eggs since this might result in defectiveness of the hatching young, which may even be hereditary since direct reaction with embryonic cells may cause mutations in the germ epithelium of the gonads, resulting in defective offspring in the second and later generations. During treatment the illumination level of the tank should be as low as possible in order to prevent unwanted toxic effects on the fishes due to photosensitisation.

Acriflavine affects some aquatic plants. *Cabomba* and *Elodea* die, whilst *Vallisneria*, *Sagittaria* and *Nitella* can stand it. Blue-green algae will die also.

For treatment of sliminess of the skin acriflavine is recommended by Schäperclaus in a much higher concentration, namely, of 1 g per 100 l, which is equivalent to 0.7 gr/Imp. gal or 0.58 gr/U.S. gal. At this high strength *Cyclochæta* and *Chilodonella* are eradicated in half a natural day (12 h), whereas for *Costia* a two-days' treatment is required. This prolonged treatment has also been reported as effective against *Gyrodactylus*.

Of course, bad effects on plants will be much more pronounced than in the lower concentration mentioned above, whereas the risk for young fish is also higher. The LC_{50} value for fry of *Catla catla*, *Labeo rotrita* and *Cirrhinus mrigala* was found to be 47.5–80 mg/l.[1]

Acriflavine has also been used as a 0.1% solution admixed to minced meat given as food to young Trout to prevent spread of *Hexamitiasis* (*Octomitiasis*), but 25% of the fishes refused to take it, whereas in the others the incidence of the disease was only reduced from 50% to 16.6%.[2]

ACRINOL (6,9-DIAMINO-2 AETHOXYACRIDINE LACTATE, RIVANOL[R], RIMAON[R], ACROLACTINE[R], ETHODIN[R], VUCINE[R])

Pale-yellow crystalline substance, slowly soluble in 15 parts of water. Chemically related to acriflavine. It is used against skin flukes and other parasites of the skin, in a concentration of 1 g in 400–500 l, up to several days' duration.

AMMONIA (NH_4OH)

Household ammonia is a solution of ammonia gas (NH_3) in water, having a strength of about 10%. It has a strong, pungent smell.

Rp.   10 parts by volume of the commercial ammonia diluted with 90 parts by volume of water. This dilution is used in preparing the bath.

M.D.S. Ammonia may be used in the treatment of skin and gill flukes. It may be used in two strengths; 1 : 2000 is the correct strength for general use, while for fishes having a strong, slimy skin, such as Goldfish, Carp, Eel and Tench, the proportion of 1 : 1000 may be used.

Fishes are bathed in the solution for 5–20 min. For very delicate fishes, ammonia treatment is not advisable, since it may sometimes produce shock. In such cases it will be better to use methylene blue.

	1	ft^3	Imp. gal	U.S. gal

	Quantity to be added (in cm^3) per:			
	1	ft^3	Imp. gal	U.S. gal
General	5	140	22$\frac{1}{2}$	18$\frac{1}{2}$
Strong bath	10	280	45	37$\frac{1}{2}$

Ammonia may not be used in planted tanks or ponds, since it has a very bad effect on plant growth, while in ponds it cannot be used owing to the short duration of treatment that is recommended.

AMMONIUM NITRATE (NH_4NO_3)

Transparent hygroscopic deliquescent crystals or white granules. Keep well closed, away from light, preferably as a 10% stock solution. For treatment add 5 ml/l, or 140 ml/ft^3, 22$\frac{1}{2}$ ml/Imp. gal or 18$\frac{1}{2}$ ml/ U.S. gal. Repeat after two days. Has been recommended against *Dactylogyrus* and for removing *Hydra* and *Planaria* infestations.

AMPICILLIN—See PENICILLIN

AQUAROL

A German commercial product advocated for treatment of tail-rot, fungus, white spot and sliminess of the skin caused by *Chilodonella* and *Costia*. Also used for eliminating *Hydra* infestation of tanks.
Fishes are bathed in a solution of 2 g in 25 l water (35 gr/ft^3). Exact duration not specified. Treatment has to be repeated three times at three-day intervals.

ARTHINOL (1% *PARA*-CARBAMIDO BENZARSONIC ACID COMBINED WITH CHLOROTETRACYCLINE HYDROCHLORIDE)

One per cent of this substance admixed to the food may be used for treatment of *Hexamitiasis*. Also see Aureomycin and Carbarsone.

ARYCIL

This is an arsenic compound, containing 36.4% As. For treatment of pox disease in Carp, 1 ml of a 1% solution is injected, intraperitoneally at first, then three injections with a 5% solution at successive days.

AUREOMYCIN[R] (CHLORTETRACYCLINE)

This is an antibiotic, isolated from cultures of *Streptomyces aureofaciens*. It is a golden-yellow crystallised substance with weak basic reaction. Solubility in water 0.5–0.6 mg/l at 25°C. Aquarium water is coloured yellowish, while a scum is formed at the surface in the course of the treatment. Aureomycin is active against many Gram-positive and Gram-negative bacteria, certain *Protozoa* (including *Ichthyophthirius*, *Oodinium*) and some viruses. It has no effect against *Proteus* and true *Pseudomonas* infections. It is effective against bacterial and some virus infections at 60 mg/Imp. gal (50 mg/U.S. gal; 13 mg/l). H. R. Axelrod recommended the use of a very heavy dose, namely, 600 mg/Imp. gal (500 mg/U.S. gal), which does not harm the fish if used only for a short time; others claimed that this dosage produces after-effects if treatment is prolonged for four days, which may be due to avitaminoses caused by the killing effect on bacteria in the intestine which synthesise vitamins necessary for the fish.

Foods containing Aureomycin increase growth rate of young fish and intensification of colours, but ill-effects due to avitaminoses (especially lack of vitamins E and K and folic acid) are likely to occur unless these vitamins are also included in the food.

One per cent of Aureomycin in the food will cure *Hexamitiasis*.

Aureomycin treatment should not be extended over a longer period than is absolutely necessary to cure the fish; four days will be a maximum for the bacteriostatic lower concentration, and not more than two days for the strong, bactericidal concentration. Generally, chloramphenicol is to be preferred. Bacteriostatic and preservative effects in sea-water are preserved by addition of citric acid.[24]

BENZALKONIUM CHLORIDE

Trade names are: *Zephirol, Zephiran chloride, Benirol, Cequartil, Drapolene, Germinol, Germitol, Roccal, Rodalon, Osvan*.

This is a cationic surface-active agent and germicide, consisting of a white or yellowish-white powder or gelatinous pieces, highly soluble in water. Solutions 1:50 000 up to 1:20 000 are used for bathing fishes for 30 min only. It may be used for skin disinfection and for treatment of sliminess of the skin and *Gyrodactylus* infections. For swabbing wounds a 1:4000 solution may be used.

In the literature there seems to be some confusion with respect to dosage and commercial names. Reichenbach-Klinke mentions 'Roccal' at a concentration of 10% solution 1 : 50 000 only, but 'Zephirol', which is chemically exactly the same substance, 1 : 4000–1 : 2000. Probably this discrepancy is due to the drugs being also sold in solutions where it is not always clear whether the absolute dosage, or the amounts of the solutions to be used, are meant. Therefore, caution with such prescriptions is needed. Do not use a bulk treatment unless a preliminary experiment has proved it safe.

BRILLIANT GREEN

This is a dye, consisting of minute, glistening, golden crystals. Chemically it is closely related to malachite green, the only difference being that it has aethyl (C_2H_5.) groups at those sites where malachite green has methyl (CH_3.) groups. It has been recommended for treatment of cotton wool disease. A stock solution is prepared by dissolving 4 gr (approx. 0.25 g) in just sufficient ethanol (alcohol) and this is added to one U.S. gal of water (0.83 Imp. gallon or 3.8 l). The fish is caught in a net and, still being in the net, is immersed in this solution for 45 sec only. It has been stated that this treatment will cure the most stubborn cases (Campbell).

However, as the very short duration of the treatment suggests, it is a drastic one, and it is recommended that experiments should be performed with lower concentrations and a longer period of treatment. In the writer's opinion, this treatment is still in the experimental stage and experience may show that it should be modified.

CALOMEL (MERCUROUS CHLORIDE; MERCURY-I-CHLORIDE) (Hg_2Cl_2)

White, heavy powder, to be protected for light. Has been used for treatment of *Hexamitiasis* by admixing it at a rate of 0.2% to the food during four days. Owing to its toxicity as a mercury compound it is not recommended any more. See Carbarsone and Fumagillin.

CARBARSONE (*PARA*-UREIDOBENZENEARSONIC ACID; *PARA*-CARBAMIDOBENZENEARSONIC ACID; N-CAR-BAMYLARSANILIC ACID; *PARA*-ARSONOPHENYLUREA) $NH_2.CO.NH.C_6H_4. AsO(OH)_2$

Also known under a great number of trade names: *Amabevan, Ameban, Amebarsone, Amibiarson, Aminarsone, Arsambide, Fenarsone, Histocarb, Leucarsone.*

White powder, slightly soluble in water. Used for treatment of *Hexamitiasis*, 0.2% of the drug is thoroughly mixed with the food and administered for four consecutive days; then treatment is stopped for three days, after which it is repeated once.

CHLORAMINE-B (SODIUM BENZENE-SULPHOCHLORAMIDE), $C_6H_5.SO_2.N(Na)Cl.2H_2O$.
CHLORAMINE-T (SODIUM *PARA*-TOLUENESULPHON-CHLORAMIDE), $(CH_3).C_6H_4.SO_2.N(Na) Cl.3H_2O$

Also known under many trade names, such as *Aktivin, Chloraseptine, Chlorazene, Euclorina, Gansil, Gyneclorina, Mianine, Tochlorine*.

In Holland both compounds are being sold under the trade name *Halamid*.

Both are a white or slightly yellowish product, Chloramine-B being a bit coarser than the other one. Must be protected from light and moisture in tightly closed bottles with glass stoppers, or in plastic flasks. The chloramines have a slight odour of chlorine.

Rp.   1 g (15 gr) dissolved in 100 cm³ of tap-water. Even in brown glass this solution should not be stored for more than a few days; use of older solution might be dangerous.

M.D.S.

Quantity of stock solution (in cm³) to be added per:			
1	ft³	Imp. gal	U.S. gal
1	28	$4\frac{1}{2}$	$3\frac{1}{2}$

Fishes are treated in this solution for 24 h. The treatment is effective against white spot, sliminess of the skin and *Gyrodactylus* infections.

A drawback of the method is some uncertainty with respect to the actual concentration, because this depends on the amount of organic substances present in the water and on the bottom, whereas increasing the amount may produce a toxic concentration if the chlorine-binding power of the water is less than assumed. It is therefore recommended to remove dirt from the bottom and eventually change the water prior to treatment. It will be even better to apply this treatment in a separate clean glass tank.

WARNING: Chloramine must not be used in contact with any bare metal, since this might lead to severe metal poisoning apart from making the drug inactive.

CHLORAMPHENICOL (CHLOROMYCETIN^R)

This is an antibiotic, originally prepared from cultures of *Streptomyces venezuelæ*, but today most of it is prepared by chemical synthesis. It is a colourless crystallised substance. Solubility in water at 25°C is 2.5 mg/l. The solutions have a neutral reaction. Aqueous solutions are very stable and are not decomposed by heating.

Chloramphenicol is very active against a number of Gram-positive and Gram-negative bacteria, against some protozoans (such as *Oodinium limneticum*, causing velvet disease, and *Ichthyophthirius*) and some viruses. It has been used successfully for treatment of dropsy, which is a combined infection by a virus and bacteria (*Aeromonas punctata*), and against other bacterial infections of fish, including furunculosis.

It should be used in a dosage not less than 25 mg/Imp. gal (20 mg/U.S. gal; 5.5 mg/l), but preferably 30–50 mg/Imp. gal (25–40 mg/U.S. gal; 6.5–11 mg/l). For treatment of dropsy and other virus infections, dosage should be increased to 60 mg/Imp. gal (50 mg/U.S. gal; 13 mg/l). For fishes of at least 10 g weight, this may be increased even to 230 mg/Imp. gal (190 mg/U.S. gal; 50 mg/l) and for bigger fishes in ponds to 370 mg/Imp. gal (310 mg/U.S. gal; 80 mg/l), for 24 h only. 10 mg/l clears *Columnaris* disease in 48 h.

For fishes of at least 10 g weight, a bath of 80 mg/l for 8 h only has been recommended by Reichenbach-Klinke / against *Aeromonas punctata* infections, or alternatively, injection of 0.1 mg dissolved in 0.1 ml of water into the body cavity.

Injection therapy has also been found effective against *Vibrio* infections in marine fishes.

Another method of application is by adding it to granulated food, at a rate of 1 gram per kilogram food (1 milligram per gram). This treatment was found effective in preventing epizootics of infectious dropsy in Carp, whereas adding it to the water (1 g/l) had no effect. Healing of Carps with manifest dropsy has been accomplished by three injections given in the intestine. Mixed with the food it may also be used against *Ichthyophonus* infections.

After-effects, such as avitaminoses, often occurring with Aureomycin treatment of fish, have not been reported from chloramphenicol. Therefore, chloramphenicol seems to be preferable for treatment of bacterial, rickettsial and virus infections of fish as compared with Aureomycin. It is effective against the same types of infection and some more, such as *Proteus* and *Pseudomonas æruginosa*.

CHLOROBUTANOL (CHLORETONE) (Cl$_3$C.C(CH$_3$)$_2$.OH)

Crystalline substance with camphor odour and taste. For medical use available in tablets. One tablet dissolved in about a quarter glass of water has been used for local treatment (swabbing) of fungus infections in fish. Use hot water for dissolving, but let it cool down to lukewarm before use.

One tablet per gallon kills *Hydra* within 15 min, but this treatment is restricted to eradication in absence of fish, since fishes would be killed, too.

CHLOROMYCETIN^R—See CHLORAMPHENICOL

COLLARGOL^R (COLLOIDAL SILVER)

This is a brownish powder. It consists of colloidal silver (Ag) and silver oxide (Ag_2O) with a derived egg albumen as a protecting colloid. Collargol contains the equivalent of about 78% silver.

Rp.   0.1 g (= 1½ gr) dissolved in 100 cm^3 of distilled water.

M.D.S. The stock solution may be used directly for touching sore spots and fungus on the skin or the eye of a fish. For bathing, the following further dilution is made from the stock solution:

Quantity of stock solution (in cm^3) to be added per:			
l	ft^3	Imp. gal	U.S. gal
1–3	28–84	4½–13½	3½–11½

Fishes are bathed in this solution for 1–3 h. Collargol may be used in treatment of fungus and bacterial diseases of fishes. It is less effective, however, than Mercurochrome or potassium dichromate, and very much inferior to phenoxethol and antibiotics.

COPPER SULPHATE (CUPRIC SULPHATE)
($CuSO_4.5H_2O$)

Blue crystals or light-blue powder. The latter is to be preferred for easier weighing. Dosages have to be very accurate because copper salts are highly toxic to fish.

It has been effectively used against *Costia*, skin flukes, fungus and *Oodinium* infections. For details see pages 56–57 and 62.

In marine aquaria, copper concentrations ranging up to 1 p.p.m. have been applied for deterring algal growth and to prevent outbreaks of *Oodinium* attacks, with no apparent ill-effects on the animals.[3]

DDT (DICHLORODIPHENYLTRICHLORETHANE); 1,1,1-TRICHLORO-2,2-*BIS* (*PARA*-CHLOROPHENYL ETHANE

Rp.
M.D.S.
Let a chemist prepare a stock solution of 10 mg of pure DDT in 100 cm^3 of 95% medicinal grade ethanol.

Quantity of stock solution (in cm^3) to be added per:			
1	ft^3	Imp. gal	U.S. gal
0.1–0.2	2.8–5.6	4$\frac{1}{2}$–9	3$\frac{1}{2}$–7

Suggested by Schäperclaus for treatment of anchor worm (*Lernæa*) infections. According to him, fishes will stand this treatment for several days.

With regard to the very high toxicity of the drug and consequent very exacting application (the final dosage being only one part in 50 to 100 millions! whereas Dr. J. C. M. de Jong found one part in 10 millions lethal[4]), the present author is not very enthusiastic about it. In many countries use of DDT is now prohibited.

For other details see:
Susan Frances King, 'Some effects of DDT on the Guppy and the Brown Trout', *U.S. Fish. and Wildlife Serv. Spec. Sci.-Report-Fish.* *399*, pp. 1–22 (1962).

DOXYCYCLINE—See OXYTETRACYCLINE

FORMALIN (FORMALDEHYDE SOLUTION) (HCHO)

Commercial formalin is a solution of formaldehyde gas in water. It is available in two strengths, namely, 32 and 40% v/v. The latter solution contains some methanol (methyl alcohol) for conservation. Since methanol is a strong poison, this solution should not be used in preparing baths for treatment of fish.

The formaldehyde solution to be used must be free from paraformaldehyde, which may be recognised as a white stuff at the bottom and/or on the sides of the bottle. The formation of paraformaldehyde (which is more toxic to fish) is accelerated by light and low temperature. Solutions should therefore be kept in a dark bottle and in a warm place. Use fresh formalin. If a small amount of paraformaldehyde is present, the solution should be filtered through a fine filter paper before use.

Formaldehyde must not be added to a tank or pond in which methylene blue or other dyes, which are adsorbed, have been used recently, since the combination might have toxic effects on the fish.

A weak formaldehyde solution may be used as a permanent bath for fish infected by skin or gill flukes (Rankin). The water temperature should be not less than 18°C (65°F). At lower temperatures there is some risk of fungus infection owing to the weakening of the mucous coat of the fish's skin. If such secondary fungus infection should occur, the water must be changed and a specific treatment for fungus started.

Rp.   (1) Stock solution for permanent bath: 1 part by volume of *British Pharmacopœia* grade formaldehyde solution is added to 99 parts by volume of water.

M.D.S. (1) 6–7 cm^3 of stock solution Rp. (1) to one litre; or 165 cm^3 to one cubic foot.

A different treatment is used to cure cases of sliminess of the skin, caused by *Costia necatrix*, if no results can be obtained by the use of salt or quinine hydrochloride treatment. For this purpose a stock solution Rp. (2) is prepared:

Rp.   (2) 10 parts by volume of 32% formaldehyde solution are diluted with 90 parts by volume of water. Be careful not to confuse this stronger solution with the stock solution Rp. (1) for permanent baths.

M.D.S. (2) A bath is prepared by further diluting the stock solution:

Quantity of stock solution Rp. (2) to be added (in cm^3) per:			
l	ft^3	Imp. gal	U.S. gal
2–5	56–140	10–25	8–21

The fishes are bathed in this solution for 15–30 min only. This treatment has to be repeated several times every two days until the fishes are completely cured.

This method of application of formalin originates from Dr. Wilhelm Roth (1922).[5] The final concentration of formaldehyde is equivalent to approx. 6.5–16 mg/l, which for the indicated bath of short duration is still a safe range, as also follows from more recent investigations by Nazarenko,[6] who found that toxic effects of formaldehyde on fish begin at 5 mg/l, whereas death occurs during the first few hours at a concentration of 50 mg/l. Toxic effects on water fleas were observed at 1 mg/l and on the green unicellular alga *Protococcus* at concentrations exceeding 5 mg/l.

Rucker, Taylor and Toney suggested the use of formalin 1:4000, which is approximately equivalent to 80 mg/l, for 1 h, for the control of most external protozoan and trematode worm parasites on most salmonids[7] and Reichenbach-Klinke mentions this same treatment against gill flukes[8]; in the light of Nazarenko's data this seems to be rather high and although it might be that *Salmonidæ* could have a higher resistance to this chemical than other fishes, the present author would advise generally to adhere to either Rankin's or Roth's prescriptions, as given before.

Recently, effective application of formalin in salmonid ponds to control 'Ich' has been reported.[9]

Formalin treatments are ineffective against *Lernæa* and other parasitic *Copepoda*.

FRIAR'S BALSAM (BALSAM TRAUMATIC; TURLINGTON'S BALSAM)

This is a balsam composed of 100 parts benzoin, 35 parts storax, 35 parts Balsam tolu, 16 parts Balsam Peru, 8 parts aloe, 8 parts myrrh, 4 parts angelica, and ethanol (alcohol) to make 1000.

It may be used as a protective wound dressing in fish. Some cotton-wool is wound round a matchstick and this is dipped in the balsam. The wound of the fish is quickly swabbed with the balsam, coating the entire area with it. It may be necessary to repeat this treatment several times to achieve a complete healing.

FUMAGILLIN (AMEBACILLIN; FUMIDIL)

This is an antibiotic, produced by the fungus *Aspergillus fumigatus*. It has a very low stability and is best stored in dark, evacuated ampoules at low temperature. It is used for treatment of *Hexamitiasis*, mixed with the food at a rate of 0.2%, for four days.

FURAZOLIDONE (3–(5-NITROFURFURYLIDENEAMINO)-2-OXAZOLIDONE)

Yellow crystals, to be protected for light. Solubility in water at pH 6 about 40 mg/l. It is decomposed by alkaline solutions.

Furazolidone is given mixed with the food for treatment of furunculosis. A dosage of 25 mg per kilogram body weight of fish per day for 14 days has been found to be sufficient for controlling mortality and prevent recurrence of the disease after withdrawal of medication.

It may be expected that this drug will also be effective against certain other bacterial infections and against *Hexamitiasis* and internal sporozoan infections.

GAMMEXANE—See LINDANE

GRISEOFULVIN (FULVICIN; FULCIN)

Antibiotic obtained from *Penicillium griseofulvum* Dierx and *Penicillium janczewskii* Zal. [= *P. nigricans* (Bainier) Thom].
  Only slightly soluble in natural water. For treatments the water should be slightly acid. Addition of 10 mg/l has been recommended for treatment of fungus infections. For treatment of fungus infections of the internal organs it could be tried as a food additive (minced meat).

HALAMID—See CHLORAMINE

HYDROGEN PEROXIDE (H_2O_2)

The common commercial solution has a strength of 3%. The liquid is colourless and does not smell. It must be kept in bottles of dark glass, since its properties are destroyed by light. The solution will gradually lose its strength.
Rp.   The commercial 3% solution may be used directly.
M.D.S. Hydrogen peroxide may only be used in fresh tap-water, in containers in which no plants, sand or other materials are present, otherwise the effective activity of the chemical is considerably decreased.

Quantity of 3% commercial solution (in cm^3) to be added per :			
l	ft^3	Imp. gal	U.S. gal
$17\frac{1}{2}$	500	80	67

In this solution fishes are bathed for 10–15 min. Treatment must be repeated several times. Hydrogen peroxide may be used for treatment of skin flukes, but it is not very effective. In cases of delicate fishes, which are not likely to stand ammonia treatment, methylene blue is more advisable. Hydrogen peroxide has also been used for treatment of cotton wool disease ('mouth fungus'). The treatment is mentioned here only for completeness.

IODINE (I_2)

The dark-brown commercial solution of iodine, used for wound disinfection, contains 10% of iodine, dissolved in alcohol.

Rp. A solution which may be used for treatment of diseased fishes is made by diluting 1 part by volume of the commercial iodine with 9 parts by volume of water.

M.D.S. The previously mentioned solution is used directly for touching sore spots, wounds or fungus. This is done by means of a small pencil or brush, or a tuft of cotton-wool, dipped in the solution. Iodine is never used for preparing baths.

ISONICOTINIC ACID HYDRAZIDE (ISONIAZID; INH)
$$NH_2.NH.CO.(C_5N)H_4$$

Also known under a great number of trade names, such as *Nidaton, Rimifon, Niadrin* and many others.

Crystalline substance. Highly effective antituberculous drug in human medicine and in tuberculosis of mink.

It is suggested for treatment of tuberculosis in fish, to be given at a rate of 3–5 μg per gram fish per day (1 μg = 0.001 mg), mixed thoroughly with the food by soaking this in a very weak solution of the drug. It is ineffective against *Mycobacterium marinum*.

Since INH is sufficiently stable in aqueous solution, it may also be tried added to the aquarium water. A concentration of 3–5 mg/l of water (0.9–1.7 gr per Imp. gal or 0.77–1.4 gr per U.S. gal) is suggested. Preliminary experiments have indicated that fishes may tolerate up to ten times this amount for several days.

KAMALA (KAMILA; KAMEELA; SPOONWOOD)

This is a plant product, consisting of glands and hairs covering the fruits of the euphorbid *Mallotus philippinensis*. $1\frac{1}{2}$–2% kamala is mixed to the food and given for two weeks to fishes suffering from adult tape worms in their intestines.

KANAMYCIN

Antibiotic, produced by *Streptomyces kanamyceticus*. It is highly effective against many bacterial infections in fish, especially against fish tuberculosis and infections by bacteria belonging to the *Pseudomonadaceæ*, such as *Pseudomonas fluorescens, Ps. putida* and *Aeromonas punctata*, and against tail- and fin-rot.

A drawback is that kanamycin generally has to be administered by intraperitoneal injection of 20 μg (0.02 mg) per gram fish, which requires special skill and is probably illegal in Britain if performed by unqualified persons, since it may be regarded to constitute some kind of surgery.

Treatment may be combined with chloramphenicol, to be added to the food at a rate of 1 mg per gram of food.

Intraperitoneal injection in cyprinid fishes is performed by inserting the hypodermic needle at the left side of the belly over the middle of the ventral fin, at about the same height as the upper juncture of the pectoral fin; the needle is inserted between two scales and two ribs at an angle of about 30° relative to the body surface, pointing from tail to head. (Fig. 10.1, page 350.)

For treatment of newts, see page 165.

More recently it has been shown that cases of tail- and fin-rot, where *Aeromonas punctata* was the principal invader, responded well to a treatment with 3.1 mg/l dissolved in the aquarium water (14 mg/ Imp. gal or 11.7 mg/U.S. gal).

LINDANE (GAMMEXANE; 1,2,3,4,5,6-HEXACHLOROCYCLOHEXANE)

This is a crystalline substance with a persistent acrid smell. Lindane is used as an insecticide. It is very poisonous to human beings. The fatal dose of the commercial product (containing about 12% of active gamma-isomer, the rest consisting of other isomers, ineffective as an insecticide) is estimated as approximately 0.4 g per kg body weight. Lindane causes hyper-irritability, convulsions and death. It is able to penetrate through the undamaged skin, causing irritation.

From this description it will be obvious that this drug should be used with the utmost caution. It has been used as an effective treatment against fish lice (*Argulus*) by Dr. Edward Hindle, in a dilution of 1 : 10 000 000. A 1% stock solution in absolute ethanol (alcohol) is prepared and 1 cm³ of this is added to 20 Imp. gal or 25 U.S. gal of water, with thorough stirring. When the solution is poured into the water, a slight milky precipitate may form which disappears almost at once when the water is stirred. After treatment the water has to be changed completely. Treatment must not be prolonged for more than 2–3 days.

With few exceptions, this treatment has only been applied to infected Carp and it is possible that other species of fish might be more susceptible to its toxic action. Pike may be killed after having been treated for 24 h with a 1 : 5 000 000 solution.

Reichenbach-Klinke has mentioned it as a cure for *Ergasilus* and other parasitic *Copepoda* of the gills, at 1–2 : 100 000 000 (half the strength given by Hindle) and even then he states that caution is required. In many countries use of lindane is now prohibited.

LIQUITOX—See PHENOXETHOL

MAGNESIUM SULPHATE (EPSOM SALT) (MgSO$_4$.7H$_2$O)

White crystals. This substance, which is used as a laxative in human medicine, has also been recommended for treatment of constipation in fish. The fish should be fasted for two days and then a pinch of the crystals may be dropped into the water in the hope that fish will swallow them. A better policy is to mix the substance with minced meat.

MALACHITE GREEN

This is a dye, consisting of green crystals with metallic lustre. It is very soluble in water and is recommended for treatment of fungus, especially fungus development on eggs.

Rp.   Stock solution: 1 g of pure malachite green, *medical grade, zinc-free*, is dissolved in 500 cm^3 of distilled water. Using a brand of dye which is intended for dyeing purposes is dangerous, because that kind is prepared as a double salt with zinc chloride, which may kill fishes in the concentrations to be used. The zinc concentration would be of the order of 1 mg/l which is already a toxic concentration for big fish; 2–2.5 mg/l would kill large Trout within a few hours.

M.D.S. From this stock solution the following quantities are added for the bath:

Quantity of stock solution (in cm^3) to be added per:			
l	ft^3	Imp. gal	U.S. gal
1–2	28–56	4.5–9	3.8–8

The lower concentration (2 mg/l) is used for treatment of eggs, while the higher concentration is used for treatment of fishes that have already developed fungus to some extent. Duration of treatment: 25 min to 1 h. As a preventive agent in fish hatcheries malachite green has met with considerable success, the percentage of hatchings being double that obtained from untreated eggs. As a curative of advanced cases of fungus in fish it has mainly been used on Pike and different species of Trout in pond management at fish breeding stations. As an alternative treatment to that mentioned above, large fishes are sometimes treated by dipping them for 10–30 sec only in a solution of one gram in 15 l of water (1 gr/l).

All treatments should be performed in subdued light, because malachite green acts as a photosensitiser.

A ten times lower concentration than indicated above ($= 0.2$ mg/l) of malachite green oxalate has been applied successfully for permanent treatment of Sunfish eggs.[10] This is in the lower limit of fungistatic activity (between 0.01 and 0.05 p.p.m. or mg/l).

In treating small aquarium fish, caution seems to be required as set forth at pages 86–87.

Malachite green may never be used in contact with zinc or galvanised iron, since it may dissolve sufficient zinc from it to produce acute zinc poisoning. It is possible, but not proved, that casualties in aquarium fish by treatment in a bare tank with soft water are due to zinc poisoning.

Investigations in Russia by Avdos'ev,[11] who used malachite green for treatment of white spot, showed the minimum effective concentration at 8–9°C to be 0.5 mg/l, whereas the maximum tolerated by Carp in permanent contact was 1.2 mg/l. The experiments involved treatments of 4500 yearling Carp and hybrid Carp × Crucian Carp with 0.5 mg/l at 5–8°C and an oxygen content of the water of 11–9.3 mg/l. After one day the water became colourless and there were still a small number of *Ichthyophthirius* parasites on the fish. Treatment was repeated and on the third day all fishes were free of white spot infection. The same three days' treatment effectively removed *Chilodonella, Cyclochæta* or relatives (see page 67 ff.) and *Gyrodactylus,* but *Dactylogyrus* proved resistant.

Hublou[12] experimented on fingerling Steelhead Trout (*Salmo gairdneri*) with *Cyclochæta* or *Trichodinella* infections. Concentrations of 1 : 200000–1 : 800000 (5–1.25 mg/l) killed the parasites in 90 min. After 30 min treatment, followed by 60 min in fresh water, complete killing of the parasites was achieved at 1 : 200 000 and 1 : 400000, whereas at 1 : 800000 approximately 90% only were killed. In a single pond 300000 Steelhead Trout were treated for 1 h at a maximum concentration of 1 : 800 000 with good success.

According to Bogdanova[13] young Salmon in waters in thè Far East often suffer from infections with another species of the *Trichodinella* group, namely: *Trichodinella* (?), *Cyclochæta* (?) *truttæ* (Mueller). Large numbers of fishes were treated with malachite green 1 : 700 000 or 1 : 100 000 for 10–15 min. The parasites were killed and washed off the fishes with streaming water. Formalin 1 : 4000 applied in the same way was as effective.

From these experiments by different investigators it would seem that for treatment of sliminess of the skin, caused by *Cyclochæta,* a 30 min treatment with a concentration of 0.5 mg/l would be adequate. This is one-quarter of the lower concentration as given above for treatment of fungus.

For treatment of white spot three days are required, fresh additions of the dye being given on the second day if the green colour has faded. A drawback of the method is the uncertainty of the correct dosage resulting from the dye being adsorbed by organic substances, especially particles of mud, thus reducing its concentration. Counterbalancing this by adding excess dye is dangerous, owing to its high toxicity. In the present author's opinion, methylene blue treatment is still to be preferred.

According to Amlacher[14] malachite green oxalate can be applied at a concentration of 0.15 mg/l in Carp culturing ponds. Ich should be eradicated in about 10 days at a water temperature of 4–10°C (39–50°F).

However, caution is required, since Trout may be killed already at 0.3 mg/l, whereas small aquarium fishes, especially *Hyphessobrycon* species, cannot stand concentrations as low as 0.1 mg/l.

For disinfection of ponds in which infestation with the Sporozoan *Myxosoma cerebralis* has occurred, addition of 10 g/m^3 (1 mg/l) has been recommended.

MEPACRINE HYDROCHLORIDE (ATEBRINE HYDRO-CHLORIDE; QUINACRINE HYDROCHLORIDE)

This is a bright-yellow crystalline substance with bitter taste. It is a very effective antimalarial drug in human medicine. The Dutch physician, Dr. C. van Dommelen, was the first to suggest its use for treatment of white spot infections in fish. In England it seems to have been used for the first time by D. C. Slater, independent of van Dommelen's publication, which was written in Dutch.

Mepacrine is more toxic than quinine and methylene blue and, therefore, it should not be used unless necessary, i.e. its use should be confined to stubborn cases which cannot be eradicated completely by the other substances. It acts as a photosensitiser.

Rp.   A stock solution is prepared by dissolving three tablets, containing 100 mg (1½ gr) each, in 350 cm^3 of water.

M.D.S.

Quantity of stock solution (in cm^3) to be added per:			
l	ft^3	Imp. gal	U.S. gal
3½	100	15	13

The total amount is not added at once, but in three equal portions, at intervals of 48 h. Treatment should not be extended over long periods. Eight to ten days should be sufficient as a maximum. The temperature of the water should be between 70° and 80°F (21° and 27°C). Use artificial aeration during treatment, but no filter with activated carbon, since the latter would remove the drug from the water. During treatment the tank should be protected for light. A warning concerning this treatment is given overleaf.

WARNING: This treatment must not be used on Guppies (*Lebistes reticulatus*); these are intoxicated and will waste away.

MERCUROCHROME^R (MERBROMIN; DIBROMO-HYDROXY MERCURIFLUORESCEIN DISODIUM SALT)

This is a red dye, a chemical compound, related to the dye eosin and containing mercury. It has strong disinfecting qualities. For disinfection of wounds the commercial solution is used, which contains 2% of Mercurochrome. Although mouldy places on the skin of strong fishes may be touched directly with this solution, it is generally advisable to use a weaker solution, which is made up by diluting one part by volume of the commercial solution with 9 parts by volume of water. This solution has a strength of 0.2% and may be used for disinfection of wounds and treatment of fungus in fish, by touching the spots with a pencil or brush, or a tuft of cotton-wool, dipped into this solution. (Also see pages 48–49.)

MERTHIOLATE (THIMEROSAL)

This is a cream-coloured, crystalline powder. It is stable in air, but not in sunlight, therefore it should be stored in dark bottles. Merthiolate is an organic mercury compound. A 1:1000 solution may be used for swabbing wounds and for local treatment of cotton wool disease ('mouth fungus'). It should not be used for bathing fish.

METHYLENE BLUE

This is a blue dye. The solid substance appears brownish-red, but in solution the colour is blue. It stains different materials with a blue colour. It is very important to use a pure grade, therefore ask your chemist for methylene blue, *medical quality.*

Rp.   A stock solution is made by dissolving 1 g (= 15 gr) in 100 cm^3 of hot water.

M.D.S. Methylene blue may be used for treatment of ichthyophthiriasis (white spot), skin and gill flukes and as a palliative medicine in all cases of diseases of the gills, where fishes suffer from difficulty in breathing. The dye is used as a permanent bath and the total quantity required is added in two parts with an interval of one day, while in very bad cases the strength may be increased during the following days.

	Quantity of stock solution (in cm^3) to be added per:			
	l	ft^3	Imp. gal	U.S. gal
	0.2–0.4 (= 3–6 drops)	6.5–12.5	1–2	0.8–1.7
In very bad cases, the strength may be increased to	0.4–0.8 (= 6–12 drops)	12.5–25	2–4	1.7–3.3

The lower concentration will not harm plants, except some of the lower plants such as *Chara* and *Nitella*, but the increased strength will have a bad effect on them. Since treatment is permanent, methylene blue may be used also in ponds. It is important, however, that the water is clean. If large amounts of dirt are present these could bind the dye so that its strength and activity would be decreased very quickly. Artificial aeration is only advisable if large bubbles are used near the surface of the water. Lack of oxygen will not occur even in tanks that contain many fishes, since methylene blue increases the respiratory capacity of fish.

For curing ichthyophthiriasis, 5–7 days of treatment are required, provided that the temperature of the water is not lower than 21–23°C. Sliminess of the skin, caused by *Chilodonella* and *Costia* and *Gyrodactylus* infections, may be cured in 3–5 days.

For treatment of velvet disease, the stronger methylene blue concentration should be used, while in very bad cases of this disease the concentration may be doubled. This strength will, however, kill several plants.

It has been stated that a very large dose of methylene blue (1 g to 100 l; which is five times the amount recommended for ordinary white spot infections) would cure neon tetra disease, but this has not been confirmed by others.

After completion of treatment, methylene blue can be removed from the water by means of an activated coal filter. Of course, changing the water will do this job, too.

Methylene blue in the higher concentration has also proved efficacious in sea-water aquaria, where quinine and mepacrine are useless. Treatment should be continued over 10 days and more, see p. 51.

It has been shown that injections with methylene blue produce a significant increase of the haemoglobin content of the blood, thus improving severe cases of anaemia.[15]

NEGUVON[R]

(2,2,2-TRICHLORO-1-HYDROXY-ETHYL) — PHOSPHONIC ACID-DIMETHYLESTER)

Neguvon is the registered trade name of the compound mentioned above, manufactured by Messrs. Bayer, Leverkusen, Germany. It has been tried with good success for treatment of several parasitical fish diseases by D. Bailösoff in Sofia, Bulgaria.[16]

In a 2–3.5% aqueous solution the fish louse *Argulus foliaceus* is killed within 50–60 sec, the skin fluke *Gyrodactylus elegans* within 15 sec, the gill fluke *Dactylogyrus vastator* almost immediately and *D. anchoratus* within 30 sec. The protozoans *Cyclochæta* (*Trichodina*) *domerguei* and *Chilodonella cyprini*, which cause sliminess of the skin, are both killed within 10–30 sec.

The drug has been tested on 4–5-month-old Carp (body weight 15–40 g), 1½-year-old Carp (weight 200–500 g, young Trout and one-year-old Trout. Solutions of 2%, 2.5% and 5% were tried on Carp for periods up to one hour and on Trout for 10–30 min. The fishes did not show any signs of distress and 20 days after having been put back in their ponds no evidence of adverse effects could be observed.

However, since the parasites are killed so very rapidly, Bailösoff recommends bathing the infected fishes for 2–3 min only in a 2–3.5% aqueous solution of the drug, at a temperature of 15°C (when trying Neguvon treatment for tropical fishes this temperature should be not lower than 20°C).

The easiest method of treatment appears to be one in which the fishes are captured in a net and, while remaining in the net, are immersed for the required few minutes in a container with the Neguvon solution. In order to avoid asphyxiation the amount of solution should be at least three times the weight of the fishes to be treated at the same time.

For treatment of ponds an addition of 1 : 1000 is recommended and the fishes are daily inspected microscopically for presence of parasites. If no more parasites can be detected after inspection of a representative sample of the fish population, the water is changed.

	Quantity to be added per :			
	l	ft^3	Imp. gal	U.S. gal
For bath of 2–3 min:	20–35 g	20–35 oz	3.2–5.6 oz	2.7–4.6 oz
For treatment of ponds:	1 g	1 oz	68 gr	57 gr

From the very rapid effect on parasites from different groups, including a crustacean, trematode worms and protozoans, Neguvon may be expected to be effective against several other infectious diseases of the skin and the gills of fishes, such as anchor worm and other parasitic *Copepoda*, velvet and pillularis diseases.

Bailösoff found that *Ichthyophthirius* in the free state is also killed, but a short treatment of several minutes was unsuccessful, as is to be expected from the fact that the parasite is covered by the epithelial growth of the proliferating skin. He has reported 'reasonable results' by treatment with a 2.5% solution for 3–60 min. The optimal conditions have still to be discovered by experiment. It is suggested to try the concentration as given for other parasites in ponds and to see what period of time is required at any given water temperature to obtain a complete cure.

Tsutsumi and Murata have found that parasites of the Family *Urceolaridæ* (*Cyclochæta* or *Trichodina* and related genera) are killed within 35 h at the low strength of 1 : 250 000.[17] This concentration is obtained by multiplying the amount of *water* in the above table for pond treatment by a factor of 250 (or reducing the amount of drug accordingly).

Neguvon has a three times lower toxicity to rats than DDT, but it may be resorbed through the undamaged skin. Therefore rubber gloves are recommended when handling a large number of fish with the drug where there is a risk of contacting the solutions with the hands.

In some countries it may be difficult or impossible to obtain Neguvon, since it is not yet sold all over the world. For information one should contact the manufacturers in Germany.

NITROFURAZONE (5-NITRO-2-FURALDEHYDE SEMICARBAZONE; FURACIN; NITROFURAL)

Pale-yellow needles, to be protected for light. Only slightly soluble in water (1 : 4200).

Nitrofurazone is effective against many Gram-negative and Gram-positive bacteria and *Sporozoa*. It is given added to the food at a rate of 0.01%, for one week to at most two weeks. This treatment has also been found effective against *Vibrio* infections, causing ulcer disease, in marine fishes.

For treatment of bacterial infections in fresh-water tanks it may be used as a permanent bath of 1 g in 50 l of water, equivalent to 1.37 gr/Imp. gal or 1.14 gr/U.S. gal, to be added in three portions at intervals of 8–12 h; total duration of treatment from three days up to three weeks. This treatment appears promising but is still in the experimental stage.

According to Dr. A. Stolk, at 1 g in 40 l it should be effective against white spot as well. Add gradually and treat for 3–20 days.

NYSTATIN (MYCOSTATIN; FUNGICIDIN)

Antifungal antibiotic, produced by *Streptomyces aureus, Streptomyces noursei* and related species. Available in tablets (intended for intra-vaginal use in female *Moniliasis*) and ointments. Crushed vaginal tablets may be admixed to minced meat to be used for treatment of internal fungus infections of fishes, whereas the ointment may be applied to fungus of the skin.

OXYTETRACYCLINE (TERRAMYCIN[R])

Antibiotic substance, produced by *Streptomyces rimosus*. In pure form it is a white finely crystalline substance; with less purity (veterinary grade) it is light yellow, whereas an entirely crude product appears brownish-red.

It has been applied successfully for treatment of *Pseudomonas* and *Aeromonas* bacterial infections in fish, by giving it in the food at a rate of 1.8 mg per gram of food, administering this food in an amount of approximately 3% of body weight each day, for 8 days. Injection therapy has also been applied, at a rate of 3 mg per 150–400 g fish.

Application by dissolving it in the aquarium water is not good policy; although it has been found reasonably effective against fish tuberculosis when given this way, it is not very stable under aquarium conditions and develops toxic properties on prolonged treatment.

It is suggested that the more recent biosynthetic derivative doxy-cycline (trade name Vibramycin[R]) may be a more effective drug because it is more stable and has a higher penetrative power in cells and tissues. It should be used in the same way as oxytetracycline, but the dosage should be 0.5 mg/g food and treatment not exceeded over 5 days.

OZONE (O_3)

Ozone is a triatomic form of oxygen, produced from the ordinary O_2 molecules by the action of ultraviolet rays or radium emanation and by silent electric discharges. It is the most powerful oxidising agent. Pure ozone is a bluish explosive gas or a blue liquid, but this can only be obtained by cooling of ozonised air to $-180°C$. Normally the reaction is reversible and in the equilibrium condition ozonised air will contain about 3% ozone.

Ozonisers have been used for longer periods of time for disin-fection and sterilisation of air and water. Recently a small apparatus has been introduced for application in aquaria, for disinfection of water, oxidation of organic material, and treatment of certain fish diseases.[18] Air from an ordinary air pump is passed through an ozoniser and introduced in a tank by a fine-bulb diffuser placed near the bottom. Solubility of ozone in water is low. For water purification special arrangements are made for circulating the water through a cylinder in which the ozoned air is released.

It has been stated that ozone treatment, applied for 1 h three to four times a day, will cure fin-rot and fungus, whereas intense ozone treatment of tanks without fish has been suggested as a means of disinfection after the occurrence of an infectious disease. Ozone treatment of live foods, such as *Tubifex* and water fleas, should prevent introduction of diseases, but this cannot apply to transmittence of internal parasites, because these cannot be reached from the outside. Therefore, it would be a serious mistake to think that such treatment could guarantee absence of parasites.

Ozone treatment of water favours growth of *Cryptocoryne*, but not of *Vallisneria*. Ozone treatment of sea-water tanks favours growth of green algae, but brown algae vanish. In cases of autumn disease ozone treatment may be very beneficial.

However, one should not employ ozone treatment without special necessity. Formerly it was thought that ozone could further good health, probably because at low concentrations (about 2 p.p.m.) in air it shows a pleasant, characteristic odour, but at higher concentrations it is irritant and injurious. Some high-pressure mercury vapour arcs act as rather effective ozonisers and this is highly objectionable, since we now know that ozone is a mutagenic and carcinogenic substance. Its apparent harmless nature when used for drinking water purification is entirely due to its instability; long before the treated water is to be consumed every excess of the ozone added will have vanished altogether. Prolonged contact of fishes with ozone in the water may be expected to produce a risk of development of tumours, especially in young fish.

PARA-CHLOROMETAXYLENOL (CHLOROXYLENOL; 4-CHLORO-3,5-XYLENOL)

Colourless crystals with phenolic smell, only very slightly soluble in water.

Rp.   A stock solution is prepared by saturating water at 20°C (about 0.033% w/v). This is done by vigorously shaking the water with the crystals and filtering off the excess.

M.D.S. Fishes affected by internal worm parasites are fed with dried food soaked in the stock solution.

Cold-water fish are also given a treatment by placing them in a bath containing 10 cm^3 of stock solution per litre of water, for 1–2 h only. The lethal dose for Goldfish is approximately 16 cm^3/l. The dosage of 10 cm^3/l appears to cause distress to tropicals, therefore these should only be fed with the soaked dried food.

Chloroxylenol has been used successfully by Ian M. Rankin for treatment of worm infections, but he has not advocated its use since he found phenoxethol to be as effective and less toxic.

PARA-CHLOROPHENOXETHOL
(2-*PARA*-CHLOROPHENOXYETHANOL)

Oily liquid. Highly effective against tail- and fin-rot. It may cure infectious dropsy, too. Further, this compound kills *Ichthyophonus* cysts, spores and plasmodia and acts more rapidly than phenoxethol.

However, whereas Rankin found this a good treatment for varieties of Goldfish and Red Swordtails, it has been shown to be extremely toxic to other species of fish, such as Guppies and Kissing Gouramis (*Helostoma temmincki*), according to a publication in Technical Bulletin 171 of the Virginia Agricultural Experiment Station, Blacksburg, Virginia, U.S.A., entitled: *Studies of the Host Range and Chemical Control of Fungi Associated with Diseased Tropical Fish.* The authors claim that any concentration which will kill fungi or inhibit their growth also kills those fishes in less than one minute (0.04% solution) and in 25–36 min in the 0.005% solution as prescribed for treatment. *Consequently, this treatment cannot be recommended any more.*

PENBRITIN[R]—See PENICILLIN

PENICILLIN (BENZYLPENICILLIN SODIUM)

White crystals, stable when kept dry, but decomposing rather rapidly in aqueous solutions. At pH 5.5–6.0 solutions will keep for a few days only when placed in a refrigerator. It is precipitated and inactivated by many metal ions. Penicillin is the most well-known antibiotic. It is active against a number of Gram-positive bacteria, but inefficient against most Gram-negative bacteria. Since most bacteria pathogenic to fish are Gram-negative, penicillin is without real value for treatment of bacterial infections in fish.

Penicillin has been stated to be effective against *Ichthyophthirius*, which is a protozoan. A dosage of 40000 I.U. per 100 l should perform a complete cure in 6 h. Further, a dosage of 100000 I.U. per 100 l has been claimed to cure fungus disease. However, penicillin cannot be recommended for treatment of diseases of fish, including treatment of those diseases for which it can be successful, since there is a very great risk of producing resistant strains of microorganisms. Penicillin has not cured one single disease of fish which could not have been cured also by other medicaments. A more promising drug seems to be the synthetic penicillin derivative Ampicillin, commercially available under the trade name Penbritin[R], which is more stable and is also effective against certain Gram-negative bacteria. 250 mg Penbritin is equivalent to 1 000 000 I.U. of penicillin. Ampicillin may be applied as a food additive (2 mg/g) against *Proteus* infections, if at the same time vitamin B-complex is added to prevent occurrence of intestinal avitaminosis.

Repeated intramuscular injections with penicillin have been reported to cure *Ichthyophonus* infections. (Also see page 191.)

Injections with a mixture of penicillin and streptomycin have been found effective against tail- and fin-rot in marine fishes.

4,7-PHENANTHROLINE-5,6-DIONE (4,7-PHENAN-THROLINE-5,6-QUINONE; ENTOBEX; Ciba 11925)

Crystalline substance, sparingly soluble in water. It is added to the food of fish suffering from *Hexamitiasis*, at a rate of one per cent of food, and given for four days.

PHENOXETHOL (2-PHENOXYETHANOL) $(C_6H_5.O.CH_2CH_2OH)$

Phenoxethol is an oily liquid with faint aromatic odour and burning taste. It is slightly soluble in water. This substance has been introduced for treatment of fish diseases by Ian M. Rankin and has proved effective against various infections, including fungus, tail- and fin-rot, some worm infections, and *Ichthyophonus* disease.

Rp.   Stock solution: 1 cm^3 of phenoxethol is dissolved in 99 cm^3 of water.

M.D.S. From this stock solution the following quantities are to be added to the water in the tank:

Quantity (in cm^3) to be added per:			
1	ft^3	Imp. gal	U.S. gal
10–20	280–560	45–90	38–75

For treatment of internal infections (worms, *Ichthyophonus*) the fishes are fed with dried food soaked in the stock solution in combination with the bath. Always use the lower concentration, unless the effect is insufficient and the fishes show no signs of sensitivity to the drug. After recovery, the water should be changed.

Phenoxethol is commercially available in special cartons containing two capsules for aquarist use. One capsule in 18 l, or 4 Imp. gal, or 4.8 U.S. gal gives the recommended strength of 1 : 10 000. The trade name is 'Liquitox'. The phenoxethol is manufactured by Nipa Laboratories Ltd. and packed for aquarists by 'The Liquifry Co. Ltd.', Dorking, Surrey, England.

PICRIC ACID (2,4,6-TRINITROPHENOL)
$(C_6H_2(NO_2)_3.OH)$

This is a yellow-coloured substance with needle-shaped crystals. In medicine it is used in the treatment of burns, while it is also used for explosives and must therefore be kept away from fire. It may be difficult to obtain pure picric acid; if such should be the case, ask your chemist to make you the solution as mentioned below, which has no dangerous qualities. Picric acid has an intensely bitter taste. It must never be brought into contact with any metal.

Rp.   A stock solution is made by dissolving 1 g ($= 15$ gr) in 100 cm^3 of hot water. If the solution is kept at low temperatures, picric acid may fall out of the solution. Then it must first be redissolved by heating the solution (which can be done without any risk even above direct fire provided its temperature is below 300°C) and shaking thoroughly. It is only explosive when dry.

M.D.S. Picric acid is an excellent chemical for treatment of different diseases of the skin, caused by worms, such as black spot and others.

Quantity of stock solution (in cm^3) to be added per:			
1	ft^3	Imp. gal	U.S. gal
2–7	56–185	9–30	7$\frac{1}{2}$–25

Fishes remain in this bath for about one hour. For delicate fishes, the strength of the bath should be lower than for strong ones. During treatment, the fish are watched carefully; if they show no signs of distress, treatment may be extended to as long as 3 h, if this should be considered necessary, according to the seriousness of the disease. After treatment, the fishes are placed in fresh, clean water.

POTASSIUM ANTIMONYL TARTRATE
(TARTAR EMETIC) $(K(SbO)C_6H_4.\frac{1}{2}H_2O)$

This is a poisonous drug, consisting of transparent odourless crystals, efflorescing on exposure to air, or white powder. It has been

Dosage to be used as a maximum per:			
1	ft^3	Imp. gal	U.S. gal
1$\frac{1}{2}$ mg	40 mg	0.1 gr	0.08 gr

suggested as a cure for worm infections in fish by the Dutch physician, Dr. C. van Dommelen. Rankin found it very effective against flukes, but has warned about the risk of poisoning effects if the dosage should not be adhered to very strictly or if the treatment should be extended for a longer period than required for recovery.

POTASSIUM DICHROMATE ($K_2Cr_2O_7$)

This is an orange-red crystallised chemical, but it can also be obtained in powdered form. If the latter is available, it is preferred, since it is easier for measuring the correct amounts.

Rp.　　For treatment of wounds, sore spots or mouldy places a 1% solution is used, which is made up by dissolving 1 g (= 15 gr) in 99 cm^3 of water. This solution can also be used for preparing a bath, by diluting it as follows:

M.D.S.

Quantity of 1% solution (in cm^3) to be added per:			
1	ft^3	Imp. gal	U.S. gal
4–5	110–140	18–22$\frac{1}{2}$	15–19

The concentrations thus obtained are 1:25 000 and 1:20 000, respectively. Fishes may be treated with this bath for several days but not longer than ten days, after which the water must be changed. Plants do not suffer from this treatment. In very bad cases, e.g. in bacterial infections, a strong bath may be used (1:10 000, i.e. double the strength as given before) for half an hour only.

Gosh and Pal determined the LC_{50} values (concentrations at which 50% of the treated fishes are killed) with fry of *Catla catla*, *Labeo rohita* and *Cirrhinus mrigala*, kept for 24 h and 48 h at 26°C and 32°C in contact with the drug.[19] This came out at 92.5–125 mg/l, which is between 2 and 3 times higher tolerance as for permanganate.

Potassium dichromate and chromate (K_2CrO_4) have been tried against *Lernæa* infections, but proved ineffective.

POTASSIUM PERMANGANATE ($KMnO_4$)

This is a violet, crystallised substance, with good disinfecting qualities. Unluckily, however, it is soon destroyed by all kinds of organic materials which may be present in the water and therefore it is difficult to get the proper strength. Its activity depends on the liberation of oxygen in a very active state, which kills parasites. If the water is alkaline or only very slightly acid, a precipitate of manganese dioxide (MnO_2nH_2O) may form, which can damage the gills of the fishes. This risk can be diminished by using artificial aeration during treatment. For treatment of aquarium fishes, potassium permanganate has lost its extreme importance as a medicine for diseases of fish since I introduced potassium dichromate instead, which has several important advantages, but for treatment of fishes in ponds potassium permanganate is still indispensable in all cases where it is impossible to change the water after treatment.

Never on any account should crystals of permanganate be added directly to a tank or a pond, but they must be dissolved first in a suitable amount of water and then this solution added with thorough stirring. It is advisable to prepare a stock solution, which must be kept in a dark bottle, since the chemical is sensitive to light.

Rp.   A stock solution is made by dissolving 1 g (= 15 gr) in 99 cm^3 of distilled water. This is a 1% solution.

M.D.S.	Quantity of stock solution (in cm^3) to be added per:			
	1	ft^3	Imp. gal	U.S. gal
For a bath of aquarium fishes, not longer than half an hour	1	28	4.5	3.5
For treatment of fully planted tanks and ponds	0.4–0.45	12.5	2	1.5–1.7

For treatment of fully planted tanks and ponds, the amount in quantity of solid permanganate is 4–5 mg/l (0.25–0.3 gr/Imp. gal or 0.2–0.25 gr/U.S. gal). If the water contains much organic material (e.g. dirt), treatment may be repeated after ten days. In clean water this could be harmful.

For treatment of velvet disease a combination of permanganate and salt has been advocated. This recommended strength is 7 g/l of salt (or 1 oz/Imp. gal or 0.8 oz/U.S. gal), and the amount of permanganate as just mentioned for treatment of fully planted tanks and ponds. After the addition of the permanganate any coal filter should be put out of operation till the next day. A change of water is made after 3–5 days to remove the excess salt.

Different species of fish have varying susceptibility to permanganate, as has been proved by the experiments of Prof. O. V. Hykes.[20] From his article, the following figures are taken: Bleak (*Alburnus lucidus*) and *Alburnus bipunctatus* endured, without any signs of distress, 27 mg/l (1.9 gr/Imp. gal = 1.58 gr/U.S. gal), but 40 mg/l

(2.8 gr/Imp. gal = 2.3 gr/U.S. gal) were lethal. Gudgeon (*Gobio gobio*) and Minnow (*Phoxinus phoxinus*) took 37 mg/l (3.7 gr/Imp. gal = 3.1 gr/U.S. gal), but 62 mg/l (4.4 gr/Imp. gal = 3.67 gr/U.S. gal) were lethal. Black Paradise Fish (*Macropodus opercularis concolor*) took only 13 mg/l (0.8 gr/Imp. gal = 0.67 gr/U.S. gal) and 22 mg/l (1.5 gr/Imp. gal = 1.25 gr/U.S. gal) were lethal. *Barbus binotatus* could stand 38 mg/l (2.6 gr/Imp. gal = 2.17 gr/U.S. gal), but died in a concentration of 45 mg/l (3.2 gr/Imp. gal = 2.86 gr/U.S. gal).

Gosh and Pal found that fry of *Catla catla, Labeo rohita* and *Cirrhinus mrigala*, kept for 24 h and 48 h at 26°C and 32°C, were for 50% killed at concentrations of 37.5–48 mg/l;[19] they, too, prefer potassium dichromate for prophylactic treatments.

From these figures it is obvious that there are great differences between the several species of fish and this must be borne in mind when using permanganate treatments. The concentrations given above for general treatment are safe, but they are not always sufficient to guarantee success. Therefore, permanganate should only be used in cases where it is impossible to substitute it. This restricts its use to ponds only.

For touching parasites on the skin, mouldy places and such, the stock solution is diluted with some parts of water and then may be used without risk, but for bathing aquarium fishes it will be better to use other treatments.

PROPYLENE PHENOXETHOL

Oily liquid, slightly soluble in water. It has been used by Rankin for treatment of bacterial and fungus infections in Goldfish varieties in the same way as phenoxethol, but the latter is to be preferred for that purpose. It may be dangerous to other species of fish.

Propylene phenoxethol in higher concentrations acts as an anaesthetic and has been used for that purpose on marine fishes to facilitate surgery. In a 0.01% solution Plaice were limp after 20 min and could recover after having been in it for 2 h, but not after 3 h. In a 0.025% solution complete anaesthesia occurred after 5 min and fishes recovered after 30 min, but not after 1 h of contact.

PYRIDOXINE (ADERMINE; VITAMIN B_6)

Generally used in the form of its hydrochloride salt. This vitamin is present in many foodstuffs, especially in yeast, liver and cereals. It is sold in tablets for medical use. Addition of $2\frac{1}{2}$ tablets per 2 U.S. qt or $2\frac{1}{2}$ tablets in every 2 l, will cure symptoms of pyridoxine deficiency, which in Angel Fish consist of a greenish colour all over the body, refusal to take *Tubifex* as food and staying in one corner.

In fishes that still take dry food, mixing this with either yeast or raw chopped liver will do the same.

PYRIDYL MERCURIC ACETATE

This drug, of technical quality, has been used successfully against bacterial infections of the gills in Salmon and Trout, and external protozoan infections in all fishes. It is ineffective against *Lernæa*.

A bath is prepared *in a non-metal container*, by dissolving the drug at a rate of 2 mg/l, or 0.136 gr/Imp. gal, or 0.11 gr/U.S. gal. Duration of treatment: *1 hour*.

Do not use this treatment on Rainbow Trout and be very careful when trying it on small aquarium fish, since it is a rather toxic mercury compound.

Fishes that have been treated with mercury compounds must not be used for human consumption, because mercury remains in their bodies for several months after withdrawal from treatment.[21] Chinook Salmon accumulated mercury after ingesting small fish which had been treated with ethyl mercury phosphate baths.

QUININE HYDROCHLORIDE

This is a white, crystallised chemical. Of several quinine compounds which have been used in practice, quinine hydrochloride is the most advisable. Quinine is used in treatment of white spot (*Ichthyophthiriasis*) and of sliminess of the skin, due to *Chilodonella*, *Cyclochæta* or *Costia*.

Rp.   A stock solution is made by dissolving 3 g (= 45 gr) of quinine hydrochloride in 300 cm³ of water.

M.D.S. For treatment of white spot:

Quantity of stock solution (in cm³) to be added per:			
1	ft³	Imp. gal	U.S. gal
3–3.5	95	15	12.5

These quantities are not to be added at once, but in three approximately equal parts at intervals of ½–1 day. Treatment must continue until the fishes have been cured, then the water must be changed, since too long a contact with quinine has a bad effect on fishes, especially on their fertility.

M.D.S. For treatment of sliminess of the skin and skin flukes:

Quantity of stock solution (in cm³) to be added per:			
1	ft³	Imp. gal	U.S. gal
2	57	9	7.5

In this solution *Cyclochæta* (*Trichodina*) is eradicated in 6 h, *Chilodonella* in 18 h and *Costia* after 24–26 h. Therefore, the addition of the required amount of stock solution in two equal portions at half a day's interval is advised and the treatment prolonged for 36–48 h after the first addition.

Quinine hydrochloride may not be used in containers of galvanised iron or zinc, since then zinc chloride can be formed, which is poisonous to fish. Quinine salts have a bad effect on plant growth; therefore it is advisable not to use quinine in fully planted tanks, but to place the fishes in a clean tank, and to use artificial aeration.

Quinine treatment must not be applied to Prussian Carp, it being highly toxic to this species.

RIVANOL—See ACRINOL

ROCCAL—See BENZALKONIUM CHLORIDE

SALICYLIC ACID ($C_6H_4(OH).COOH$)

This is a white crystalline substance. A saturated solution at room temperature contains one part in 500 parts of water. For general use in treatment of diseased fishes, this chemical cannot be recommended, since it has an irritative effect on the mucous coat of the skin and the gills, but it is the most effective medicine against stubborn cases of *Dactylogyrus*, when other chemicals have no effect.

Rp.   A stock solution is made by dissolving 1 g (= 15 gr) in 1 l of water (or 8.5 gr in 1 pint of water). It is advisable to use hot water in making the solution.

M.D.S.

Quantity of stock solution (in cm^3) to be added per:			
1	ft^3	Imp. gal	U.S. gal
10–12	280–340	45–55	37.5–46

Fishes are bathed in this solution for not longer than half an hour. During this treatment they are carefully watched and, if they show any signs of distress, they should be removed immediately and put into fresh water.

SALT (SODIUM CHLORIDE) NaCl

A description of this household chemical seems superfluous. It may be used as an effective treatment for a great number of diseases, although it is not such a panacea as some aquarists seem to think. Salt may be used in treatment of sliminess of the skin, in early stages of skin flukes (*Gyrodactylus*) and as an additional treatment in several cases of bacterial diseases. Fishes may be treated by bathing them in a strong solution for a short period or treatment may be permanent by using gradually increasing strengths.

M.D.S. (1) Short bath:

Quantity of salt to be added per:			
l	ft³	Imp. gal	U.S. gal
15–30 g	15.5–31 oz	2.5–5 oz	2–4 oz

This is a strength of $1\frac{1}{2}$–3%. In this solution diseased fishes are bathed for 15–30 min. Generally, treatment must be repeated several times at intervals and, therefore, continuous treatment is preferable, which is done according to the following scheme originating from Dr. Wilhelm Roth (*'Die Krankheiten der Aquarienfische und ihre Bekämpfung'*, Stuttgart, 1922), but restricted to three additions only, after investigations by Prof. Schäperclaus, proving that higher concentrations are not necessary for curing the sensitive infections and are too harmful to certain fishes.

M.D.S. (2): Permanent bath:

	Quantity to be dissolved per:			
	l	ft³	Imp. gal	U.S. gal
First day:	7 g	6 oz	1 oz	0.8 oz
Second day: Change half of the water by using a solution which contains	11 g	13 oz	2 oz	1.5 oz
Third day: Change half of the water by using a solution which contains	13 g	13 oz	2 oz	1.75 oz

Fishes may be kept for an indefinite period in this solution. Gradual addition of salt is necessary to allow the fish to adapt itself to this strong solution. Replacement in fresh water must also be done gradually, by changing about one-third of the salt solution by fresh water at intervals of at least one day. After four changes the fishes may be put into fresh water. It is not advisable to use this permanent salt treatment in a community tank, since such a strong salt solution will have a bad effect on plant growth. Salt treatment should not be carried out in the presence of galvanised iron or zinc otherwise severe zinc poisoning could occur.

This same treatment can be used for small ponds infested with anchor worms (*Lernæa*), provided the water temperature is not below 14°C (57°F). This salt concentration will kill the hatching nauplii (larval stages). Treatment should continue for 2–3 weeks during which period the water should be repeatedly changed and resalted after a few days.

According to investigations in Israel[22] Carps are killed in 60 min in a 2.5% salt solution, whereas *Lernæa* became numbed in 25 min and in the field recovered after 30 h. The LC_{50} value for fry of the Indian Carps *Catla catla*, *Labco rohita* and *Cirrhinus mrigala*, kept for 24 h and 48 h at 26°C and 32°C, came out to be 0.55–0.75%.[19] Therefore, the prolonged salt treatment should not be used on young fry.

SILVER NITRATE (AgNO₃)

This is a crystallised substance and must be protected from light. If touched with a wet finger, the skin is attacked and becomes covered with a black layer, due to the formation of metallic silver, which may combine with sulphur, present in the proteins of which the skin consists.

Rp.   A solution is made by dissolving 1–2 g (= 15–30 gr) in 100 cm³ of distilled water. If water from the tap were used, a white precipitate would be formed.

M.D.S.   The solution is used directly to treat mouldy places of the skin of a fish or on the eye. Silver nitrate is the best medicine for treatment of eye fungus, while it may be used with good success in tail-rot, too. A pencil or brush, or a tuft of cotton-wool, is dipped into the solution and with this the affected places are touched, holding the fish in the hand. After this treatment, the same places are touched with a 1% solution of potassium dichromate to avoid damage to the fish, which could result from too long a contact with the chemical. In doing this, a red precipitate will be formed (silver dichromate) which does not harm the fish. The fish is then placed in a 1 : 25 000–1 : 20 000 solution of potassium dichromate until complete recovery has been obtained. This is necessary to avoid new infections. If no potassium dichromate solution is at hand with which to touch the places after treatment with silver nitrate, the fish must be placed for 5–10 min in a 1–2½% salt solution and then into fresh water, to which potassium dichromate may afterwards be added.

STILBAMIDINE

This drug has been suggested by Dr. C. van Dommelen for treatment of sliminess of the skin. However, actual experience is lacking, so that one should be very cautious in using it. A few worthless fish should be treated to see what happens before risking a whole stock. Stilbamidine is toxic. The recommended dosage is 150 mg/100 l, or 0.1 gr/Imp. gal, or 0.08 gr/U.S. gal. The drug is decomposed by light, therefore the tank must be protected from strong light during treatment. Use artificial aeration.

STREPTOMYCIN

This is an antibiotic produced by *Streptomyces griseus*. It is a highly efficient anti-tuberculous drug in human medicine.

Schäperclaus has suggested its use for treatment of bacterial infections in fish, either by injection (Fig. 10.1) of 10–20 μg per

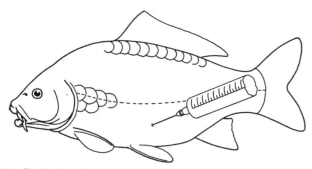

Fig. 10.1. Positioning of syringe and hypodermic needle for injection therapy of a fish. Syringe and needles must be sterilised by heating them for 10 min in boiling water before use (after Amlacher)

gram fish (1 μg = 0.001 mg) or by adding 10 mg/l of water (0.7 gr/Imp. gal or 0.56 gr/U.S. gal). The most appropriate form appears to be the hydrochloride salt, $C_{21}H_{39}N_7O_{12}.3HCl$.

It has been found ineffective against *Mycobacterium marinum* and in cases of Exophthalmus where unidentified Mycobacteria were found, but good results have been obtained with injection therapy of marine fishes suffering from ulcer disease due to *Vibrio* infections.

SULPHADIAZINE

One of the modern sulpha drugs, experimentally used for treatment of bacterial infections in fish. To be used in the same way as sulphanilamide.

Sulphadiazine is also a white, crystalline powder. It is only slightly soluble in acid water (130 mg/l at pH 5.5 at a temperature of 37°C, which temperature is too high for fish); much more soluble in alkaline water (2 g/l at pH 7.5 and 37°C). Therefore, it can only be used in a sufficient dosage in neutral or alkaline waters.

Also see sulphisoxazole.

SULPHAGUANIDINE $(NH_2).C_6H_4.SO_2.NH.C(=NH).NH_2$

One of the modern sulpha drugs, used for treatment of furunculosis and other bacterial infections in fish. It occurs in needle-shaped crystals; solubility about 1 g in a litre of water at 25°C or 1 g in 10 cm³ of boiling water.

Use of a combination of sulphaguanidine with the other sulpha drug, sulphamerazine, is recommended. During three days a mixture of 12 g of sulphamerazine with 6 g of sulphaguanidine per 100 lb (45.4 kg) of fish per day should be given in the food. This should be followed by giving 6 g of sulphamerazine and 4 g of sulphaguanidine per 100 lb of fish in the food daily for seven days.

For treatment of small aquarium fish, dry food could be soaked in a 1 : 1000 solution and dried again. Also see sulphisoxazole.

SULPHAMERAZINE (PERCOCCID)

One of the modern sulpha drugs, experimentally used for treatment of bacterial infections in fish. To be used in the same way as sulphanilamide.

Solubility about 1 g in 6.25 l of water at 20°C. In acid water its solubility is much less, while in slightly alkaline water solubility is greater.

The sodium salt (sulphamerazine sodium) is much more soluble (1 g dissolves in 3.6 cm³ of water), but since this salt has a rather strong alkaline reaction itself, when dissolved in water (due to hydrolysis) it should only be used if the aquarium water is acid, otherwise an undue rise of pH could occur.

Sulphamerazine itself (free base) is used against furunculosis in Salmonid fish, combined with sulphaguanidine (see there). Otherwise it is given mixed with the food at a rate of 175 mg per kilogram fish per day.

Sulphamerazine sodium has also been reported to be effective as a cure for worm cataract. It should be given orally for 2–3 weeks, confined to diseased fish only. Worm cataract cannot be transmitted from fish to fish, so there would be no reason for treatment of all the inhabitants of the aquarium in which the infection has occurred.

WARNING: Do not use sulphamerazine for treatment of Brown Trout. See Sulphisoxazole.

SULPHANILAMIDE

White, crystalline powder. Solubility in water 2.6 g/l at 10°C; 4.2 g/l at 15°C; 6 g/l at 20°C; 7.5 g/l at 25°C. It is an antibacterial drug, one of the so-called sulpha drugs.
Dosage: 100–250 mg/l; 2.8–7 g/ft^3; 6.8–17 gr/Imp. gal; 5.6–14 gr/U.S. gal.

Sulphanilamide has been stated to be effective against fungus, and for treatment of bacterial infections. Treatment should not be extended for more than five days, otherwise toxic reactions may occur, resulting in renal damage, anaemia and leukopenia. Generally three days should be sufficient if the drug is effective at all, but nowadays it is recommended to use sulphisoxazole instead, which is the least toxic of sulpha drugs for treatment of fishes.

SULPHISOXAZOLE (GANTRISIN; GANTROSAN; SULFAZIN; SULPHAFURAZOLE; a.o.) (3,4-DIMETHYL-5-SULPHANILAMIDO-ISOXAZOLE)

Modern sulpha drug. Prism-shaped crystals. Solubility in water at pH 6.0 is 3.5 g/l. Used for treatment of bacterial and related infectious diseases in fish, especially against infectious kidney and liver disease (see page 202), where treatment has to be prolonged over very long periods in which the other sulpha drugs show a growth-retarding effect in some species of fish, especially Brown Trout. For this species, sulphisoxazole is the sulpha drug of choice. Of all sulpha drugs, sulphisoxazole has been found to be the most active against *Cytophaga psychrophila* (causing 'cold-water' disease) and furunculosis infections of fish and to be the least toxic compound.[23] It even showed growth-stimulating properties. Peak concentrations in the blood are reached within 12 h of the initial dose, whereas sulphamezathine requires 2–4 days. On the other hand, sulphisoxazole is eliminated most rapidly from the blood, followed by sulphadimethoxine and sulphamezathine (sulphamethazine).

Sulphisoxazole is given mixed with the food, at a rate of 8–10 g per 100 lb (45.4 kg) of fish per day. Duration of treatment for ordinary infections could be 7–10 days. For treatment of infectious kidney and liver disease, see page 202. In marine fishes good results have been obtained in cases of ulcer disease due to *Vibrio* infections.

TERRAMYCIN[R]—See OXYTETRACYCLINE

TRYPAFLAVINE—See ACRIFLAVINE

TRYPARSAMIDE

This is an organic arsenicum compound and rather toxic. It must be kept in tight containers, protected from light and preferably at a temperature not exceeding 20°C (68°F). In human medicine it is used against syphilis and African trypanosomiasis.

Tryparsamide has been suggested for treatment of sliminess of the skin, caused by *Costia necatrix*, by the Dutch physician Dr. C. van Dommelen. However, actual experience is lacking, so that one should exercise the utmost caution and not use it on a whole batch of fish before having experimented with a few worthless ones. The recommended dosage is 1 g in 100 l, or 0.6–0.7 gr/Imp. gal, or 0.5–0.55 gr/U.S. gal.

The tank must be protected from strong light during treatment and treatment must not be continued any longer than is necessary to obtain a cure. After treatment, a complete change of water must be made. There are reasons to believe that this treatment might be effective against sleeping sickness in fish, caused by *Cryptobia* and *Trypanosoma* species.

VIBRAMYCIN[R] (DOXYCYCLINE)—
See OXYTETRACYCLINE

ZEPHIROL—See BENZALKONIUM CHLORIDE

REFERENCES

1 GOSH, A. K. and PAL, R. N., 'Toxicity of four therapeutic compounds to fry of Indian Major Carp', *Fish Technol. (India)* **6**, 120–23 (1969)
2 AMLACHER, E., *Taschenbuch der Fischkrankheiten*, p. 157, Fischer-Verlag, Jena (1961)
3 DEMPSTER, R. P. and SHIPMAN, W. H., 'The use of copper sulfate as a medicament for aquarium fishes and as an algaecide in marine mammal water systems', *Occas. Pap. Calif. Acad. Sci.* **71**, 1–6 (1969)
4 DE JONG, J. C. M., *Het Aquarium* **19**, 39 (1948–49)
5 ROTH, W., *Die Krankheiten der Aquarienfische und ihre Bekampfung*, Stuttgart (1922)
6 NAZARENKO, I. V., 'Vliyanie formal'degida na vodnye organizny', *Tr. Vses. Gidrobiol. Obshchestva Ak. Nauk. S.S.S.R.* **10**, 170–74 (1960)
7 RUCKER, R. R., TAYLOR, W. G. and TONEY, D. P., 'Formalin in the hatchery', *Progr. Fish-Cult.* **25**, 203–07 (1963)

8 REICHENBACH-KLINKE, H. H., *Krankheiten und Schädigungen der Fische*, Stuttgart (1966)

9 CONRAD, J. F. and WYATT, X., 'Control of Ichthyophthirius in rectangular circulating ponds', *Progr. Fish-Cult.* **32**, 235 (1970)

10 MERRINER, J. V., 'Constant-bath malachite green solution for incubating sunfish eggs', *Progr. Fish-Cult.* **31**, 223–25 (1969)

11 AVDOS'EV, B. S., 'Novye metody primeneneniya malakhitogo zelenogo pri ikthiofteriazise karpoo', *Rybnoe Khoz.* **38**, 27–29 (1962)

12 HUBLOU, W. F., 'The use of malachite green to control *Trichodina*', *Progr. Fish-Cult.* **20**, 129–32 (1958)

13 BOGDANOVA, E. A., 'Malakhitovaya zelen'i formalin-effektivnye sredstva bor'bys trikhodiniazisom', *Rybnoe Khoz.* **38**, 30–31 (1962)

14 AMLACHER, E., 'Die Wirkung des Malachitgrüns auf Fische, Fischparasiten (*Ichthyophthirius, Trichodina*) Kleinkrebse und Wasserpflanzen', *Deutsche Fisch-Ztg.* **8** (1961)

15 TACK, E., 'Beiträge zur Erforschung der Forellen-Seuche', *Allg. Fischerei-Ztg.* **85**, 634–35 (1960)

16 BAILÖSOFF, D., 'Neguvon—ein wirksames Mittel zur Bekämpfung der Karpfenlaus und sonstiger parasitärer Fischkrankheiten', *Deut. Fischerei-Z.* **10**, 181 (1963); SCHÄPERCLAUS, W., 'Einige Ergänzungen zu dem Aufsatz von Bailösoff über die Bekämpfung von Karpfenläusen und anderen Hautparasiten mit Hilfe von "Neguvon" (Trichlorphon)', *Deut. Fischerei-Z.* **10**, 183–84 (1963)

17 TSUTSUMI, T. and MURATA, M., 'Anwendung eines geringtoxischen organischen Phosphorpräparates bei der *Cyclochæta*-Krankheit', *Vet. Med. Nachr.*, 414–16 (1963)

18 SANDER, E., 'Ozone—its application to aquarium-keeping', *Pet-Fish Monthly* **1**, 9–10 (1966)

19 GOSH, A. K. and PAL, R. N., 'Toxicity of 4 therapeutic compounds to fry of Indian Major Carp', *Fish Technol. (India)* **6**, 120–23 (1969)

20 HYKES, O. V., *Water Life* **IV**, 313 (1938)

21 RUCKER, R. R. and AMEND, D. F., 'Absorption and retention of mercurials by Rainbow Trout and Chinook and Sockeye Salmon', *Progr. Fish-Cult.* **31**, 197–201 (1969)

22 SHILO, M., SARIG, S. and ROSENBERGER, R., 'Ton scale treatment of *Lernæa* infected Carps', *Bamidgeh* **12**, 37–42 (1960)

23 AMEND, D. F., FRYER, J. L. and PILCHER, K. S., 'Studies of certain sulfonamide drugs for use in juvenile Chinook Salmon', *Progr. Fish-Cult.* **31**, 202–06 (1969)

24 YONE, Y., FUZINO, S. and TOMIYAMAT, T., *Bull. Japanese Soc. Sci. Fish* **26** (5), 514–19 (1960). Japanese with English summary

INDEX

INDEX

[Bold type indicates the more important pages. Illustrations are indicated by the addition of an asterisk.]

357